A Practical Operative Guide for

Total Knee and Hip Replacement

A Practical Operative Guide for
Total Knee and Hip Replacement

Second Edition

Ajit Kumar Mehta
MBBS D Ortho MS (Ortho)
Senior Consultant Orthopedic Surgeon
Orthopedic and Joint Replacement Center
Jagjivan Ram Hospital
Mumbai, Maharashtra, India

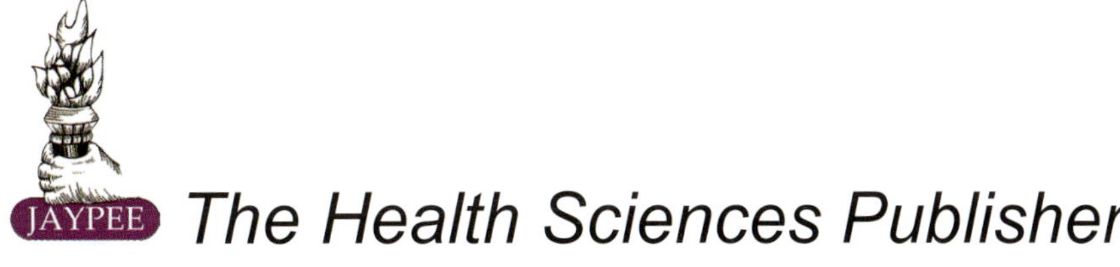

New Delhi | London | Philadelphia | Panama

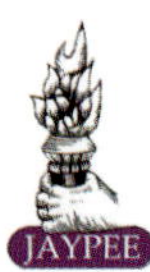

Jaypee Brothers Medical Publishers (P) Ltd

Headquarters

Jaypee Brothers Medical Publishers (P) Ltd
4838/24, Ansari Road, Daryaganj
New Delhi 110 002, India
Phone: +91-11-43574357
Fax: +91-11-43574314
Email: jaypee@jaypeebrothers.com

Overseas Offices

J.P. Medical Ltd
83 Victoria Street, London
SW1H 0HW (UK)
Phone: +44 20 3170 8910
Fax: +44 (0)20 3008 6180
Email: info@jpmedpub.com

Jaypee-Highlights Medical Publishers Inc
City of Knowledge, Bld. 237, Clayton
Panama City, Panama
Phone: +1 507-301-0496
Fax: +1 507-301-0499
Email: cservice@jphmedical.com

Jaypee Medical Inc
The Bourse
111 South Independence Mall East
Suite 835, Philadelphia, PA 19106, USA
Phone: +1 267-519-9789
Email: jpmed.us@gmail.com

Jaypee Brothers Medical Publishers (P) Ltd
17/1-B Babar Road, Block-B, Shaymali
Mohammadpur, Dhaka-1207
Bangladesh
Mobile: +08801912003485
Email: jaypeedhaka@gmail.com

Jaypee Brothers Medical Publishers (P) Ltd
Bhotahity, Kathmandu, Nepal
Phone +977-9741283608
Email: kathmandu@jaypeebrothers.com

Website: www.jaypeebrothers.com
Website: www.jaypeedigital.com

Inquiries for bulk sales may be solicited at: jaypee@jaypeebrothers.com

A Practical Operative Guide for Total Knee and Hip Replacement

First Edition : 2008
Second Edition : **2015**

ISBN: 978-93-5152-482-3

Printed at Ajanta Offset & Packagings Ltd., New Delhi.

Dedicated to

My parents

and

My teachers

Preface to the Second Edition

Total knee and hip replacement surgeries are special operations which require highest order of aseptic precaution, surgical skill and good team with almost fixed preoperative, peroperative and postoperative techniques and protocols with some modifications according to the individual case. We are strictly following the protocols and steps which are mentioned here. The first edition of this book (2008) had been written after gaining the experience in more than 800 cases of total knee and hip replacement surgeries with successful outcome. The second edition of this book (2015) has been revised after gaining experience in more than 3,000 total knee and hip replacement surgeries and vast experience with management of various complications.

Extension of chapters like total knee replacement (TKR) by navigation system, important points and total hip replacement (THR) in difficult situations, bone cement, ultrasonic system for cemented and uncemented revision surgeries, complications and revision THR, physiotherapy in TKR and THR has been made. In revision THR, we have used uncemented modular revision stem with distal fixation (solution revision stem or REEF) in addition to cemented C-stem and uncemented Summit stem. To make these special surgeries easier, diagrammatic and some more original photographs have been included. Outline of TKR by navigation system has been mentioned. Basic principles and technique remain the same as conventional technique, only the assessment of tibial and femoral resections is made by morphing the hip center, femoral mechanical axis, whiteside line, tibial mechanical axis, various femoral and tibial landmarks and surfaces. Ligament balancing and patellar tracking are being seen on computer. TKR with navigation system is more useful in patients with arthritis of the knee and extra-articular femoral and/or tibial deformity, retained hardware or intramedullary implants.

Various techniques of postoperative analgesia like patient-controlled analgesia (PCA) have been added in addition to epidural analgesia.

In place of unicondylar knee replacement for medial compartment osteoarthritis, we are performing high tibial osteotomy (HTO) by hemicallotasis (HCO) using dynamic axial fixator (DAF) with the principle of neohistogenesis and gradual correction of varus deformity. The chapter of high tibial osteotomy by hemicallotasis has been separated from second edition of this book and published as a separate book titled *Step by Step High Tibial Osteotomy by Hemicallotasis*—parts of dynamic axial fixator, technique of fixator application and audiovisual presentation for education to medial compartment osteoarthritis patients for easy and better understanding of the steps.

Postoperative pain management has been described after TKR and THR. Management of complications like supracondylar fracture femur and infection following TKR have been included. Technique of revision TKR and THR has been mentioned. Whenever planned for arthrodesis of the knee following infected TKR, the technique has been described with limb reconstruction system (LRS).

A patient's guide to arthritis and joint replacement and ultrasonic cement removal system for revision joint replacement surgeries have been added.

Technically well-performed joint replacement surgeries and postoperative good physiotherapy give excellent results. Long-term success of joint replacement depends on restoration of the normal alignment of the lower limb, thereby, bringing the transverse axis of the knee parallel to the ground in anatomic two-legged stance and restoring normal weight distribution across the joint.

Ajit Kumar Mehta

Preface to the First Edition

Severe arthritis of the knee and hip is a painful disabling condition which cripples millions of people around the world and make them dependent on others even for activities of daily living. Due to increase in the life-expectancy, there is increase in the disease of advancing age like painful and disabling arthritis of knee and hip joints which require total knee and hip replacement (TKR and THR). A successful total knee and hip replacement not only provides relief from pain and disability but also makes a person fit to perform most of normal activities with some modification in life style. Total knee and hip replacements are extremely reliable and universally-accepted procedures that improve the quality of life significantly.

Total knee and hip replacement surgeries are special operations which require highest order of aseptic precaution, surgical skill and good team with almost fixed preoperative, peroperative and postoperative techniques and protocols with some modifications according to the individual case. We are strictly following the protocols and steps which are mentioned here. This book has been written after gaining the experience in more than 800 cases of total knee and hip replacement surgeries with successful outcome. It is very important to select the patients, educate them about the surgery, physiotherapy and postoperative protocols. Before doing the surgery plan properly, if required template, assess the difficult situations like FFD more than 30°, stiff knee (flexion <30°), large medial or lateral defects (i.e. severe varus or valgus deformity), post-HTO. Keep in mind the important points, sequential soft tissue release, cementing technique and avoid silly mistake in TKR. In cases of THR, look for acetabular dysplasia, posterior osteophytes, protrucio acetabuli, coxa magna, fractured acetabular floor, bony ankylosis of hip, adductor tightness, poor bone stock and plan properly before surgery. We have used the cruciate-substituting fixed-bearing PFC sigma knee implants and rotating platform high flexed (RPF) design for TKR. C-stem for cemented THR and Summit-tapered hip system for uncemented THR have been used. Whatever the implants used the basic principle remains the same. In this book the important points have been explained and demonstrated by the original photographs which will be helpful for the beginners. As these surgeries require highest order of aseptic precaution, so I have mentioned about the operation theater setup specification. It is advisable to have an adequate exposure of these surgeries before starting independently because there is no scope for even a small error which may jeopardize the activities of daily living (ADL) of the patients and early implant failure resulting into revision surgeries which are more difficult and less survival of the joint. Patients are coming for better quality of life so they cannot accept any error or complication. **It is also important to note that till joint is not operated the joint remains the patient's joint but once operated it becomes the surgeon's joint and hence the operating surgeon has to look after the joint whatever the problem arises.**

Postoperative pain management has been described after TKR and THR. Management of complications like periprosthetic fracture and infection following TKR have been included. Technique of revision TKR has been mentioned. Whenever planned for arthrodesis of the knee following infected TKR, the technique has been described with limb reconstruction system (LRS). Patient's guide to arthritis and joint replacement has been added.

We have used high tibial osteotomy by hemicallotasis using dynamic axial fixator for medial compartment osteoarthritis of knee with the principle of neohistogenesis and gradual correction of varus deformity in place of unicondylar knee replacement surgery with excellent result. The selection criteria and technique of HTO using dynamic axial fixator has been described for desired outcome.

Ajit Kumar Mehta

Acknowledgments

First of all I thank Prof Sudhir Kumar, New Delhi under the guidance of whom I really learnt the discipline of orthopedics during the tenure of my senior residency at BP Koirala Institute of Health Sciences, Dharan, Nepal. I take this opportunity to thank Dr SS Vengsarkar, Honorary Consultant and Dr JP Jain, Ex-HOD who have continuously guided while performing total joint replacement surgeries. I gladly acknowledge my debt to Dr Mangal Parihar who took the trouble of reading over sections of the manuscript and offering helpful comments. I sincerely thank him for his timely valuable suggestions. My special thanks to Dr VK Ramteke, Ex-Director General of Indian Railway Health Services, Ministry of Railways, Delhi, India, who has taken keen interest in developing this center during his tenure as Chief Medical Director and under guidance of whom, the best possible treatment is being provided to the patients.

My special thanks to my younger brother Mr Binay Mehta, Director, Dedicated Academy, who has encouraged and inspired me to write this book for the benefits of the beginner orthopaedic surgeons in total joint replacement surgeries. I am thankful to my wife Mrs Kiran Mehta who has taken care and my son Aman Raj who has spared time for me whenever I remained busy.

I am also very much thankful to anesthesiologists, especially Dr Reena Parampil, Dr Atul Sharma, Dr Dinesh Sahu, Dr Chandrakant Patel, Dr Ashish Korgaonker and Dr Anand Nirgude for writing the postoperative pain management in patients of TKR and THR.

My sincere thank to Dr Ashok Kumar Malviya and Dr Vipin Maheshwari from Ratlam, Madhya Pradesh, India for valuable comments and suggestions. My special and extended thanks to Dr Vipin Maheshwari for contribution of tibial flare index and thorough reading over manuscripts and grammatical corrections.

I am also thankful to physiotherapist Mrs Mrinalini S Bapat for valuable contribution of chapter on physiotherapy in TKR and THR and pre- and postoperative care of the patients.

I am very much thankful to Shri Jitendar P Vij (Group Chairman), Mr Ankit Vij (Group President) and Mr Tarun Duneja (Director-Publishing) of M/s Jaypee Brothers Medical Publishers (P) Ltd, New Delhi, India, and their Mumbai Branch Manager, Mr CS Gawde and Senior Sales Executive, Mr YT Bist (Mumbai Branch), who approached me for publishing the second edition of this book and their subsequent cooperation.

Contents

Introduction

1

CHAPTER

CHAPTER OUTLINE

- History and Clinical Examination
- Investigations
- Radiographic Classification of Osteoarthritis of Knee
- Physiotherapy, Education and Training
- Medicines to be Started
- Medicines to be Stopped Prior to Surgery
- Informed Consent for Surgery
- Patient and Relatives' Signature for Risk/Benefit Ratio
- Preoperative Planning for TKR
- Applied Anatomy
- Types of Total Knee Replacement
- Preparation of the Patient for Surgery and Arranging Blood

Introduction

Patient is preferably admitted 2–3 days prior to surgery for the purpose of:

1. History and clinical examination.
2. Investigations.
3. Physiotherapy, education and training.
4. Medical fitness and PAC (Preanesthetic checkup).
5. Informed consent for surgery and high-risk consent if associated with medical illness.
6. Patient and relative's signature for risk/benefit ratio.
7. Preoperative planning and templating.
8. Preparation of the patient for surgery and arranging blood.

However, all these purposes can be fulfilled on OPD basis and can be admitted one day prior to surgery.

History and Clinical Examination

Painful severe disabling arthritic joint with or without deformity, not responding to nonsurgical treatment, adversely affecting activities of daily living, ADL (such as ability to walk, climbing of stairs, performing job, care for self, knee bending activities, sleep pattern, sexual function) and quality of life.

Types of Patients according to Pain and Function (Krackow)

1. *No useful activities*: Marked difficulty even in routine essential activities.
2. *Minimal useful activities*: Moderate difficulty in indoor activities, just able to get outside house.
3. *Major limitations of activities*: Mild difficulty in indoor activities, major difficulty in outdoor activities.
4. *Moderate limitations of activities*: Can perform indoor activities but limited long distance walking.

Review of previous medical records: History of local injection, arthroscopy, HTO or any surgery.

Past history of trauma, medical/surgical illness.

Treatment history: Note the name of the medicines.
Socioeconomic condition.

General Examination

Normal higher functions, record—Pulse, BP, pallor, jaundice, edema, lymphadenopathy, chest, CVS, abdomen, assess the chest expansion and cardiopulmonary status in cases of spondyloarthropathies.

Local Examination

Knee Joints

	Right knee	Left knee
Skin condition		
Swelling		
Quadriceps wasting		
Local temperature		
Tenderness		
Crepitus		
Fixed flexion deformity (FFD)		
Hyperextension		
Varus/Valgus deformity		
Ligament laxity		
Range of motion (ROM)		

1. Intercondylar distance.
2. Intermalleolar distance.
3. Distal pulsation (Posterior tibial and dorsalis pedis artery), neurological deficit, look for varicose veins and calf tenderness.

Examination of Adjacent Joints

Hips, ankles and spine.

Hip Joints

	Right hip	Left hip
Skin condition		
Swelling		
Wasting		
Level of anterior superior iliac spine (ASIS)		
Lumbar lordosis		
Local temperature		
Tenderness		
Femoral pulsation		
Deformity (FFD, fixed adduction, abduction or rotation)		
Movements:		
• Flexion		
• Extension		
• Adduction		
• Abduction		
• Internal rotation (IR)		
• External rotation (ER)		
Adductor tightness		

Limb length discrepancy, gait, Trendelenburg's test, squatting, cross-legged sitting.

Note: **If the ipsilateral hip and knee joints are involved then hip should be operated first** to decide the mechanical axis and to get adequate movement of hip required during total knee replacement.

Investigations

1. X-rays
   i. Both knee joints—anteroposterior (AP) (standing or stress) and Lateral views (in 20° of flexion)
   ii. Patella skyline view
   iii. Both hip joints with upper 2/3rd thigh and 15° internal rotation—AP view
   iv. Involved hip with upper 2/3rd thigh—lateral view
   v. Both ankle joints—AP view
   v. Preferably take full length lower limbs standing X-ray (from both hips to both ankles)—AP view
   vi. LS spine—AP and lateral view
   vii. X-ray chest— posteroanterior (PA) view
   viii. X-ray cervical spine—AP and lateral view [for ankylosing spondylitis (AS)].
2 Routine:
   i. Blood—Hb, PCV, TLC, DLC, ESR, blood group, PT, PTT, INR, platelet count, blood sugar (fasting and PP), LFT (S. bilirubin, SGOT, SGPT, S. protein), S. alk. phosphatase, RFT (BUN, S. creatinine), S. uric acid, S. electrolytes (Na^+, K^+), RAF and CRP [for rheumatoid arthritis, (RA)]
   ii. Routine examination of urine
   iii. ECG.
3. Special—HIV, HbsAg, AntiHCV, VDRL.
4. Others—PFT and HLA B_{27} (for ankylosing spondylitis, AS), 2D ECHO, thallium scan, USG, CT, MRI, DEXA scan, color Doppler, bone scanning, arthroscopy, thyroid function tests, lipid profile, etc., if indicated.

Radiographic Classification of Osteoarthritis of Knee

Ahlback's classification: This reflects the anatomic and pathologic progression of medial compartment osteoarthritis and useful to decide the method of treatment.

Grade	AP view (stress X-ray)	Lateral view in 20° of flexion
1	Reduction of joint space	
2	Obliteration of joint space	
3	Tibial plateau attrition <5 mm	Posterior part of plateau intact
4	Attrition 5–10 mm	Attrition extending to posterior margin of the plateau
5	Severe subluxation of the tibia	Anterior subluxation of tibia >10 mm

In grade 1, there is reduction in height of the medial articular cartilage **(Fig. 1.1)**. In grade 2, there is loss of articular cartilage down to bone **(Fig. 1.2)**. In grade 3, there is anteromedial bone attrition of the tibial plateau **(Fig. 1.3)**. In grade 4, the lesion includes the posterior margin of the plateau; the progression from grade 3 to grade 4 is associated with rupture of the anterior cruciate ligament **(Figs 1.4A and B)**. In grade 5, there is anterior subluxation of the tibia more than 1 cm **(Fig. 1.5)**. The amount of tibial subluxation is measured as the distance between vertical lines drawn from the posterior edge of the medial femoral condyle and the posterior margin of the medial tibial plateau. Osteophytes should be ignored in the measurement.

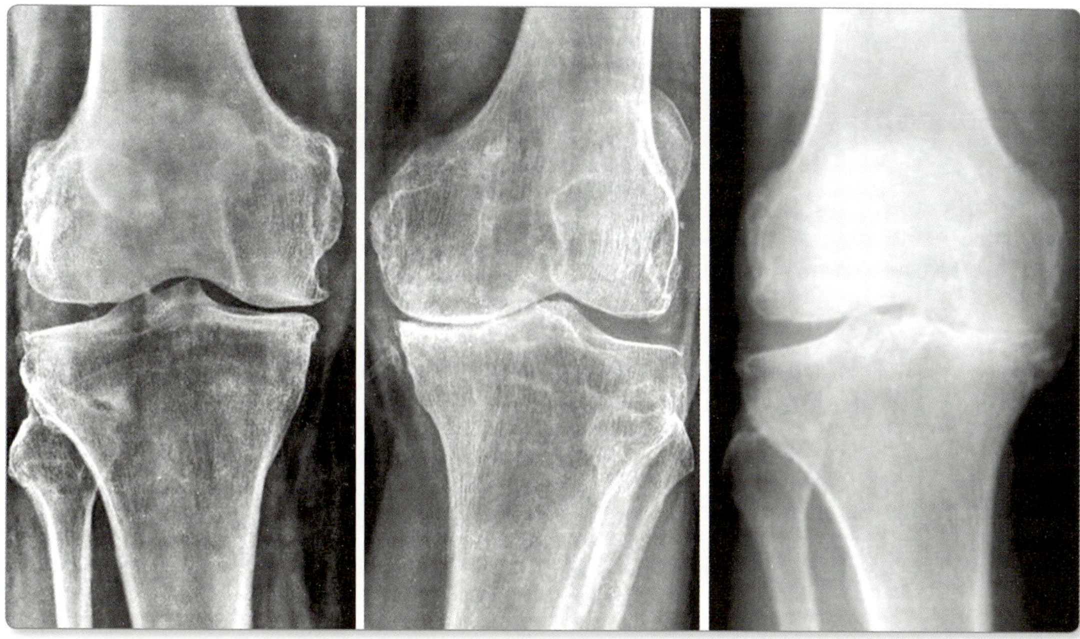

Fig.1.1 Grade 1 **Fig.1.2** Grade 2 **Fig.1.3** Grade 3

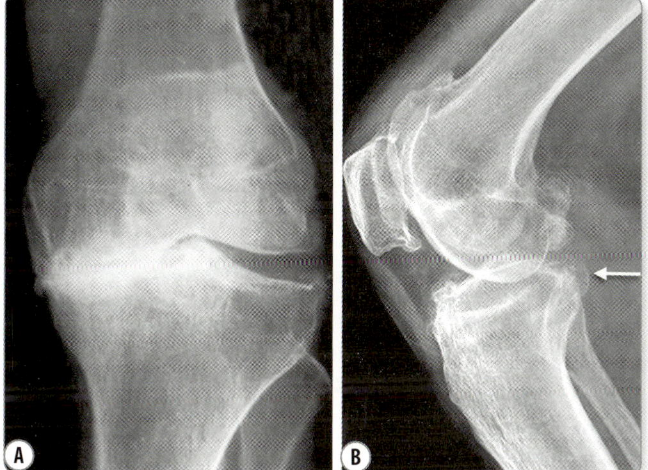

Figs 1.4A and B Grade 4

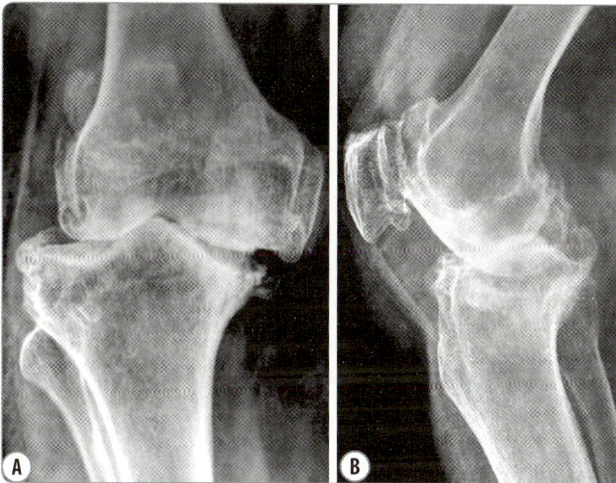

Figs 1.5A and B Grade 5

Grade 1, 2 and 3 are suitable for high tibial osteotomy (HTO) or unicondylar knee replacement and grade 4, 5 for total knee replacement (TKR).

Physiotherapy, Education and Training

1. Quadriceps exercise and knee bending exercise, active ankle and toes movement, straight leg raising exercise.
2. Education about surgery and postoperative protocols:
   - i. Avoid squatting or sitting on floor, jogging or running, local massage or heat therapy, cross-legged sitting.
   - ii. Use of western type of toilet.
   - iii. Sit on high chair approximately 20 inches height.
   - iv. Training to come out from the bed without flexing at hip in case of hip replacement surgery and abduction exercise of hip.

Medicines to be Started

In cases of osteoporosis where DEXA scan shows T score < –2.5, **following medicines are started:**

1. Injection Arachitol 6 lakhs unit IM weekly or 3 weekly for 3 injections.

2. Injection Deca-durabolin 25 mg IM weekly or 3 weekly for 3 injections.
3. Tablet Shelcal 500 mg BD.
4. Tablet Alpha—D_3 OD.
5. Osteofos 70 mg once weekly at least 30 minutes before breakfast in the morning with a full glass of water (not less than 200 mL). Alternatively, in postmenopausal woman, injection Ibandronate sodium 3 mg/3mL intravenously every 3 months or injection Zolendronic acid 5 mg/100 mL infusion bottle once per year.
6. In cases with severe osteopososis, injection teriparatide 20 μg daily self-injection is taken subcutaneously in thigh or abdominal wall at the same time each day and to be continued for 1½ year.

Medicines to be Stopped Prior to Surgery

1. If the patient is taking **Aspirin and/or Thienopyridine platelet inhibitors Clopidogrel (Clopid) and Ticlopidine,** they should be stopped at least one week prior to surgery and can be restarted after one week after surgery.
2. If the patient is taking **Methotrexate** [disease modifying antirheumatic drugs, (DMARD)] **or Abatacept** in rheumatoid arthritic cases, it should be stopped at least one month prior to surgery. It can be restarted one month after surgery.
3. If the patient is taking **Infliximab** for the treatment of spondyloarthropathies, it should be stopped at least two months prior to surgery and can be restarted after three months of surgery.

Informed Consent for Surgery

I, the undersigned Shri/Smt./Kum. .... Age ....S/O, W/O, D/O of Shri .... give consent of my free will for me/my ward's operation under General/Spinal/Epidural/Local or any other type of anesthesia, combined or supplemented, as required to be administered by anesthesiologist working in the hospital.

I also grant my consent to the doctor to use assistance of any other doctors as they feel needed, for any type of surgery, i.e. elective or emergency.

I also consent to the administration of blood/blood products, if necessary and understand the risks involved in it.

I have been explained and I have fully understood:

1. The necessity of operation/procedure.
2. The alternative methods of treatment.
3. The nature of operation.
4. The procedure of operation.
5. The consequences of operation.
6. The risks and complications of the operation.
7. The procedure of administration of anesthesia.
8. The risks and complications of anesthesia.
9. The allergic/unexpected reaction likely to any drug being used.

I have been explained the **additional risks** involved in the procedure because of my pre-existing medical problems of ....

I authorize the hospital to dispose off the tissues and parts removed during operation.

I shall not hold the hospital and doctors responsible in whatever manner for any consequence that may arise out of and in the course of my treatment/operation and administration of drug or injection, etc.

This has been explained to me in the language I understand.

Signature of patient

Signature of relative
Name
Relation
Date

Witness

Patient and Relatives' Signature for Risk/Benefit Ratio

Risk/benefit ratio about the surgery, postoperative limitation and protocols have been explained to the patient and relatives in their own language. They are willing for surgery.

Benefits: After complete recovery from the surgical procedure, patient will have painless, mobile and stable joint with normal limb alignment.

Risks: Complications like infection, deep vein thrombosis, limb length discrepancy, neurological deficit can occur. Wear-out and loosening of implant can happen later on.

Limitations: These are to avoid squatting or cross-legged sitting on floor, jogging or running, sports activities, local massage or heat therapy.

Protocols: Patient has to use western type of toilet life-long, regular quadriceps exercise, control of weight and regular follow-up as per advice.

Signature of patient   Signature of relative   Witness

Preoperative Planning for TKR

It is essential to prepare for the case and to anticipate situations that may arise during surgery for a successful outcome.

The goal of total knee replacement is to restore the joint line by inserting a prosthesis that is of the same thickness as the bone and cartilage that was removed and thus to relieve pain and normalize range of motion while providing stability through the gait cycle.

1. Full length lower limbs standing X-ray (from both hips to both ankles)—AP view.
2. Identify angle between mechanical and anatomical axis for distal femoral cut.
3. Lateral X-ray is required for sizing of femoral component with the help of templates.

Usually templating is not required for primary TKR but it is recommended if there is severe deformity with large defect, post-high tibial osteotomy (HTO) and revision TKR.

Vertical axis of body: This extends from the centre of gravity to the ground. Draw a vertical line from the center of symphysis pubis. In normally aligned lower limb, this will intersect perpendicular to the transverse knee and ankle axes **(Fig.1.6)**.

Mechanical axis of the lower limb: Draw a line from the center of head of femur to the center of the ankle. Normally, this line should pass through the base of lateral tibial spine (Fujisawa point) **(Fig.1.6)**. Because the hips are more widely separated than the knees and ankles, this mechanical axis is in 3° of valgus from the vertical axis of the body, i.e. 3° mechanical axis valgus **(Fig. 1.6)**. If this line passess through the center of the knee joint, then it is called neutral mechanical axis. Thus this line passes near or through the center of knee in the normally aligned lower limb which allows even load sharing between the medial and lateral condyles. Mechanical axis of lower limb also called Mikulicz line or load bearing axis or load line. The Mikulicz line (mechanical axis or load bearing axis or load line) intersects the total width of the tibia plateau lateral from the eminentia at a point at 62% to 66% of the distance from the medial border, called the Fujisawa point.

Jakob and Murphy have elaborated the method of passage of the mechanical axis based on the amount of cartilage space remaining on the medial side as determined from varus stress radiographs. When the mechanical axis passes through the center of the knee, the medial compartment bears 70% of the load. When the mechanical axis is moved into 4 degrees of valgus, the load is 50% medial and 50% lateral. When the mechanical axis is moved into 6 degrees of valgus, the load is 40% medial and 60% lateral.

Mechanical axis of the femur: Draw a line from center of head of femur to the highest point of the femoral notch. Draw another line perpendicular to this mechanical axis at the highest point of femoral notch.

Normally, mechanical axis of lower limb passes slightly lateral to the centre of knee and mechanical axis of femur in 3 degree mechanical axis valgus **(Figs 1.6 to 1.8)** or coincident in neutral mechanical axis.

Anatomic axis of femur: Draw a line from pyriform fossa to the highest point of the femoral notch. It is in 6° of valgus from mechanical axis of femur and 9° of valgus from vertical axis of body **(Fig. 1.6)**.

Mechanical/anatomic axis of the tibia: Draw a line from the midpoint between the tibial spines (i.e. center of proximal tibia) to the center of ankle. Draw another line perpendicular to the tibial axis at the level of upper tibial surface. The mechanical axis of the tibia is in 3 degrees of varus from the vertical axis of the body **(Fig. 1.6)**.

Anatomic axis of tibia is a line that bisects medullary canal while mechanical axis of the tibia is the line from center of proximal tibia to center of ankle. Usually mechanical axis and anatomic axis of tibia are coincident. If there is tibial deformity then mechanical and anatomic axis are not the same.

Determine the angle between mechanical and anatomical axis of the femur. Determine the angle between the lines perpendicular to the mechanical axis of femur and mechanical axis of tibia. The aim is to make these two lines parallel (i.e. converting the trapezoidal space into rectangular space) and hence to achieve 3 degree mechanical axis valgus or at least neutral mechanical axis of lower limb.

Normally, the anatomic axes of the femur and the tibia (fimorotibial angle, FTA) form a valgus angle of 6° ± 2°.

Hip-Knee-Ankle (HKA) angle: It is the angle between mechanical axes of femur and tibia. An HKA angle of less than 180 degree is defined as varus. Normal HKA angle is 183 to 185 degree which is measured on the medial side of the knee. As a convention, the HKA angle may be expressed as its angular deviation from 180°. Varus deviations are negative and valgus deviations are positive. The normal alignment of the lower limb is 3 to 5 degree positive (+ 3 to + 5).

In a normal knee, the tibial articular surface is in approximately 3° of varus with respect to the mechanical axis and the femoral articular surface is in a corresponding 9° of valgus. Since the tibia is cut perpendicular to the mechanical axis, hence the femoral cut is done at 9°–3° = 6° i.e. 5° to 7° valgus of the anatomic axis of femur to get the distal cut perpendicular to the mechanical axis of femur. Thus the tibial tray is implanted perpendicular to the mechanical axis of the tibia and the femoral component is implanted in 5° to 7° valgus of the anatomic axis and thus perpendicular to the mechanical axis of femur.

Long-term success of joint replacement depends on restoration of the normal alignment of the lower limb, thereby bringing the transverse axis of the knee parallel to the ground in anatomic two-legged stance and restoring normal weight distribution across the joint **(Fig 1.8)**.

In osteoarthritis of knee, following changes occur in the axes **(Fig. 1.7)**—

1. Mechanical axis of lower limb passes through the medial compartment or medial to the knee joint (Normally passes through lateral joint at Fujisawa point).
2. Hip-knee-ankle (HKA) angle <180 degree when measured on the medial side (Normal HKA angle is 183 to 185 drgree).
3. Anatomic axis and mechanical axis varus angles (Normal 3 to 5 degree mechanical axis valgus and 8 degree anatomic axis valgus).

Varus malalignment of lower limb is due to mechanical axis deviation (MAD) which is usually attributed to femoral or tibial osseous defomitties or both and also due to ligament laxity. The initiation of osteoarthritis occurs when healthy cartilage experiences some condition (traumatic or chronic) that causes kinematic changes during amulation at the knee to shift the load-bearing contact location of the joint to a region not conditioned to the new loading. The rate of progression of osteoarthritis is associated with increased load during ambulation. Noyes has classified the varus deformities as "primary varus" that is caused by a bony varus deformity arising from the tibia and femur. A "double varus" deformity develops when there is secondary loss of articular cartilage of the knee along with degeneration of menisci (intra-articular varus). In later stage, the "triple varus" is being contributed by laxity of the posterolateral ligament complex causing a hyperextension varus deformity.

As the varus deformity progress, there is maltracking of patella which leads to arthritis of patellofemoral joint and

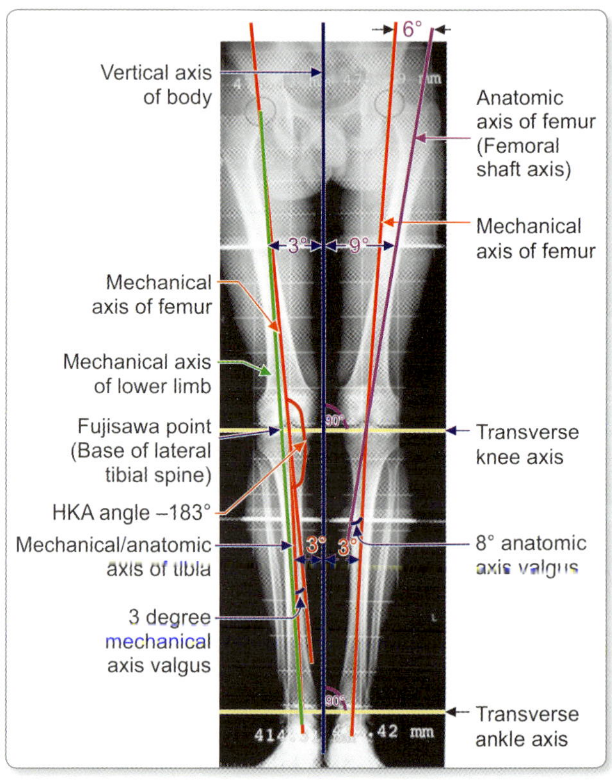

Fig. 1.6 Normal alignment of lower limbs

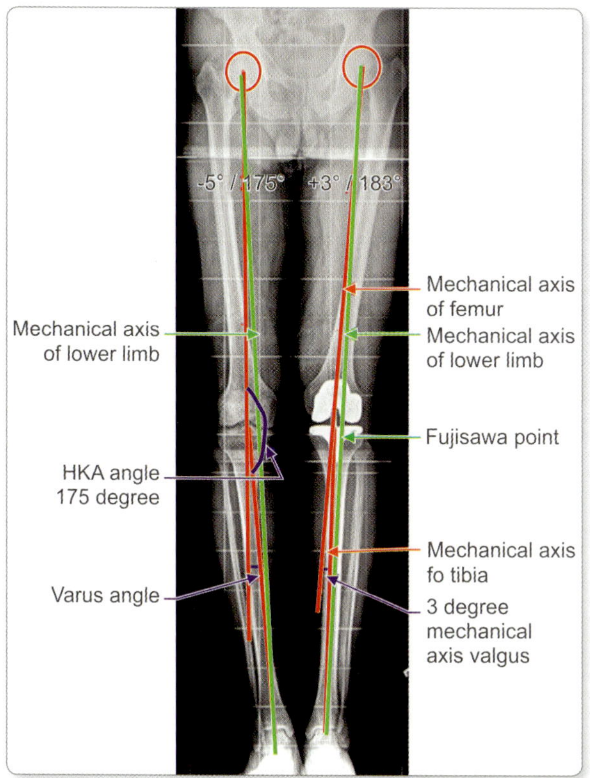

Fig. 1.7 Osteoarthritis right knee with varus angle and left knee after total knee replacement with restoration of 3 degree mechanical axis valgus and mechanical axis passes through Fujisawa point

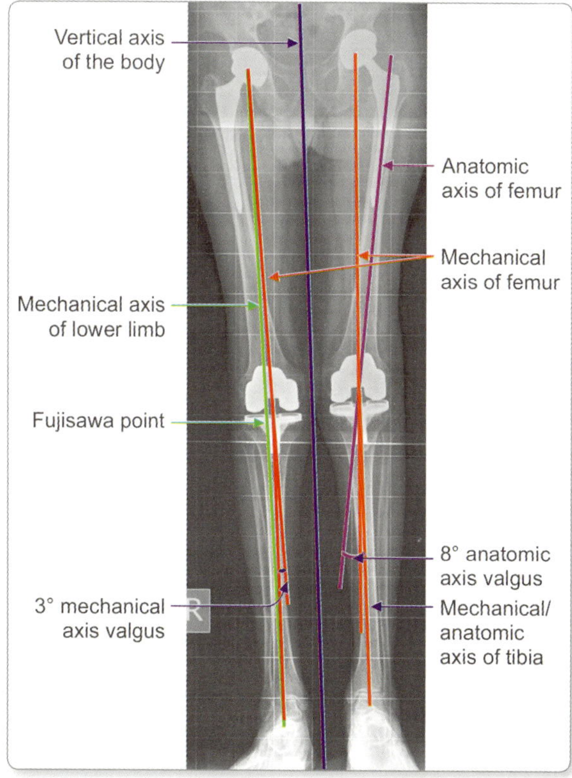

Fig. 1.8 Restoration of normal alignment of lower limbs after bilateral TKR and THR (3 degree mechanical axis valgus, 8 degree anatomic axis valgus and mechanical axis of lower limb passes through Fujisawa point)

gradually progresses to arthritis of lateral compartment (i.e. triple compartment osteoarthritis). Ultimately, there is failure of ACL and PCL with stretching of lateral collateral ligament which leads to subluxation of knee joint **(Fig. 1.1 to 1.5)**.

During knee replacement surgery, the damaged joint is resurfaced by using tibial and femoral cutting jigs in such a way that the mechanical axis reverts back to normal level, i.e passes through Fujisawa point and 3 to 5 degree mechanical axis valgus **(Fig. 1.7 and 1.8)**.

Applied Anatomy

Knee Joint

It is made of three joints:

1. Medial condyloid joint between medial condyle of femur and corresponding medial meniscus and condyle of tibia (Medial compartment).
2. Lateral condyloid joint between lateral condyle of femur and corresponding lateral meniscus and condyle of tibial (Lateral compartment).
3. Patellofemoral joint between patella and femur.

The femur and tibia are connected together by the following ligaments:

1. Articular capsule (capsular ligament).
2. Ligamentum patellae.
3. Oblique popliteal ligament.
4. Tibial collateral ligament.
5. Fibular collateral ligament.
6. Anterior cruciate ligament.
7. Posterior cruciate ligament.
8. Medial and lateral menisci.
9. Transverse ligament—connects the anterior convex margin of the lateral meniscus to the anterior end of the medial meniscus.
10. Coronary ligament—portions of the capsule which connect the periphery of each meniscus with the margin of the head of the tibia.

Other structures are synovial membrane, lateral patellofemoral plicae, infrapatellar fat pad and bursae around the knee joint.

Arrangement of Neurovascular Structures around the Knee

The arrangement of neurovascular structures can be linked to the points on the face of a clock as shown in **Figure 1.9**:

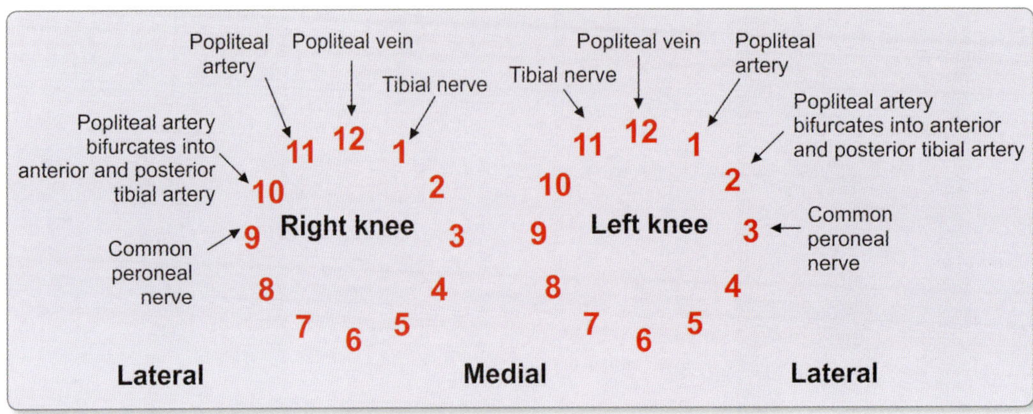

Fig. 1.9 Arrangement of neurovascular structures

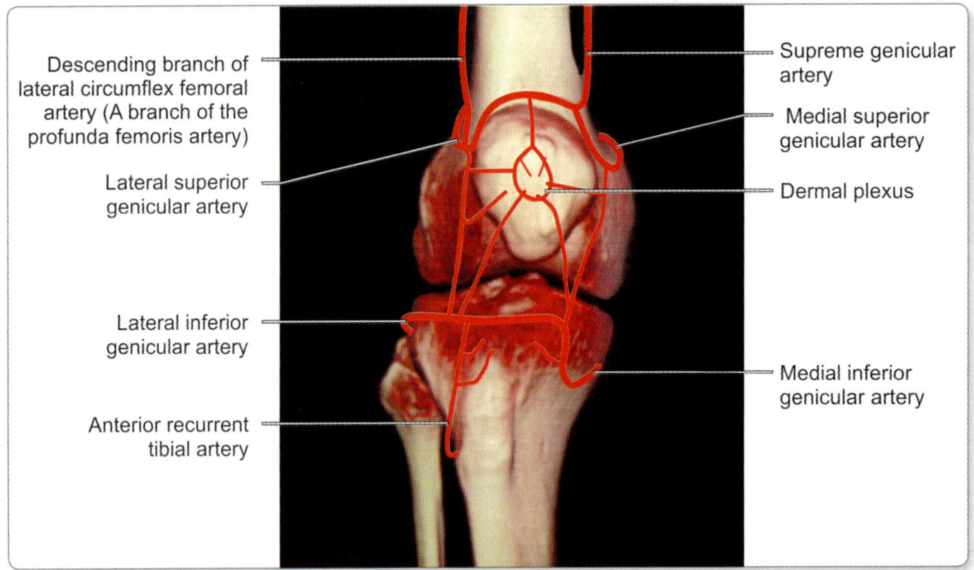

Fig 1.10 Blood supply to knee joint

Popliteal vein: It lies directly in the midline posteriorly at 12 O' clock position.

Tibial Nerve: It lies just medial to popliteal vein at the 11 O' clock position in left knee and 1 O'clock position in right knee.

Popliteal artery: It lies just lateral to popliteal vein at 1 O' clock position in left knee and 11 O' clock position in right knee.

Bifurcation of popliteal artery: The popliteal artery bifurcates below the joint line into anterior and posterior tibial arteries at the 2 O' clock position in left knee and 10 O' clock position in right knee.

Common peroneal nerve: It lies further laterally against the neck of fibula, distal to the joint line at the 3 O' clock position in left knee and 9 O' clock position in the right knee.

Damage to neurovascular structures may occur between 11 O' clock and 3 O' clock positions in left knee and between 9 O' clock and 1 O' clock position in right knee. Careful surgical technique and knowledge of the neurovascular anatomy at the knee will help in avoiding neurovascular injury during TKR.

Blood Supply to the Knee (Fig. 1.10)

The blood supply to the knee arises predominantly from the peripatellar anastomotic ring which is formed by the contributions of:

1. The superior and inferior genicular arteries (medial and lateral) which are branches of popliteal artery.
2. The supreme genicular artery which is the branch of superficial femoral artery.
3. The anterior recurrent tibial artery.
4. A branch of the profunda femoris artery.

Anterior knee circulation is dependent on the dermal plexus which originates from arterioles travelling with the midline subcutaneous fascia. Hence, during midline skin incision, do not undermine the skin and raise the skin flaps deep to the fascial layer to avoid skin necrosis. The blood supply from the medial side is generally more significant than that arising from the lateral side. Consequently, when faced with more than one parallel longitudinal incision, the lateral incision should be selected.

Lateral inferior genicular artery is usually cut during surgery and requires coagulation by electrocautery.

Movements of Knee Joint

1. Flexion and extension.
2. Internal and external rotation in certain position of the joint.

The movements of flexion and extension at knee joint differs from those in a typical hinge joint. The axis around which motion takes place is not a fixed one but shifts forward during extension and backward during flexion and the commencement of flexion and the end of extension are accompanied by rotatory movements associated with the fixation of the limb in a position of great stability.

Types of Total Knee Replacement

In a normal knee, anterior cruciate ligament (ACL) is an important stabilizer but in a prosthetic joint ACL is not necessary for adequate functioning and PCL is more important to prevent posterior shift or sag of tibia in order to maintain relative position of femur and tibia, and thereby also to maintain adequate quadriceps function. When PCL is not working or has to be sacrificed to correct severe deformities, it must be substituted in the prosthesis by a Spine-Cam mechanism. TKR is of 3 types depending on the degree of mechanical stability provided by the design of the artificial knee—

1. Nonconstrained (Cruciate-retaining or CR design).
2. Semiconstrained (Cruciate-substituting or posterior stabilized or PS design).
3. Constrained (hinged design).

Nonconstrained (Cruciate-retaining or CR design): In this implant, the artificial components are not linked to each other and have no stability built into the system. Stability relies on intact PCL. Here ACL is sacrificed but PCL is retained. In CR design, lateral distal femoral condyle of femoral component is longer in anteroposterior direction than the corresponding medial condyle. This disparity creates unequal rolling distances (i.e. differential rolling) and facilitates external rotation of femur when flexion begins and vice versa internal rotation of femur to bring about screw-home movement in final degree of knee extension. As the flexion increases, center of femur moves posteriorly relative to tibia and this shift can be as much as 8 mm on 0–120 degree flexion. This is known as femoral rollback in flexion and is an important part of normal knee biomechanics which is guided mainly by PCL and lateral collateral ligaments. This rollback is duplicated when CR design prosthesis is used. Femoral rollback is facilitated by less dished surface geometry of posterior part of tibial polyethylene. Hence tibial articular surface of CR prosthesis is flat looking as compared to the sagittal profile of corresponding femoral component.

Semiconstrained (Cruciate-substituting or posterior stabilized or PS design): This type of artificial knee has some stability built into it in the form of Spine-Cam mechanism. Here both ACL and PCL are sacrificed. In PS femoral component medial and lateral femoral condyle have same length anteroposteriorly and hence differential rotaion does not occur. The tibial articular surface is more dished and deeper to allow controlled motion between femur and tibia. Spine-Cam mechanism is a mechanical substitution for PCL and consists of a post in the middle of tibial polyethylene and a metal stabilizing bar (cam) in intercondylar area of femoral prosthesis. Both are so positioned that the stabilizing bar (cam) is posterior to tibial post. Polyethylene tibial post has an extension to prevent medial or lateral displacement of post around either of femoral condyle when knee is flexed beyond 90 degree. In order to accommodate polyethylene tibial post and femoral cam, the middle of posterior stabilized femoral component has a dropped box built in, which requires removal of some bone from intercondylar area of femur to accommodate this box. We are using PFC sigma cruciate-substituting fixed bearing and cruciate-substituting mobile bearing (rotating platform high flexed TKR, i.e. RPF) knee implants.

Constraint or hinged variety implants are rarely used as a first choice of surgical options. In this case, the two components of the knee joint are linked together with a hinged mechanism. This type of knee replacement is used when the knee is highly unstable and the person's ligaments will not be able to support the other type of knee replacements. It is useful in the treatment of severely damaged knees particularly in very elderly people undergoing a revision replacement procedure. The disadvantage of this type of knee joint is that it is not expected to last as long as the other types.

A unicondylar knee replacement replaces only half of the knee joint. It is performed if the damage is limited to one side of the joint only with the remaining part of the knee joint being relatively spared. Here only that area of the knee joint is replaced which is severely damaged. However, even with only half of the joint destroyed, many surgeons prefer doing a total knee replacement believing this is a better procedure than the half-knee (unicondylar) replacement. But equally, there are surgeons who believe it is more appropriate to perform a unicondylar knee in the right circumstance.

In place of unicondylar knee replacement for medial compartment osteoarthritis (MCOA), we are performing high tibial osteotomy (HTO) by hemicallotasis HCO) using a dynamic axial fixator (DAF) in younger patients and total knee replacement in elderly.

Preparation of the Patient for Surgery and Arranging Blood

Arrange 2 units of blood for replacement of each knee or hip joint.

2 days prior to surgery: Thorough bath with antiseptic soap (e.g. dettol soap).

1 day prior to surgery:

1. Thorough bath with antiseptic soap (e.g. dettol soap) in the morning.
2. Injection Enoxaparin sodium (Clexane), a low molecular weight heparin (LMWH), 40 mg/0.4 mL SC (subcutaneously) at 8.00 AM (1st dose, 24 hours prior to surgery).
3. Injection TT (Tetanus toxoid) 1 amp. IM stat if not immunized previously or immune status is not known.
4. Injection Xylocaine sensitivity test.
5. Scrubbing of the part by betadine scrub in the evening.
6. Soap water enema at 5.00 PM.
7. Injection Dexona (Dexamethasone) 4 mg IV at 8.00 PM (1st dose, 12 hours prior to surgery).
8. Tablet Reglan 1 tab at bed time.
9. Tablet Rantac 1 tab at bed time.
10. Tablet Alprax (0.25 mg) 1 tab at bed time.
11. NBM (Nil by mouth) after 10.00 PM.

On the day of surgery:

1. Injection Cefotaxime 1 g IV just before sending the patient to OT.
2. Injection Amikacin 500 mg IV just before sending the patient to OT. In cases where BUN and serum creatinine are on higher side, use Augmentin 1.2 g IV in place of injection Amikacin.
3. Injection Dexona (Dexamethasone) 4 mg IV 2nd dose, just before sending the patient to OT.
4. Part preparation—Shaving and antiseptic dressing from umbilicus to toes including private parts on the operative side of limb and up to lower thigh on the other side. Shaving should be done on the day of surgery just before sending the patient to OT to avoid colonization of bacteria. Operative side limb is wrapped in a sterile towel or sterile polyethylene drape.
5. Side room in OT: Premedication (Injection Reglan and injection Glycopyrrolate/Atropine) and change of clothes.
6. Patient is taken on OT table.
7. Anesthesia: Preferably spinal + epidural
8. Bladder is catheterized.

Note:

1. If the patient is diabetic and on hypoglycemic agents, switch over to insulin prior to surgery. Withhold morning dose of insulin and send fasting blood sugar.
2. If the patient is hypertensive and on antihypertensive medicines, give antihypertensive medicines with sips of water in the early morning.
3. Alternative low molecular weight heparins (LMWH) are Dalteparin (Fragmin), Nadroparin (Fraxiparine), Tinzaparin (Innohep), Reviparin (Clivarin), Parnaparin (Fluxum), Fondaparinux sodium (Arixtra).

Recently one of the following oral anticoagulant can be used:

i. Rivaroxaban (Xarelto).
ii. Apixaban (Eliquis).
iii. Dabigatran (Pradaxa).

The dose of Rivaroxaban (Xarelto) is 10 mg once daily. The initial dose should be taken within 6 to 10 hours of completing surgery, provided that hemostasis has been established. Treatment duration is two weeks for TKR and five weeks for THR. It can be taken with or without meal. Coagulation monitoring is not required. There should be 18 hours gap between last dose of Xarelto and removal of epidural catheter and the next dose has to be given 6 hours after the removal of catheter followed by every 24 hourly.

The dose of Apixaban (Eliquis) is 2.5 mg twice daily. The initial dose should be taken 12 to 24 hours after surgery. The treatment duration is 10 to 14 days for TKR and 32 to 38 days for THR. It can be taken with or without food.

Dabigatran (Pradaxa) is started 110 mg stat 1–4 hours postsurgery on day 1. From day 2, it is given 220 mg (110 mg capsule × 2) up to 10 days for TKR and 35 days in THR. In patients more than 75 years, moderate renal impairment and patients taking Amiodarone and Verapamil, effective lower dose is 75 mg OD on day 1 started within 1–4 hours and 150 mg (75 mg capsule × 2) once daily.

Total Knee Replacement (Cruciate-substituting Fixed Bearing TKR)

2 CHAPTER

CHAPTER OUTLINE

Tourniquet Application

Tourniquet is applied in upper-third of thigh after pulling the thigh muscle down to minimize the catching of quadriceps under tourniquet. Recheck the ligament laxity under anesthesia. If varus/valgus deformity is correctable under anesthesia, it means that much soft tissue release is not required **(Figs 2.1A and B)**.

Positioning

A small sand bag is fixed with elastoplast at the junction of middle-third and lower-third of the table. The patient is brought down towards the foot end of the table so that the fixed sand bag lies beneath the knee. In an obese patient, the level of knee should be kept slightly proximal to the fixed sand bag. On full flexion of knee, the fixed sand bag will

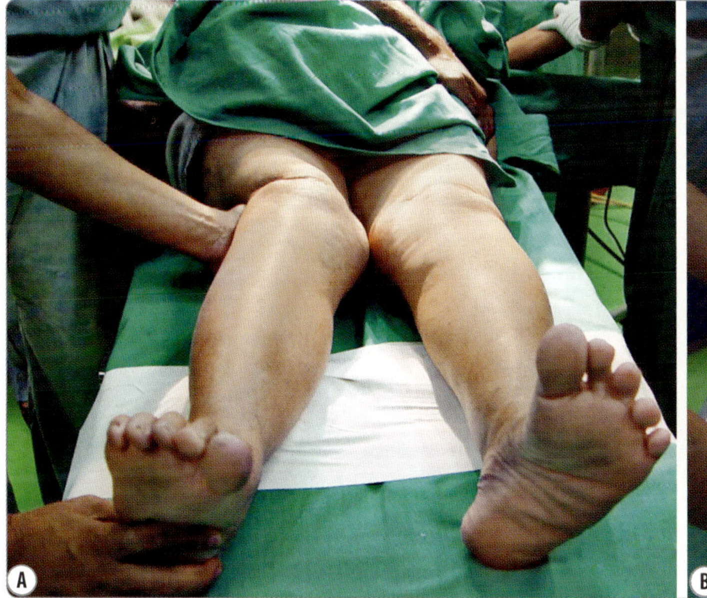

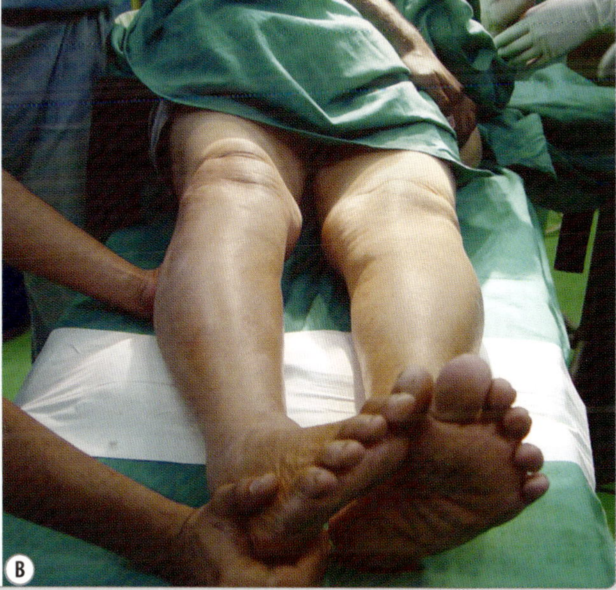

Figs 2.1A and B (A) Valgus stress; (B) Varus stress

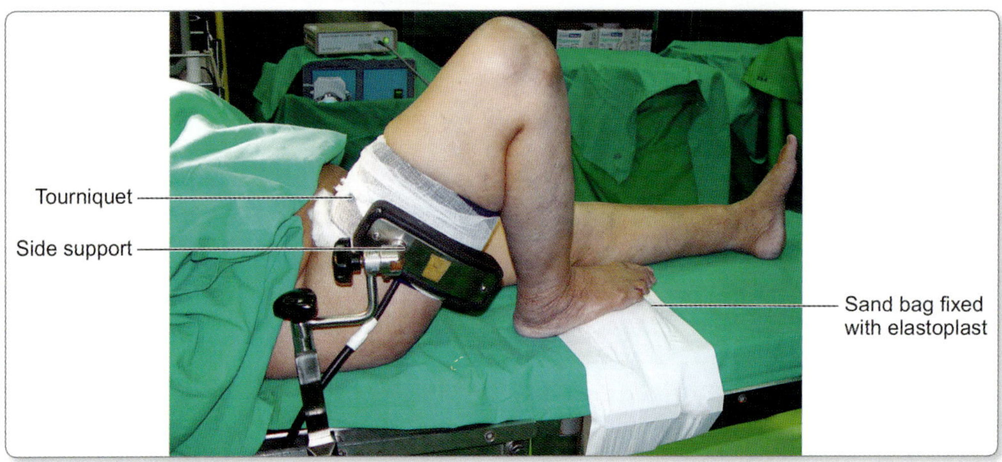

Fig. 2.2 Side support and perpendicular position of leg on full flexion of knee

support the foot. A side support is applied to support the upper third of the thigh. In this position, the leg becomes perpendicular to the table **(Fig. 2.2)**. Electrocautery pad is kept under the back of the patient. Cover the chest and abdomen of the patient with warm clothes or body warmer to avoid hypothermia in elderly as the operating room temperature is kept 20–22°C. Keep the operating table at lower most level.

Scrubbing

Keep one sterile polyethylene drape below the operative limb on the table. One attendant will hold the limb from heel and other will scrub it by betadine scrub from thigh to toes for 3 to 5 minutes. Wipe out the scrub with sponge and apply sprit on the limb from thigh to toes. While scrubbing is going on, the operating surgeon and three assistants get prepared and wear the body exhaust system **(Fig. 2.3)**. Apply betadine solution over the limb from thigh to toes. The polyethylene drape is removed from the table.

Draping

Take four sterile polyethylene drapes (100 × 150 cm) and apply two below the limb on the table and two above covering the proximal third of thigh with tourniquet. Apply one big towel below the limb on the table and one above covering the proximal third of thigh and spread proximally. Both the sheets are fixed by towel clips snugly with skin on medial and lateral aspect of thigh. The surgeon holds the leg with a sponge and applies betadine solution over the heel and foot. Make the heel and foot dry by wiping with dry gauze piece. Apply two 8.5 number gloves on the foot and then apply double layered stockinet on the limb and fix the stockinet by towel clips with sheets in upper part of thigh. Put curtain in the proximal part. Apply U-drape and then two side sheets which are fixed by two towel clips in the proximal part and one towel clip near the thigh in posterior aspect. Finally apply the hole-sheet. Keep two suction drains and electrocautery on proximal part of draping in a towel bag. Elevate the limb and apply Esmarch's bandage from toes to upper thigh. Flex the knee beyond 90° to avoid the catching of quadriceps muscle under tourniquet. Inflate the cuff of tourniquet up to 400 mm Hg. Extend the knee. Slit the stockinet from thigh to tibial tubercle by help of forceps and scissors. Fold the slit margins of stockinet inwards to expose the knee. Wipe out the area with spirit or betadine solution and dry with dry gauze piece. Apply InteguSeal (sterile, film-forming cyanoacrylate liquid, provided in a ready-to-use applicator) microbial sealant to the operative field to lock the skin pathogens and thus prevent contamination of the incision site. With a sterile marking pencil or methylene blue, mark the outline of patella, tibial tubercle, one mark 3 fingerbreadths (6 cm) proximal to the upper pole of patella in the thigh. Draw one straight line over the center of patella joining the proximal mark in thigh up to 1 cm medial to the tibial tubercle. Flex the knee at 90° and apply one large Ioban (60 × 45 cm) over the knee. Extend the knee and apply another large Ioban (60 × 45 cm) over lower part of leg and whole foot to cover it completely **(Fig. 2.4)**. Put the sand bag beneath the knee to keep the knee flexed at 30° to 60° **(Fig. 2.5)**. Put two sponges over the Iobans on knee and leg and press them so that the Ioban sticks completely to the skin. Remove the two sponges and every member of surgical team will wear the second pair of gloves.

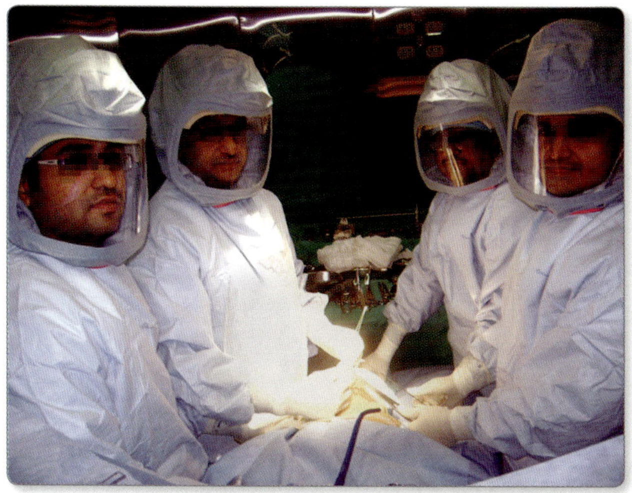

Fig. 2.3 Body exhaust system

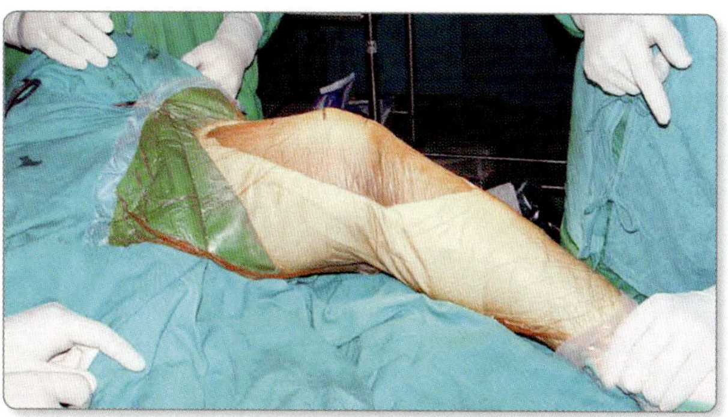

Fig. 2.4 After draping

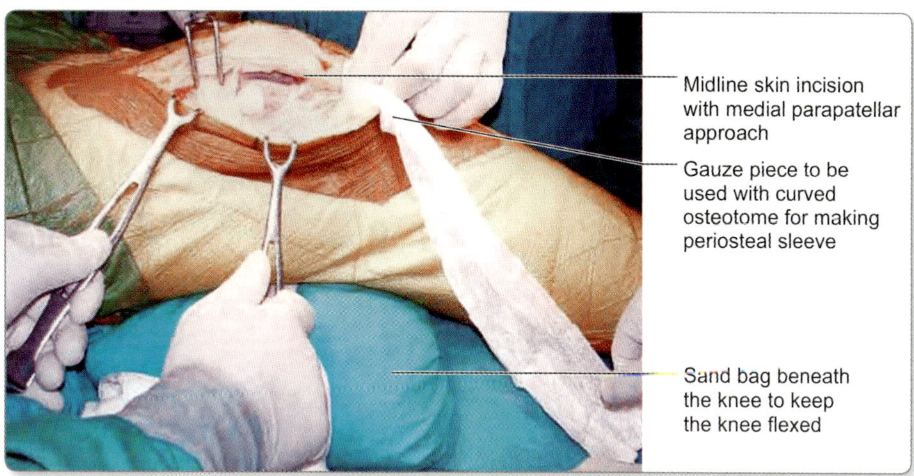

Fig. 2.5 Midline skin incision and medial parapatellar approach

Incision

Give a midline skin incision (with BP blade No. 22) extending from 3 fingerbreadths (6 cm) above the upper pole of patella to 1 cm medial to the tibial tubercle as per skin marking. Do not undermine the skin. Raise the skin flaps deep to the fascial layer to avoid skin necrosis. Take 2nd knife (BP blade No. 24) to expose the knee by medial parapatellar approach staring at the junction of medial 1/3rd and lateral 2/3rd of the tendon of rectus femoris, curve the incision medially and ½ cm away from the medial boarder of patella to 1 cm medial to the tibial tubercle **(Fig. 2.5)**. For right knee, the incision is from above-downward and for the left knee it is below-upward. Suck the synovial fluid by suction.

Exposure of Knee

Using a curved osteotome and gauze piece, make a periosteal sleeve between soft tissue and bone on the anteromedial and medial aspect of tibial condyle while flexing and externally rotating the leg. By the help of electrocautery, do a preliminary essential soft tissue release along the margin of medial tibial plateau and tibial condyle. Remove osteophytes from the tibia and femur by nibbler to reduce the Bowstring effect. Evert the patella, remove osteophytes from the patella. Straighten the leg and remove the infrapatellar fat pad and do localized synovectomy from supracondylar region. Synovial tissues from supracondylar region may be sent for histopathological examination.

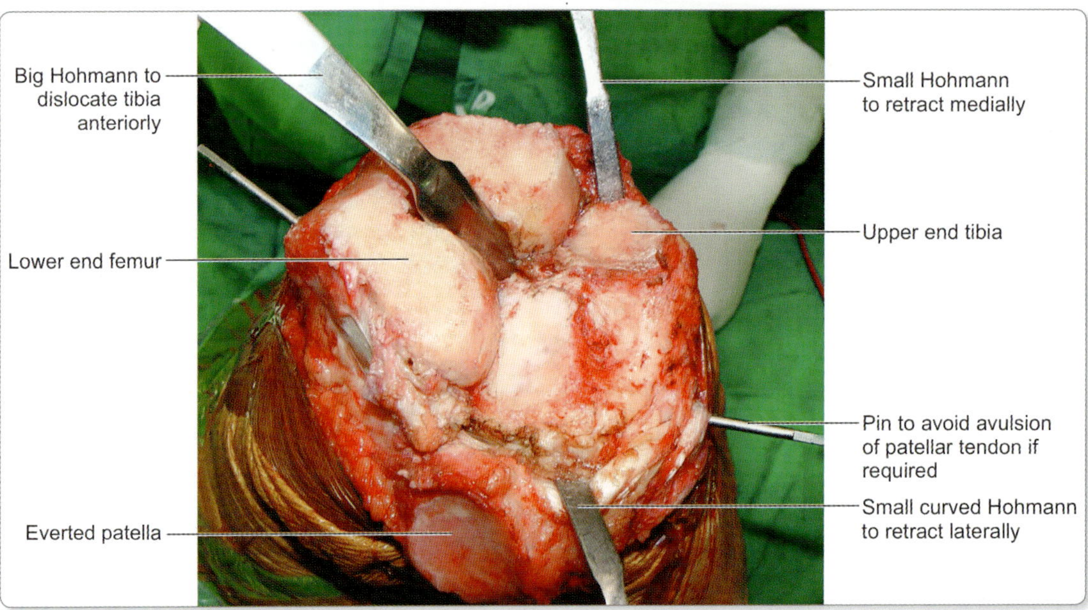

Fig. 2.6 Exposure of knee

Remove the sand bag from beneath the knee, evert the patella and gradually flex the knee. While everting the patella and flexing the knee, care should be taken to avoid avulsion of patellar tendon from the tibial tubercle. In case of tight patellar tendon, apply a pin over the insertion of patellar tendon. Apply a small curved Hohmann on the lateral aspect of tibial condyle to retract the everted patella. Release lateral patellofemoral plicae. Apply a small Hohmann on the medial aspect of tibial condyle to retract the medial collateral ligament and soft tissues on the medial side. Remove the remaining infrapatellar fat pad. Excise the medial and lateral menisci, ACL and PCL. Leave a stump of PCL behind to prevent injury to the popliteal vein which lies directly posterior in the midline. Flex the knee gradually till the leg becomes perpendicular to the table. One assistant should hold at the ankle to keep the knee flexed fully. Another assistant will lift the thigh and surgeon will apply a big Hohmann on the posterior aspect of upper part of tibia to dislocate it anteriorly. Excise the remnant of meniscus parallel to the posterior margin of the tibia after pulling it anteriorly and leaving a portion of the medial and lateral menisci peripherally to avoid the risk of vascular injury. While removing medial meniscus, leave about 2 mm part of medial meniscus to avoid damage to the medial collateral ligament. Slightly release the PCL from the tibial attachment by electrocautery **(Fig. 2.6)**.

Tibial Cut

Keep the knee fully flexed so that the leg remains perpendicular to the table. Apply the tibial alignment device with either 0° or 3° sloped tibial cutting block. **Usually take** a 3° **posterior sloped tibial cutting block** (The posterior slope of tibia is 10° and 7° slope is already given in the tibial insert so required posterior slope is 3°). 0° posterior sloped tibial cutting block is taken if there is fixed flexion deformity (FFD), post high tibial asteotomy (HTO) or post-trauma and 5° if there is residual tightness in flexion after cutting with 3° posterior sloped tibial cutting block and even after addressing the posterior osteophytes, soft tissues and loose bodies. The malleolar clamp of the tibial alignment device is positioned immediately proximal to the malleoli and the platform is raised to the level of condyles. In the lower part, adjust 0° slope on tibial alignment device, shift the tibial alignment device 1 mark medial (3 mm) to keep it in the center of the leg (as the midline of the tibia is approximately 3 mm medial to the transaxial midline). In the upper part, align the platform with the medial 1/3rd of the tibial tubercle and medial margin of the lateral intercondylar eminence with extremities of the cutting surface against the anterior cortex **(Fig. 2.7)**.

Take the tibial stylus with slotted mark on the outrigger and insert the foot plate of tibial stylus into the slot of tibial cutting block with height set at 0 mm on the more involved condyle while keeping the tip of outrigger at the center of tibial plateau or 8 mm on less involved condyle and maximum up to 10 mm. Fix the tibial cutting block with two Steinmann pins (3.2 mm) introduced through the central holes marked with square. If bone is hard, make 2.5 mm drill holes before putting the pins. Check the amount of cut with the help of visualization guide. Put the oscillating saw (1.25 mm thick saw blade, No. 519.115) in the slot of tibial cutting block and cut the tibia perpendicular to the tibial

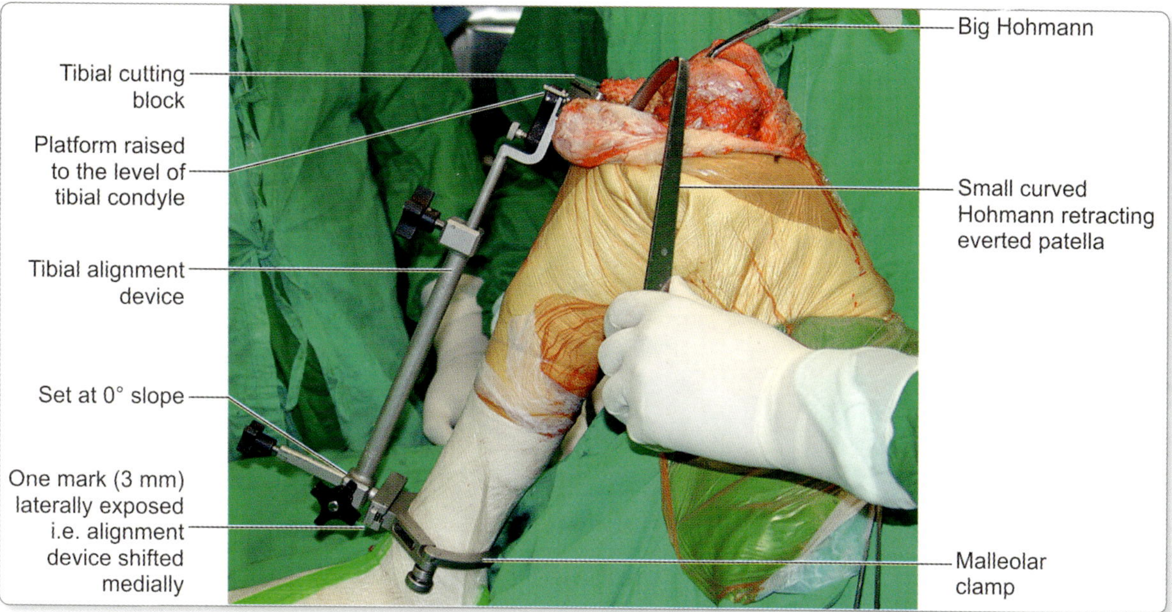

Fig. 2.7 Position of tibial alignment device

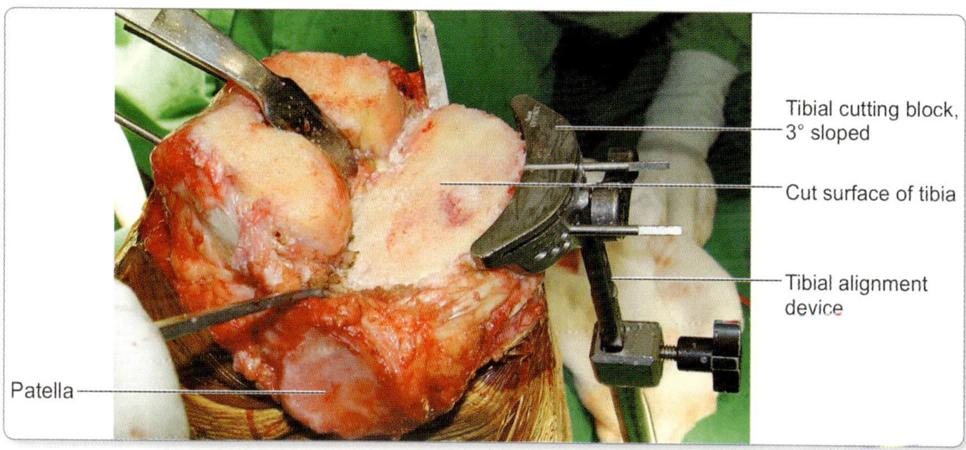

Fig. 2.8 Cut surface of upper tibia perpendicular to the tibial axis

axis **(Fig. 2.8)**. Lift the resected part of tibia with osteotome. Hold it with a Kocher and remove it from soft tissues on posterior and lateral aspect with help of electrocautery keeping adjacent to the resected bone. Remove the tibial alignment device and tibial cutting block. Put the trial tibial tray over the upper surface of resected tibia and determine the size of the tibial tray. The trial tibial tray should rest on the cortex. It should not overhang otherwise it will cause friction to the collateral ligaments and it should not be undersized otherwise it will sink.

If the defect in tibia is more, cut 10 mm tibia on less involved condyle and built up the residual defect either by bone cement when the defect is less than 5 mm or by screws and bone cement/bone graft/metallic wedge when the defect is more than 5 mm. Less than 2 mm residual tibial defect may be included in tibial resection. For this, re-apply the same tibial cutting block at +2 mark hole and resect the 2 mm tibia by oscillating saw.

Femoral Cut

Remove the posterior Hohmann and push the tibia back. Remove the osteophytes from the femoral notch by nibbler **(Fig. 2.9)**. Find out the insertion point for the femoral drill at the midline of the femoral notch 7–10 mm anterior to the origin of the PCL. While palpating the distal femoral shaft, pass an 8 mm femoral drill about 5–7 cm in the medullary canal keeping the drill in the line of femur to avoid penetration of the cortices **(Fig. 2.10)**.

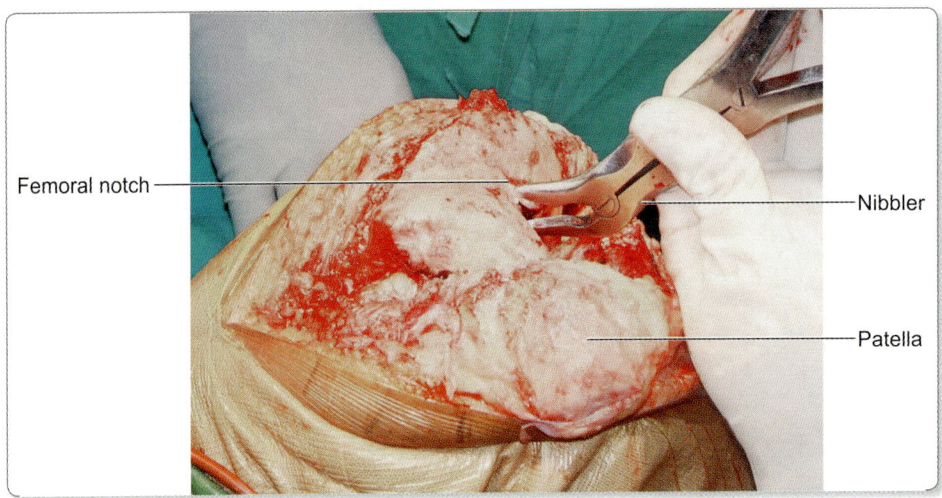

Fig. 2.9 Removing osteophytes from femoral notch by nibbler to find out the entry point for femoral canal

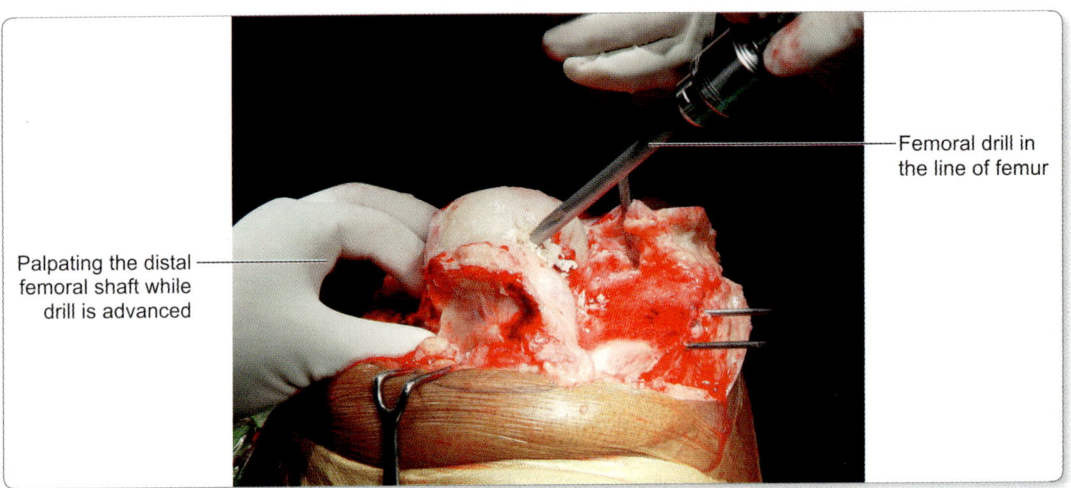

Fig. 2.10 Drilling with 8 mm femoral drill in femoral canal

While bringing out the drill from medullary canal, widen the canal to minimize the intramedullary pressure to avoid fat embolism. After removing the drill, wash the femoral canal with 100 mL normal saline to remove the fat globules to avoid possible fat embolism. Pass the fluted intramedullary rod with help of T-handle in medullary canal of femur after attaching the femoral locating device fixed at 5° or 7° valgus on operating side (R or L). Usually select 7° valgus in varus knee and 5° in valgus knee. The alignment tower is assembled onto the femoral locating device and alignment rod is passed through the upper hole and advanced towards the hip. Keep the alignment rod of 2 fingerbreadths medial to the anterior superior iliac spine (i.e. center of the hip). Check the rotational alignment that the posterior part of medial condyle is exposed more than the posterior part of lateral condyle (slight external rotation) and the calibrated outrigger is centered at the femoral trochlea **(Fig. 2.11)**. Also check that the posterior surface of femoral locating device is perpendicular to the mechanical axis of the tibia in 90° of flexion. Fix the assembly by hammering on medial and lateral self-attached pins. The distal femoral cutting block is assembled onto the calibrated outrigger by depressing the button located on the right proximal end. Adjust the distal femoral cutting block at 9 mm marked on the calibrated outrigger (as the thickness of femoral component is 9 mm). Remove the alignment tower with alignment rod. The

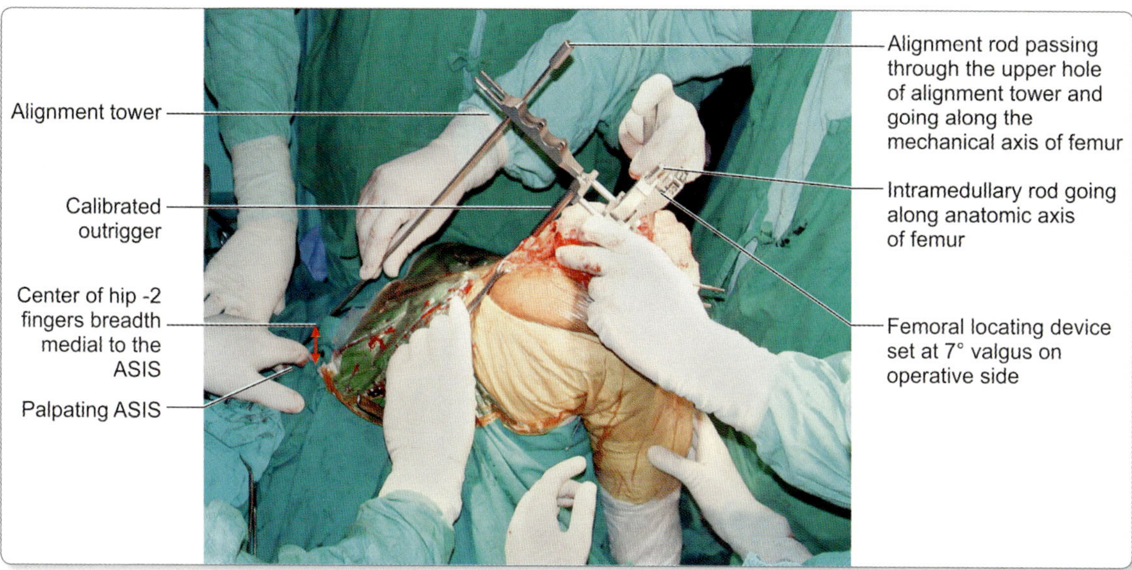

Fig. 2.11 Femoral locating device set at 7° valgus with alignment tower and alignment rod

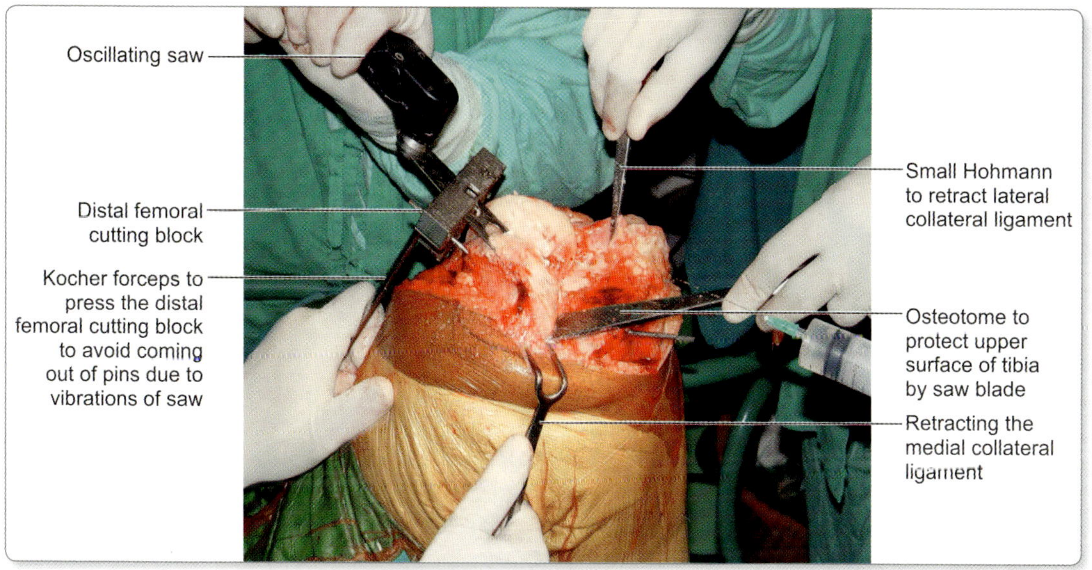

Fig. 2.12 Cutting distal femur and protecting the upper surface of tibia by osteotome

outrigger and distal femoral cutting block is lowered onto the anterior cortex by depressing the button on left hand side of the locating device. Fix the distal femoral cutting block with two pins in the square marked holes. If bone is hard, make 2.5 mm drill holes before passing the pins. If required, the distal femoral cutting block can be adjusted at 11 mm or maximum up to 13 mm. But extra cutting of femur will lead to elevation of the joint line which should be avoided as the joint line elevation will lead to patella baja and cause increased stress across the patellofemoral joint. Remove the intramedullary rod with femoral locating device by pulling the T-handle. Check that the distal femoral cutting block is in slight valgus position. Check the amount of cut with the help of visualization guide. The distal part of lateral condyle is exposed more than the distal part of medial condyle in varus knee and vice versa in valgus knee. The assistant will retract the medial and lateral collateral ligaments and press the distal femoral cutting block by Kocher forceps to avoid coming out of pins and/or block due to vibrations of saw. Make the distal cut by oscillating saw (1.25 mm thick saw blade No. 519.115) passed through the slot in distal femoral cutting block. While cutting, another assistant should protect the upper surface of tibia by osteotome **(Fig. 2.12)**. Usually the cut part of lateral condyle is more than the cut part of medial condyle in varus knee and vice versa in valgus knee. Remove the distal femoral cutting block.

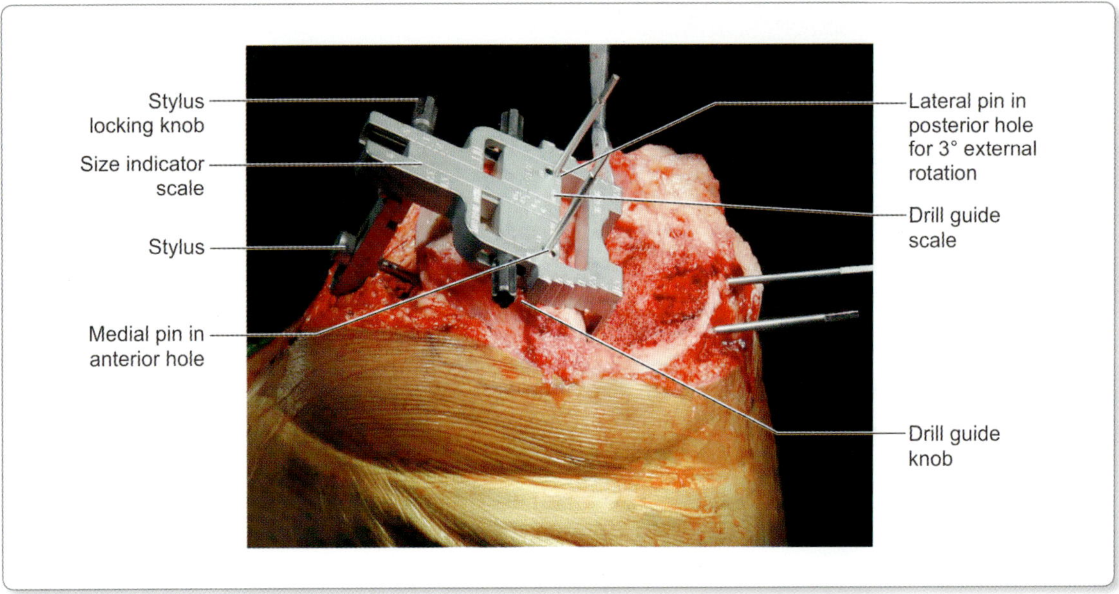

Fig. 2.13 Fixation of femoral sizing guide by two pins, lateral in the posterior hole and medial in the anterior hole to keep the AP and chamfer cutting block in 3° external rotation

Put the spacer block between cut ends of femur and tibia in extended position of the limb. Check the mediolateral stability and extension gap. If it is unstable, add further 1 mm shim with spacer block. The space between cut ends of tibia and femur should be rectangular (i.e. rectangular extension gap). This can also be checked by lamina spreader but care should be taken in osteoporosed bone to avoid compression of bone. Further soft tissue release can be done at this stage at the posteromedial aspect of upper tibia if there is tightness on medial aspect. Put the alignment rod through the hole in spacer block and check the alignment that center of hip, knee and ankle are in one line. Remove the alignment rod, spacer block and pins from femur and tibia.

Flex the knee fully. Lift the thigh. Put the femoral sizing guide (anterior reference guide) over the center of the distal femoral surface and is seated flush. The skids of femoral sizing guide are positioned against the posterior condyles and determine the rotational alignment. If the posterior part of either condyle is deficient, then rotate the femoral sizing guide in such a way that it lies perpendicular to the mechanical axis of the tibia (Chapter 3, Fig. 3.48).The stylus is allowed to move freely within the guide and moved proximal to the articular surface (in supracondylar region). At the appropriate level where the stylus is not impeded, turn the stylus locking knob clockwise until tight to fix its position. Adjust the drill guide scale at appropriate size as determined by stylus and fix it by tightening the two knobs. The surgeon should hold the femoral sizing guide firmly and assistant will put pins (or drill), one in the posterior hole on lateral side and another in the anterior hole on medial side to keep the AP and chamfer cutting block in 3° external rotation (3° inbuilt external rotation femoral sizing guide) **(Fig. 2.13)**.

This 3° external rotation is further confirmed by joining the centers of lateral and medial epicondyles (transepicondylar axis, the lateral epicondyle is lower than the medial epicondyle), Whiteside line (Determine the anteroposterior axis by drawing a line between the bottom of the sulcus of the femur and the top of the intercondylar notch and make posterior femoral cut line perpendicular to this axis) and putting the spacer block between upper cut surface of tibia and posterior surface of AP and chamfer cutting block in 90° flexion of knee (i.e. parallel upper cut surface of tibia and posterior surface of AP and chamfer cutting block). **This 3° external rotation will cut more posterior part of medial condyle (8 mm lateral and 10–11 mm medial resection) and thus compensate the 3° varus slope of tibia as the tibia is cut perpendicular to the tibial axis**. This will make rectangular space between upper surface of tibia and posterior cut surface of femur while knee is flexed at 90° (i.e. rectangular flexion gap) and thus keeping the equal tension on medial and lateral ligaments. Remove the pins and sizing guide. Put the AP and chamfer cutting block of appropriate size seated into the pins holes, hammer it to flush and fix it with two pins. If required, drill with 2.5 mm drill bit to avoid avulsion of epicondyles while passing the pins. Check that the AP and chamfer cutting block is slightly externally rotated. Check the amount of cut by the help of visualization guide both anteriorly and posteriorly. Be sure that there is no notching on the anterior cortex of femur otherwise notching will reduce the strength of femur by 40% and liable to supracondylar

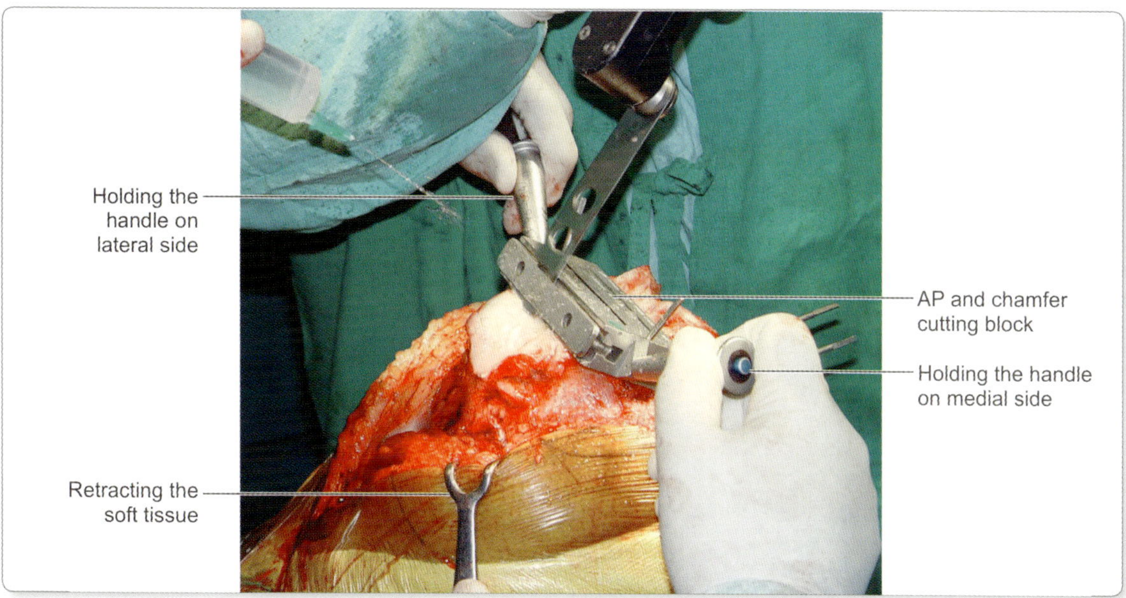

Fig. 2.14 Anterior cut

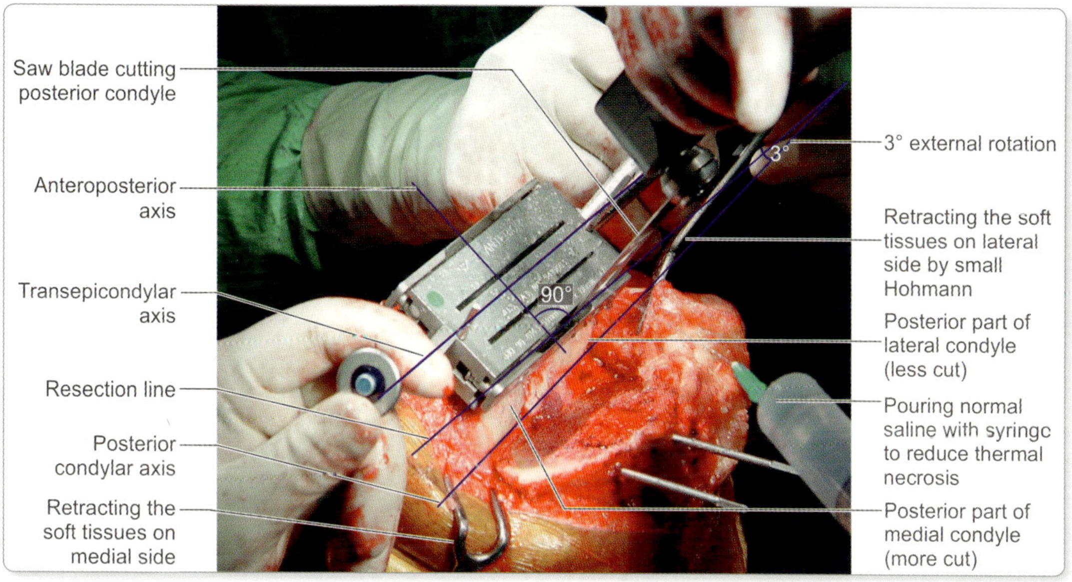

Fig. 2.15A Posterior cut is perpendicular to anteroposterior axis (APA) or parallel to transepicondylar axis (TEA) and 3° externally rotated relative to posterior condylar axis (PCA)

fracture. Posterior part of medial condyle is exposed more than the posterior part of lateral condyle. By the help of oscillating saw (1.25 mm thick saw blade, No. 519.115) make an anterior, posterior and chamfer cuts through the appropriate slots of AP and chamfer cutting block while assistant will retract the soft tissues and hold the handles attached on AP and chamfer cutting block on both sides **(Figs 2.14 to 2.16)**. While making the posterior cut, slightly tilt (about 5°) the tip of saw blade away from the femoral notch and keeping the tip inside the posterior condyle to avoid inadvertent injury to neurovascular structures at 11, 12 and 1 O'clock position. Sudden loss of resistance to saw blade will confirm the posterior cut. The chamfer cuts may be further checked by open chamfer. Pouring of normal saline by syringe during each cut will reduce the thermal necrosis due to vibration of the saw **(Fig. 2.15A)**.

While cutting the posterior chamfer the assistant should protect the upper surface of tibia by osteotome **(Fig. 2.16B)**. Remove the pins and AP and chamfer cutting block. The assistant will lift the thigh and the cut portions

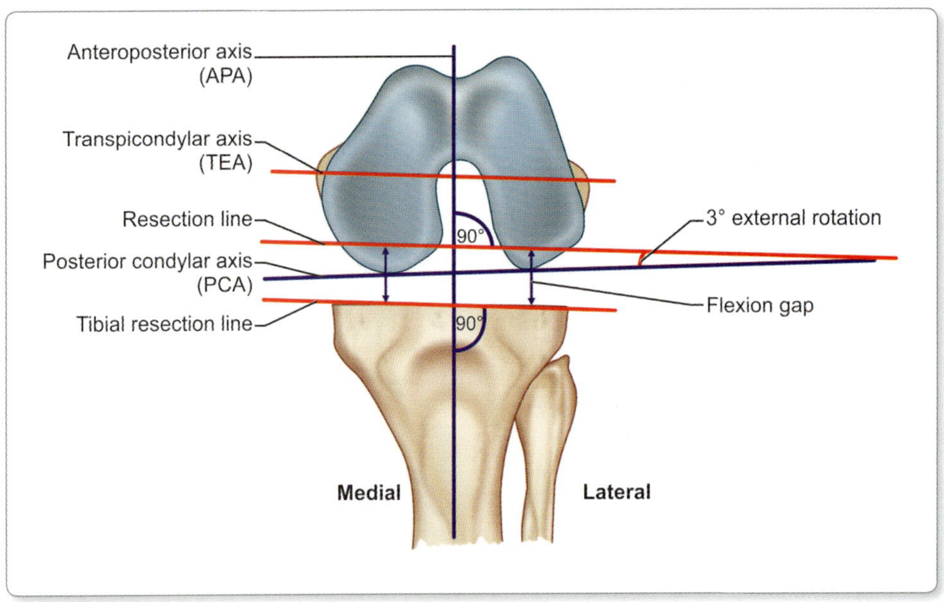

Fig. 2.15B Diagrammatic picture showing APA, TEA, PCA and resection line 3° external rotation and perpendicular to the anteropostrior axis (APA)

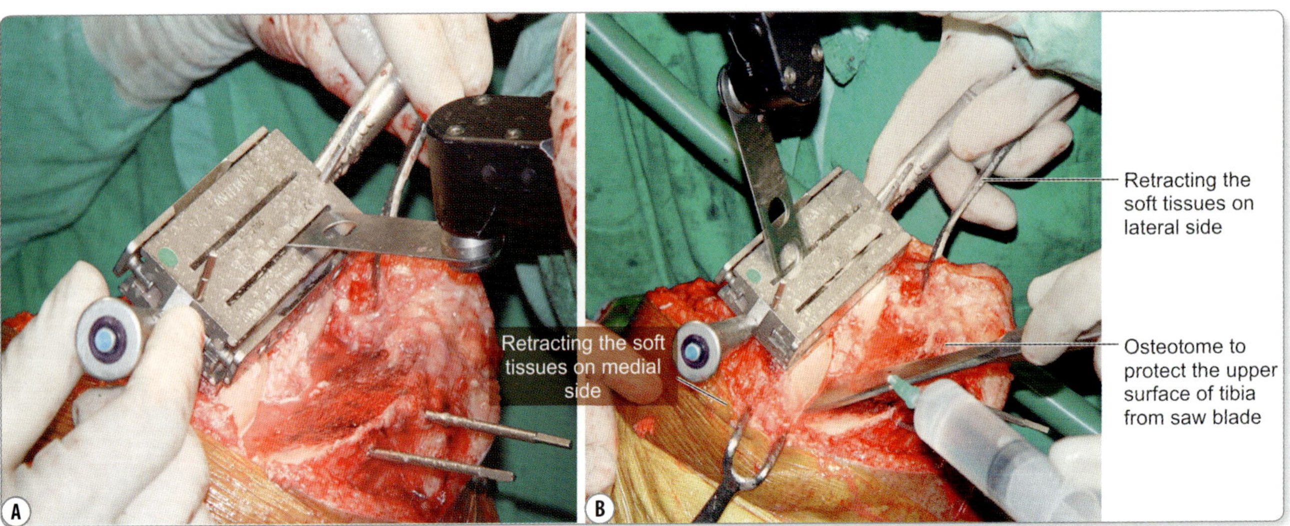

Figs 2.16A and B (A) Anterior chamfer cut; (B) Posterior chamfer cut

of posterior condyles of femur are levered by osteotome to bring them out. With the help of forceps, hold the cut portion of posterior condyle of femur and remove with the help of electrocautery. The size of posterior cut on the medial condyle is more than the lateral condyle. Remove the cut portions of bone during AP and chamfer cuts. Check the flexion gap with spacer block kept between upper surface of tibia and posterior surface of condyles while keeping the thigh and leg at 45°- 45°. Check the mediolateral stability. The flexion and extension gaps are roughly equal. If the extension gap is too tight, extension will be limited and if the flexion gap is too tight, flexion will be limited. Laxity of either gap can lead to instability. So balance the flexion-extension gap. If the extension gap is smaller than the flexion gap, remove more bone from the distal femoral cut surface or release the posterior capsule from the distal femur. If the flexion gap is smaller than the extension gap, remove more bone from the posterior femoral condyles by making appropriate cuts for the next smaller available femoral component (i.e. downsizing the femoral component but avoid anterior femoral notching). If the flexion and extension gaps are equal, but there is not

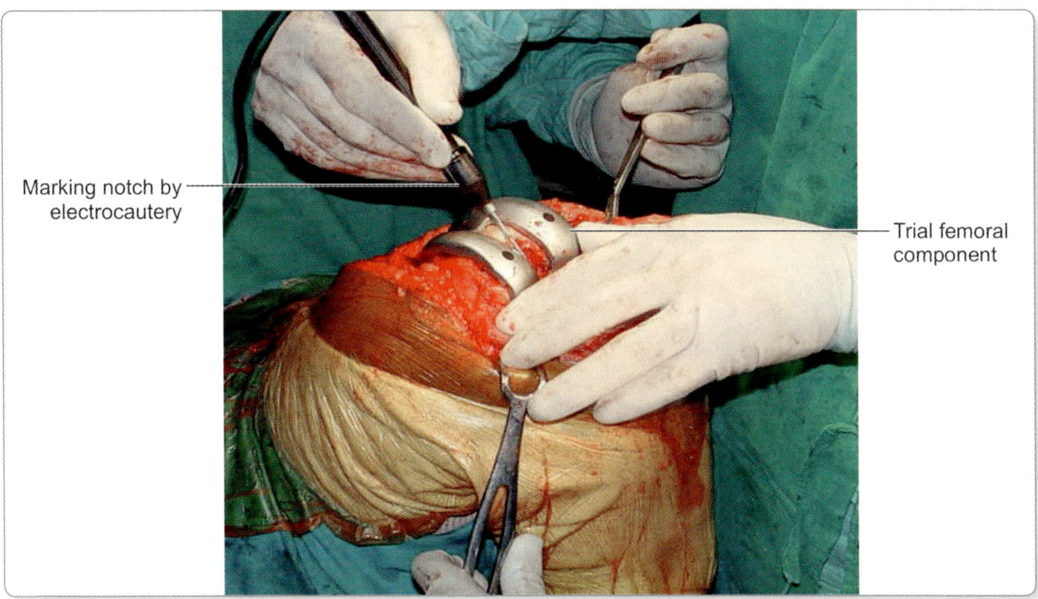

Fig. 2.17 Marking of notch by electrocautery for box cutting

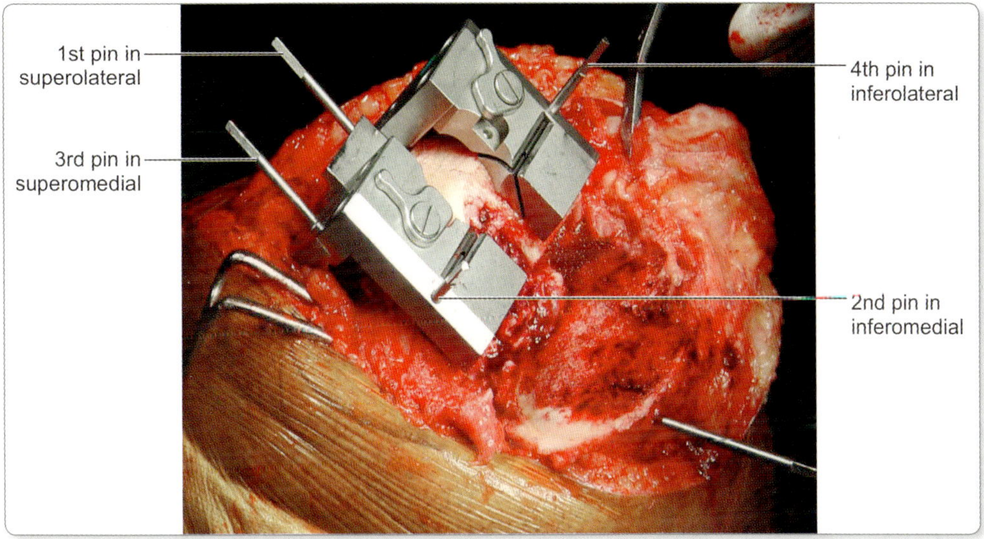

Fi.2.18 Fixation of femoral notch cutting guide by 4 pins

enough space for the desired prosthesis, remove more bone from the proximal tibia, because bone removed from the tibia affects the flexion and extension gap equally. When the flexion and extension gaps are equal but lax, add shim with spacer block and larger tibial polyethylene insert is required to obtain stability.

The assistant will lift the thigh. Apply the trial femoral component over the distal end of the femur while keeping it lateralized for better patellar tracking. Make the trial femoral component well-flushed with femur by femoral impactor and hammer. Mark the notch by electrocautery **(Fig. 2.17)**.

Lift the thigh and remove the trial femoral component with the help of radius-ulna punch and hammer. Apply the appropriate size femoral notch cutting guide over the distal femur centered about the two marks as made by the electrocautery and check that guide is seated flush upon the cut anterior and distal surfaces. Fix it with 4 pins after making 2.5 mm drill holes. Sequence of putting pins is as shown in the **Figure 2.18** (1st pin in superolateral, 2nd pin in inferomedial, 3rd pin in superomedial and 4th pin in inferolateral, i.e. contralateral) to avoid rotation or tilt of femoral notch cutting guide.

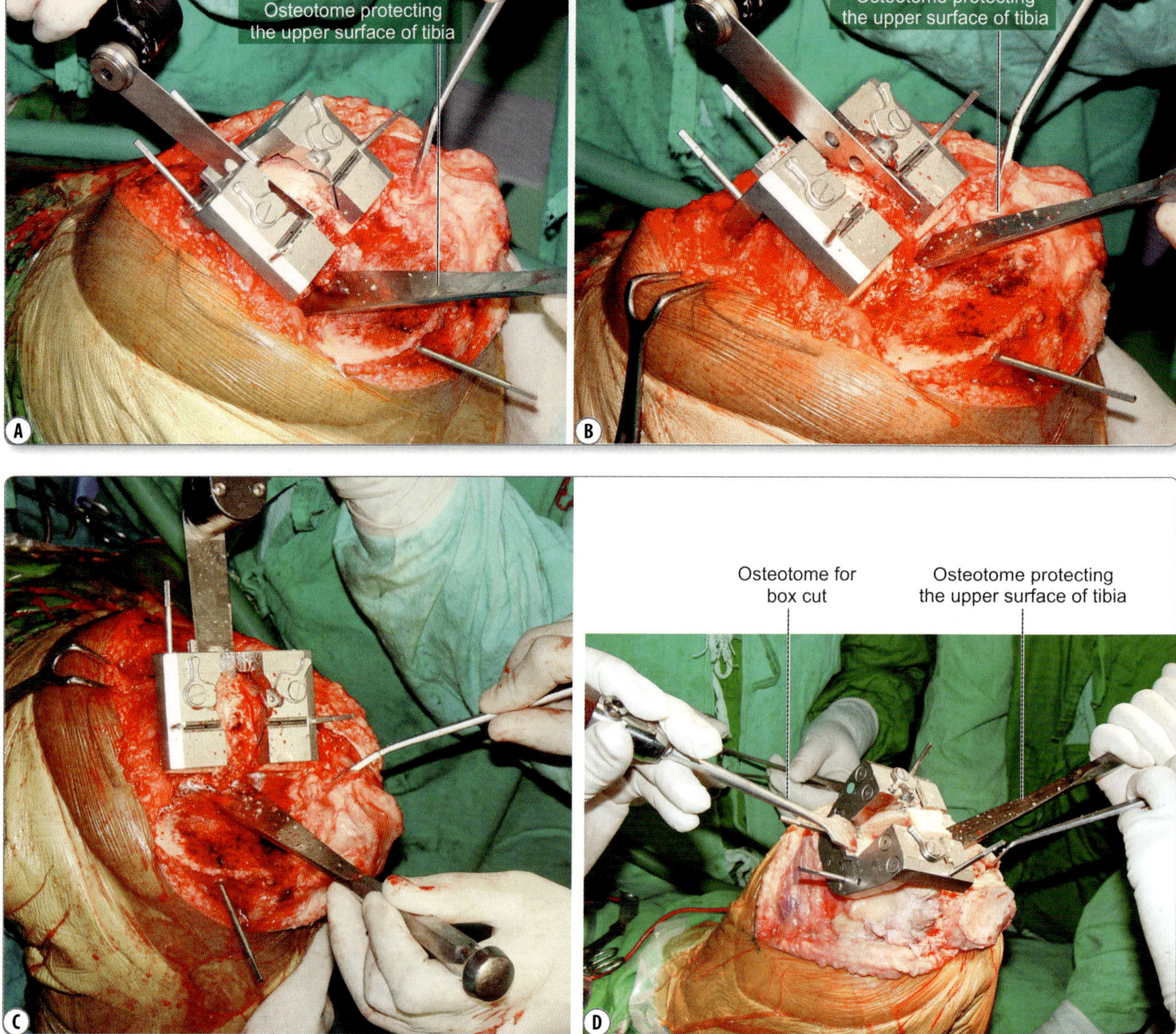

Figs 2.19A to D (A) Box cut by saw (towards lateral condyle); (B) Box cut by saw (towards medial condyle); (C) Box cut by saw (superior transverse cut); (D) Box cut by osteotome

Cut the box (notch) by reciprocating saw or oscillating saw (0.9 mm thick saw blade, No. 519.107) as marked **(Figs 2.19A to C)**. Protect the upper surface of tibia by putting osteotome **(Figs 2.19A to D)**. Finally cut the box by osteotome **(Fig. 2.19D)**. Hold the bone piece with Kocher forceps and remove it by electrocautery keeping near the cut part of bone. This bone piece is used for closing the medullary opening in the femur. Make the box smooth by bone file **(Fig. 2.19E)**. Remove the pins and notch cutting guide. Lift the thigh and remove the osteophytes or elevations if any on the posteromedial and posterolateral angles of box cut. **Figure 2.19F** shows femur and tibia after all cuts.

Fix the trial box with trial femoral component. For making the femoral component box assembly, place the two outrigger tabs of the box trial into the recesses of the posterior condyles, insert the anterior tabs into the recesses of the anterior flange and turn the angled screw, located in the side of box until tight. Put the femoral component box assembly on the distal end of femur, press it by palm and gently hammer it with the help of femoral impactor till flushed with femoral condyles **(Fig. 2.20)**. The accuracy

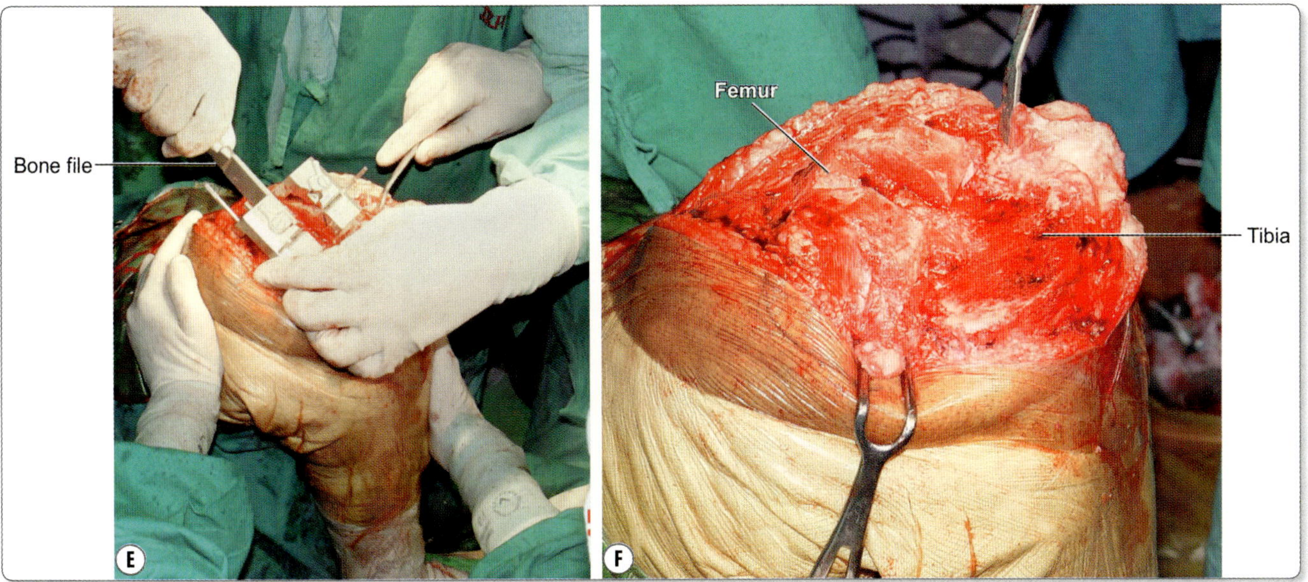

Figs 2.19E and F (E) Smoothening the box (notch) with bone file; (F) Cut surfaces of femur and tibia

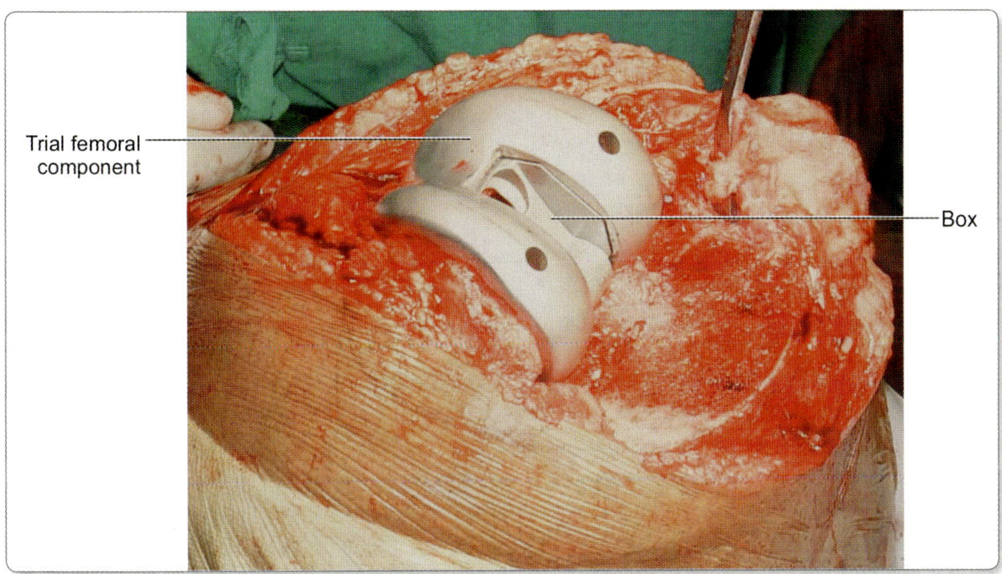

Fig. 2.20 After applying trial femoral component with box

of the cuts is evaluated and all appropriate modifications must be made at this time. If the component tends to rotate posteriorly, the AP cuts may require adjustment and if there is lateral rocking, the depth of notch is inadequate.

Flex the knee fully. Apply the big Hohmann on the posterior aspect of upper tibia to dislocate it anteriorly and small Hohmann on the lateral aspect of upper tibia. Take the appropriate size trial tibial tray with tibial tray alignment handle and appropriate size 8 mm trial tibial insert and keep on the upper cut surface of tibia. Remove the big and small Hohmannns. Reduce the joint and carefully extend the knee fully. For reduction, one assistant will hold the ankle and other will lift the thigh. The surgeon will hold the alignment handle with trial tibial tray and insert and push it posteriorly and downward and simultaneously extend the knee. The tibial tray will take its own position according to kinematics of the knee. Check that the alignment handle is slightly externally rotated (3°) in relation to tibial tubercle. Check the mediolateral stability in full extension, midflexion and flexion at 90°. The medial or lateral compartment should not open more than 2 mm on either side in full extension and in 90° flexion. If it is more, then take a thicker trial tibial insert.

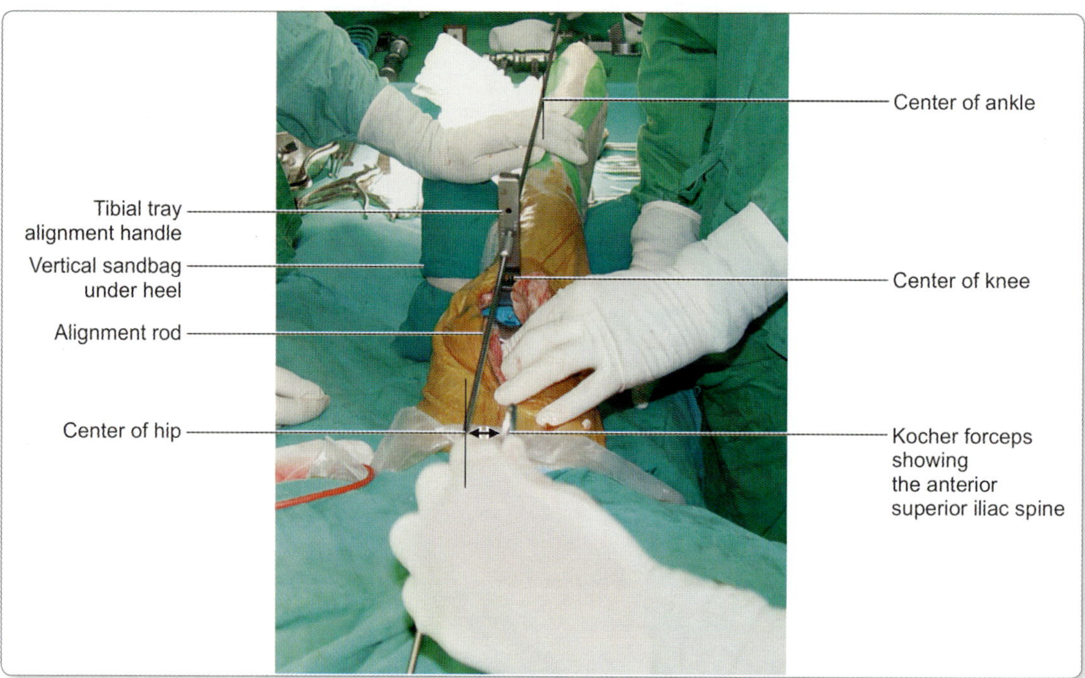

Fig. 2.21 Center of hip, knee and ankle in one line with all trial components

Thus the insert that gives the greatest stability in flexion and extension and allows full extension, is selected. If the knee is not straight even with 8 mm trial tibial insert, then further release the soft tissues at this stage on the posteromedial aspect of upper tibia and posterior aspect of femoral condyles. Extend the knee and keep the vertical sand bag under the heel. Check the alignment with alignment rod passing through the hole in the tibial tray alignment handle attached with the tibial tray. This will pass through the centers of hip, knee and ankle **(Fig. 2.21)**. Usually the femoral component and tibial tray are of the same size but sometimes one size down or up may be selected as per requirement.

Remove the alignment rod. Mark by electrocautery over the anterior aspect of upper tibia in center and on medial according to the marks on the center of tibial tray alignment handle and trial tibial tray, respectively. Remove the tibial alignment handle.

Resurfacing of Patella

Measure the thickness of the patella by caliper keeping at anterior cortex and median ridge of everted patella **(Fig. 2.22)**. Normal anteroposterior patellar dimension is 22–26 mm. Synovial tissue is cleared by electrocautery to the level of the insertions of the quadriceps mechanism and the patellar ligament. Excise the synovium from the superior pole of patella to prevent patellar clunk syndrome. Set at minimum 14 mm mark on the calibrated column of patellar cutting guide to retain patella of minimum 14 mm for 22 mm thick patella (resection: 8 mm, 32 mm patellar size), 15 mm for 23 mm and 24 mm thick patella (Resection: 8.5 mm, 35 mm patellar size), 16 mm for 25 mm thick patella (resection: 9 mm, 38 mm patellar size) and 26 mm thick patella (resection: 1.5 mm, 41 mm patellar size). Hold the patella with patella cutting guide positioned with the prongs of the fork deep to the prepatellar bursa and against the anterior patellar cortex with serrated jaws at the superior and inferior margins of the articular surface. The switch is placed to the lock position and the jaws closed to firmly engage the patella. The assistant will hold the patellar cutting guide. Support the patella by Kocher forceps from opposite side. Check the amount of cut by visualization guide **(Fig. 2.23)**.

Cut the patella by oscillating saw (1.25 mm thick saw blade No. 519.115) through the slot in patellar cutting guide maintaining the blade flush to the cutting surface **(Fig. 2.24)**. The patellar cut should be parallel to the anterior surface of patella **(Fig. 2.25)**. Remove the cut portion of patella by electrocautery keeping it close to patella. The patellar template (32 mm, 35 mm, 38 mm or 41 mm) is selected that most adequately covers the resected surface without overhang. Keep it superiorly and medialized for better patellar tracking **(Fig. 2.26)**. The template is positioned onto the cut surface with the handle positioned on the medial side of the everted patella, such that two drill holes lie at the medial side, one at the lateral. Assistant will support the patella by Kocher forceps. Hammer the patellar template, hold it firmly and drill the holes for pegs of patellar buttons **(Fig. 2.27)**. Apply the patella trial **(Fig. 2.28)** and check the patellar tracking. The patella trial should stay without holding it.

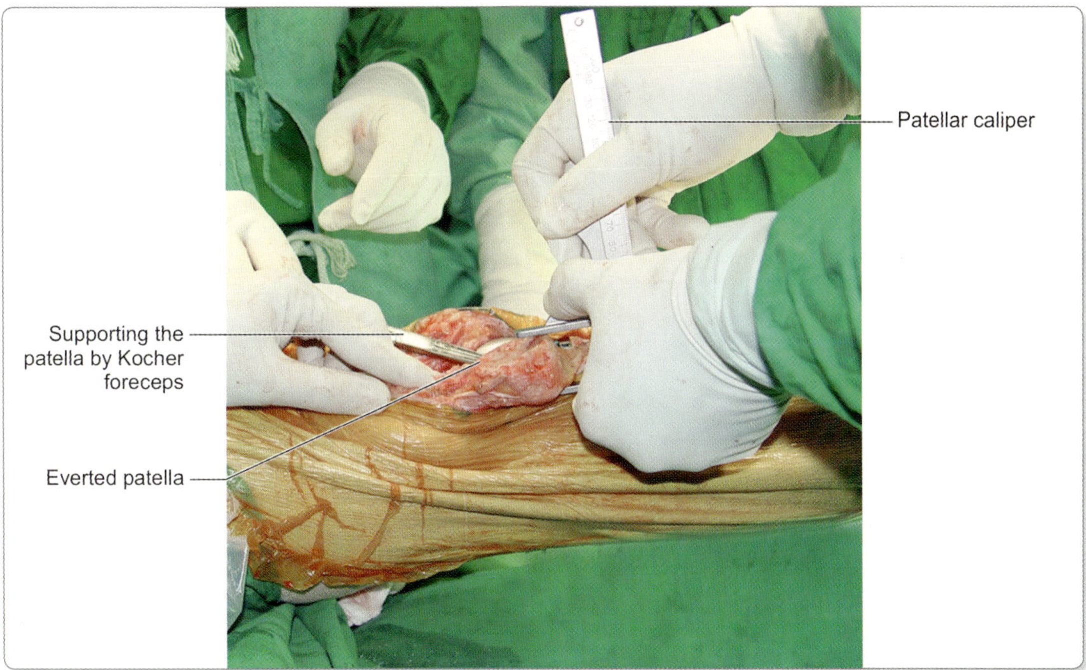

Fig. 2.22 Measuring the thickness of patella by calipers

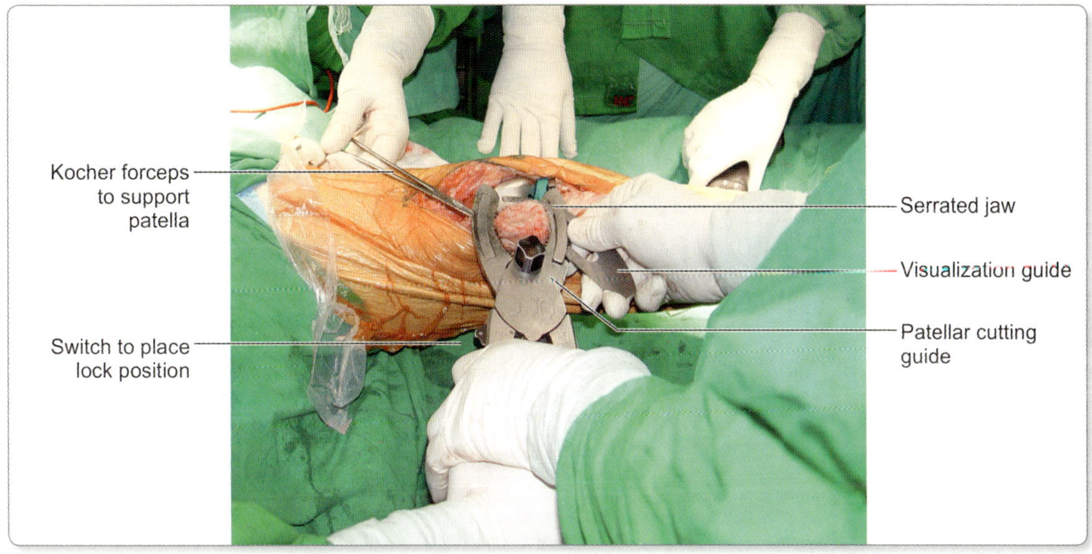

Fig. 2.23 Holding the patella by patellar cutting guide at minimum 14 mm and checking the cut by visualization guide

If it is not staying, the final check should be done after release of the tourniquet. Staying of patellar tracking can also be tested by putting one suture knot in the parapatellar incision in the quadriceps tendon at the level of upper pole of patella and flexing the knee. If the suture knot is not breaking, then further lateral release is not required. Remove the trial patellar component.

Tibial Preparation

Flex the knee and the assistant will hold the ankle to keep the knee fully flexed. Remove the trial tibial insert by tibial insert extractor and trial tibial tray but trial femoral component box assembly is left in position. Apply a big Hohmann on the posterior aspect of upper tibia to dislocate the tibia anteriorly and a small curved Hohmann on the lateral aspect of upper tibia to retract the everted patella. Put the trial tibial tray with alignment handle on the cut surface of tibia. Tally the two electrocautery marks on tibia with central and medial marks on tibial tray keeping the trial tibial tray slightly externally rotated (3°) in relation to tibial tubercle. Fix the trial tibial tray with two short fixation pins **(Fig. 2.29A)**. If bone is hard then drill with 2.5 mm drill bit before applying the short fixation pin. Remove the

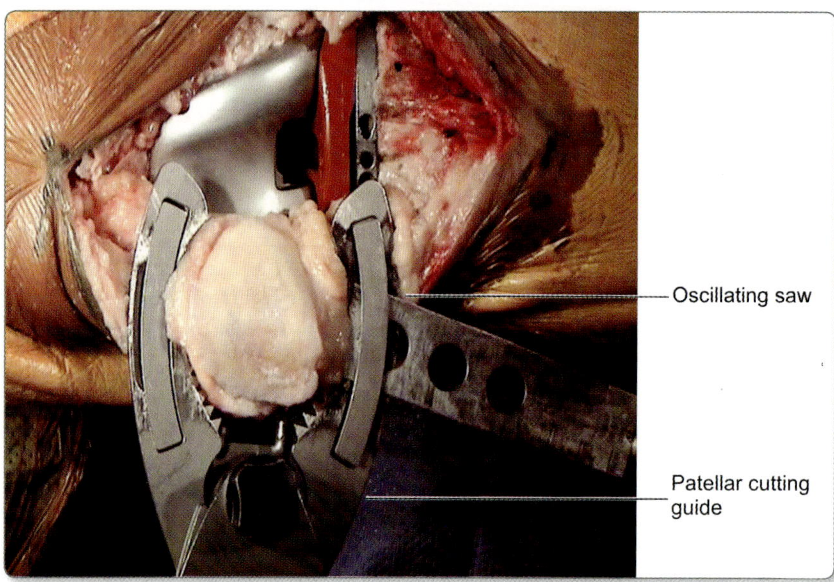

Fig. 2.24 Cutting the patella by oscillating saw through the slot in patellar cutting guide

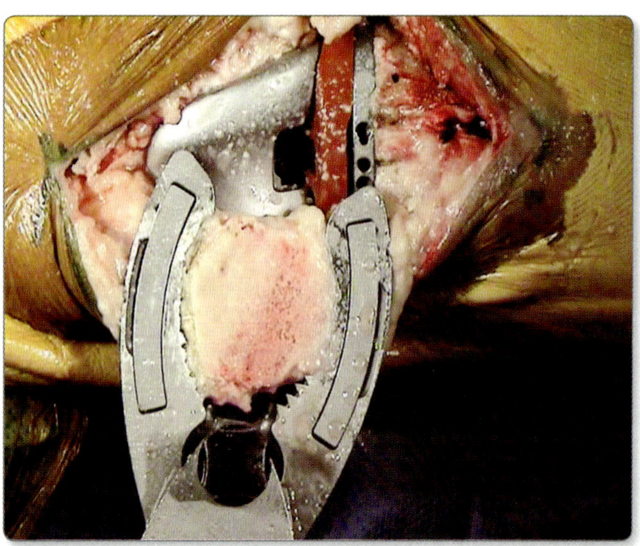

Fig.2.25 Resurfaced patella

alignment handle from tibial tray. Apply the appropriate size modular punch guide with drill bushing on tibial tray (13 mm punch guide and drill bushing for 1.5 to 3 size tibial tray and 15 mm for 4 to 6 size tibial tray). The matching drill (13 mm drill for 1.5 to 3 size tibial tray and 15 mm drill for 4 to 6 size tibial tray) is fully advanced through the drill bushing into the cancellous bone **(Fig. 2.29B)**. Remove the drill bushing. Widen the drilled area by oscillating saw **(Fig. 2.29C)** and osteotome **(Fig. 2.29D)** to avoid shattering of upper tibia. The appropriate size modular tray keel punch is subsequently positioned through the guide and impacted with hammer until the shoulder of the punch is in contact with the guide **(Fig. 2.29E)**. The modular tray keel punch is subsequently removed with slap hammer moving up. Remove the short fixation pins by plier and trial tibial tray. Remove the small and big Hohmann and trial femoral component box assembly. Make some drill holes by 2.5 mm drill bit in the hard area of the bone for better penetration of the cement **(Fig. 2.30)**. Wash the medullary canal of femur with 100 mL normal saline and suck the fluid by suction from the medullary canal. Make a bone peg with bone piece of box cut and close the hole in the medullay canal of femur. Thoroughly cleanse the cut surfaces of bones with pulse lavage (Normal saline mixed with gentamicin). Make the area dry with sponge. Apply fresh sheets beneath the limb and above the thigh. Following things are kept ready on the sheets beneath the limb: Mosquito artery forcep, patellar clamp, small curved Hohmann, one knife, two curettes (2 mm and 4 mm), femoral punch and hammer.

Cementing

Store the bone cement in outer shelf of refrigerator (not in freezer compartment) for at least 24 hours before use. For cementing with two packets, take out the gentamicin bone cement (CMW1—one packet of 40 g and another packet of 20 g) from refrigerator about ½ hour before cementing and kept in operation theatre at 20°–22° C temperature. If the cementing has been planned with one packet bone cement of 40 g, then take out the cement from refrigerator just before cementing to avoid early setting. Cementing with one packet should be done after gaining experience.

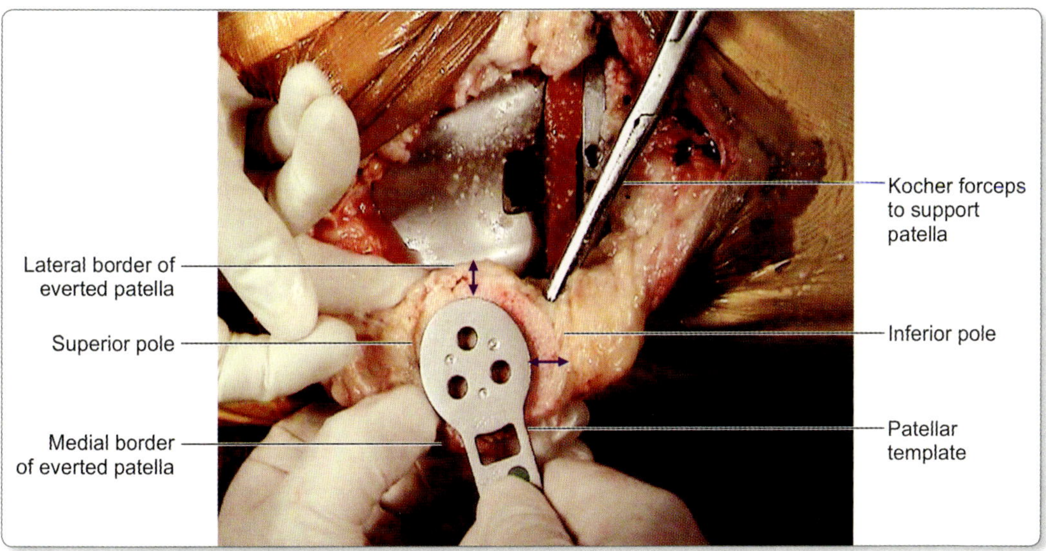

Fig.2.26 Position of patellar template—Superiorly and medialized

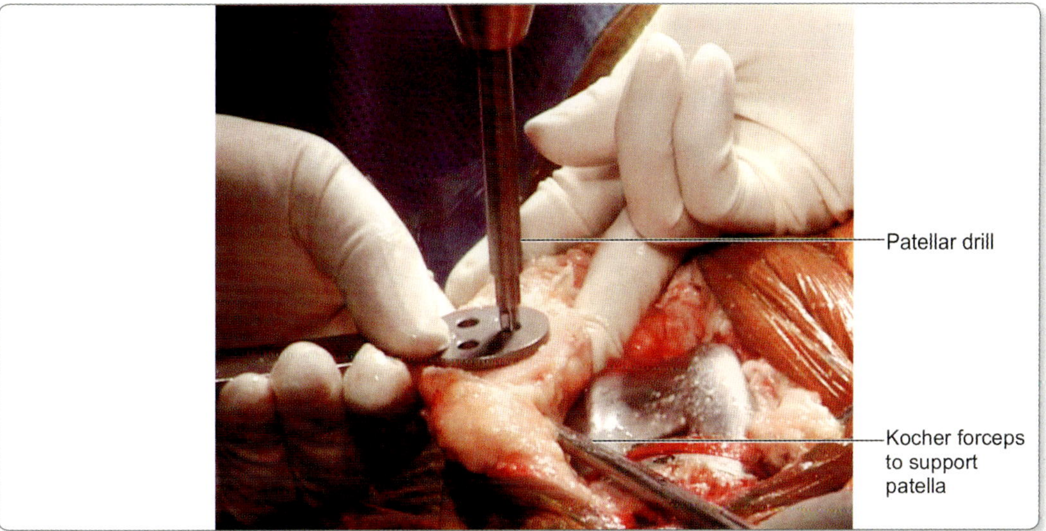

Fig.2.27 Patellar drilling

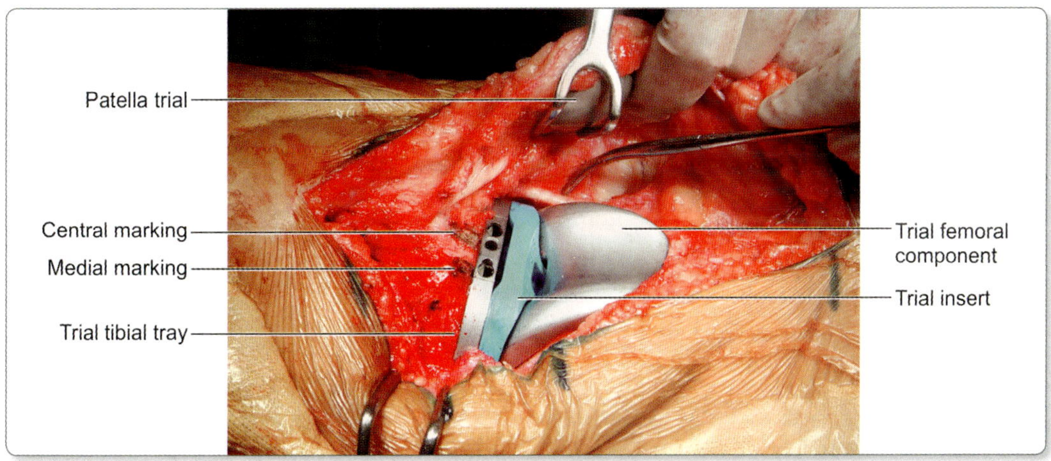

Fig. 2.28 With all trial components

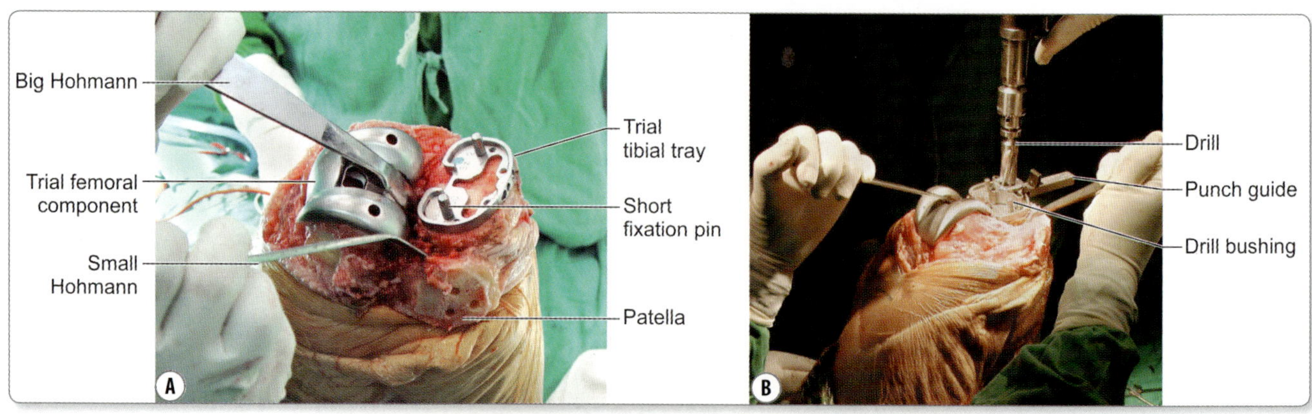

Figs 2.29A and B) (A) After fixing trial tibial tray; (B) Drilling

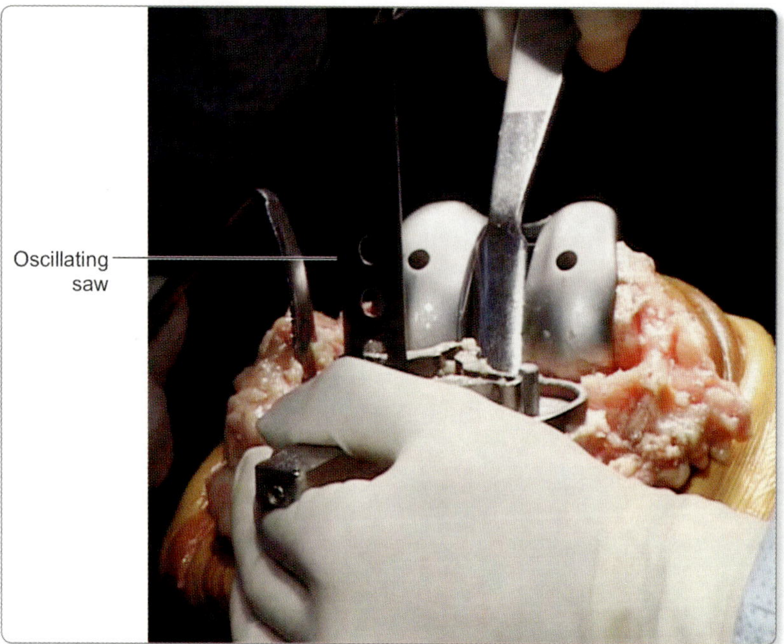

Fig. 2.29C Widening by oscillating saw

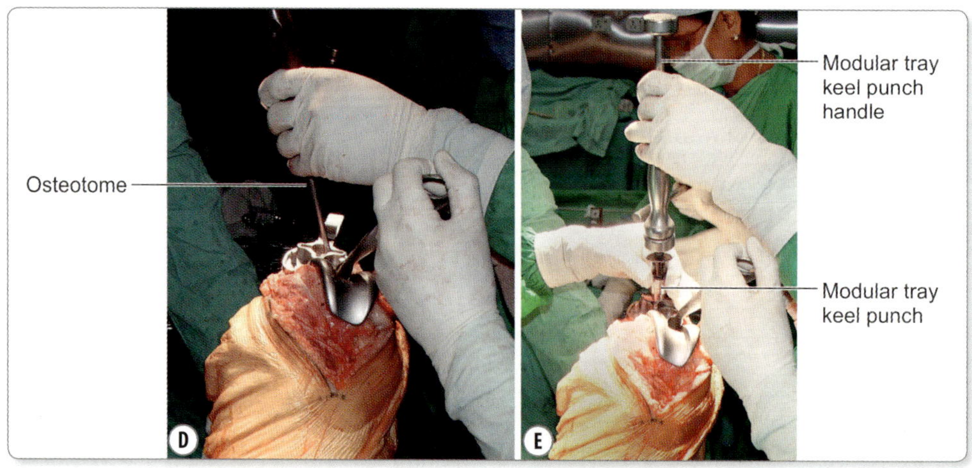

Figs 2.29D and E (D) Widening by osteotome; (E) Broaching with modular tray keel punch

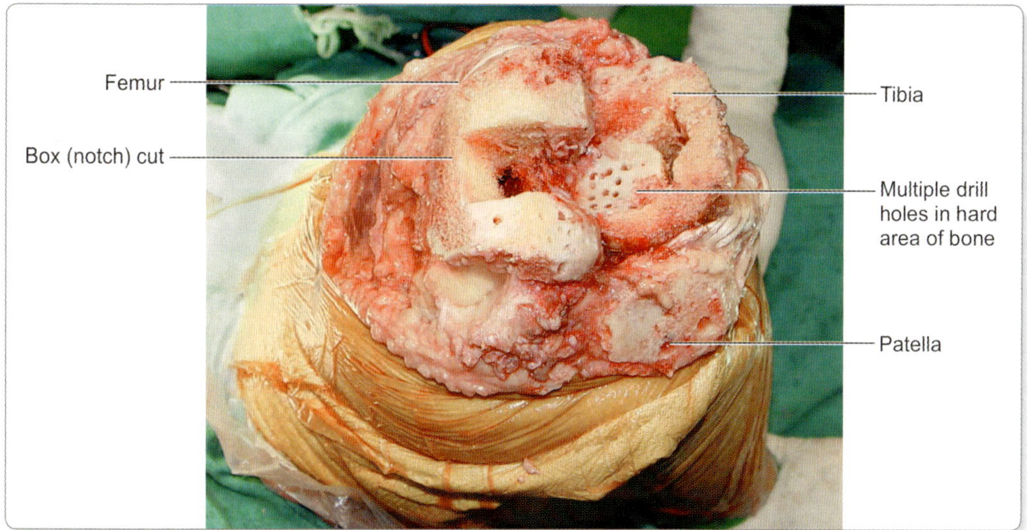

Fig. 2.30 After final cuts and tibial preparation

The advantage with one packet bone cement is that the femoral and tibial components are pressurized against each other simultaneously. Anesthetist gives injection Efcorlin (Hydrocortisone succinate) 100 mg IV just before cementing. Change gloves. The circulating nurse will open the packets of implants and bone cement. Take the appropriate size and side (left or right) of femoral component, appropriate size of tibial tray and patellar implant on the same trolley on which the bone cement has been taken. The universal handle is assembled onto the universal tibial tray inserter and assembled onto the tibial tray.

Cementing with two packets of bone cement (40 g and 20 g)—Mix 40 g cement in a stainless steel bowl with a spoon slowly to avoid mixing of air. When wrinkling will start in cement at about 3 minutes, apply the cement on under surface of femoral component up to the posterior aspect. Apply cement on patellar implant. One assistant will hold the ankle to keep the knee flexed and other will support the patella. Take small amount of cement and apply on the patella. Find out the three drill holes on resurfaced patella by mosquito artery forcep. Put the patellar implant on resurfaced patella. Press it with thumb and fingers so that the three pegs of patellar implant will go into the three holes in the patella. The patellar clamp is positioned with the silicon O-ring centered over the articular surface of the patellar implant and the metal backing plate against the anterior cortex. When snug, the handles are closed and held by the ratchet until the cement sets. The assistant will hold the patellar clamp and remove the extruded cement by 2 mm curette. Apply the small curved Hohmann on the lateral aspect of upper tibia to retract the patella. Apply bone cement on the cut surfaces of femur. Another assistant will lift the thigh and the surgeon will put the femoral component on the cut surface of femur and pressurize it first with thumb and palm and then with femoral impactor and gentle blows of hammer for equal distribution of pressure. Take care that the femoral component should not tilt posteriorly. To avoid posterior tilting of the femoral component, the assistant will put the index finger in anterior part of the notch of femoral component and pull it anteriorly and upwards towards the thigh while the surgeon is impacting the femoral component. Remove the extruded cement by knife to avoid pulling out of cement from under surface of femoral component **(Fig. 2.31)**. Remove the extruded cement from the posterior aspect of femoral component by 2 mm curette. The assistant will hold the femoral impactor and pressurize it with manual pressure. When the bone cement sets at about 10 minutes, put normal saline to avoid thermal damage to the tissues. Do not hammer when cement is setting otherwise there will be fragmentation of the cement.

In the meanwhile the surgeon will start mixing the 2nd packet (20 g) of cement. When wrinkling will start in the cement, apply the cement on the under surface of tibial tray. Put wet gauze piece over the femoral component to avoid scratching by Hohmann. Apply big Hohmann on the posterior aspect of upper tibia to dislocate it anteriorly. Make the upper surface of tibia dry by gauze piece. Take some amount of bone cement and apply on the cut surface of tibia. Put the tibial tray in proper orientation on the upper surface of tibia and deliver several gentle blows over the top of the universal handle with hammer for equal distribution of pressure **(Fig. 2.32)**.

The assistant will remove the extruded cement from the posterior aspect of tibial tray by 4 mm curette. While holding the universal handle, the surgeon will remove the

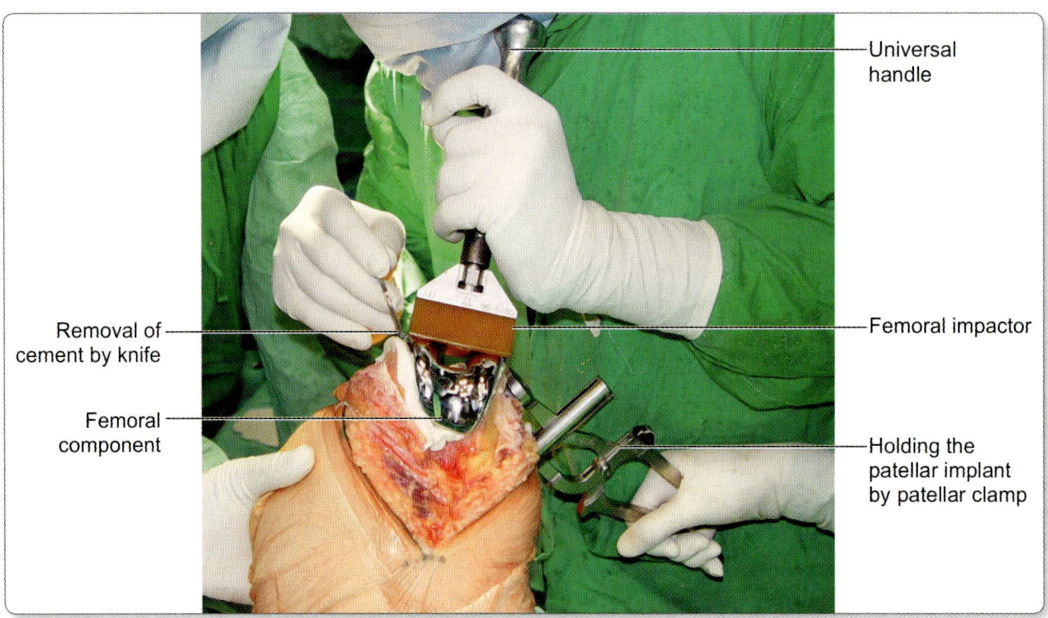

Fig. 2.31 Implantation of patella and femoral component and removal of cement by knife

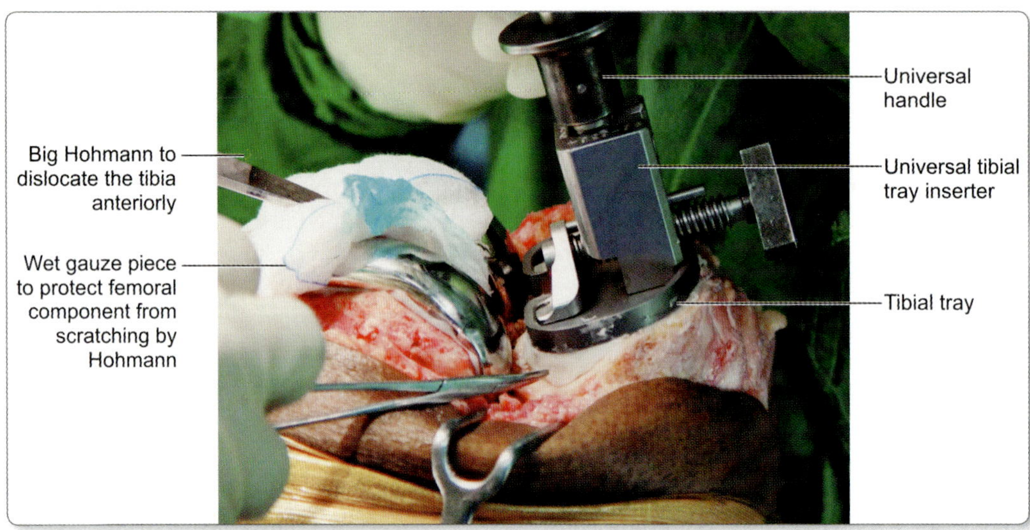

Fig. 2.32 Implantation of tibial tray

extruded cement from medial, lateral and anterior aspect of tibia by knife. While cement is setting, remove the universal tibial tray inserter with universal handle. Put the trial tibial insert (whatever the thickness has been determined during final trial) in the tibial tray and reduce the knee **(Fig. 2.33)** and extend it. For reduction, one assistant will hold the ankle and other will lift the thigh and the surgeon will press the top of upper tibia downward and posteriorly and simultaneously extend the knee. Keep the vertical sand bag under the heel. Put one sponge over the knee and apply controlled pressure over the knee till it becomes straight (i.e. no FFD) taking care not to cause supracondylar fracture. The assistant will hold the ankle dorsiflexed to counteract the action of gastrocnemius over knee. There is pressurization of cement under tibial tray over the fixed femoral component.

Remove the extruded cement by 2 mm curette. When the cement sets, put normal saline to avoid thermal damage. Check the stability—mediolateral in full extension, midflexion and in 90° flexion and anterior drawer. On testing the mediolateral stability, the joint should not open more than 2 mm. If it is more than 2 mm, apply thicker trial tibial insert, check the stability and determine the appropriate thickness of tibial insert but there should be no FFD. For testing the nil flexion deformity, extend the knee and keep

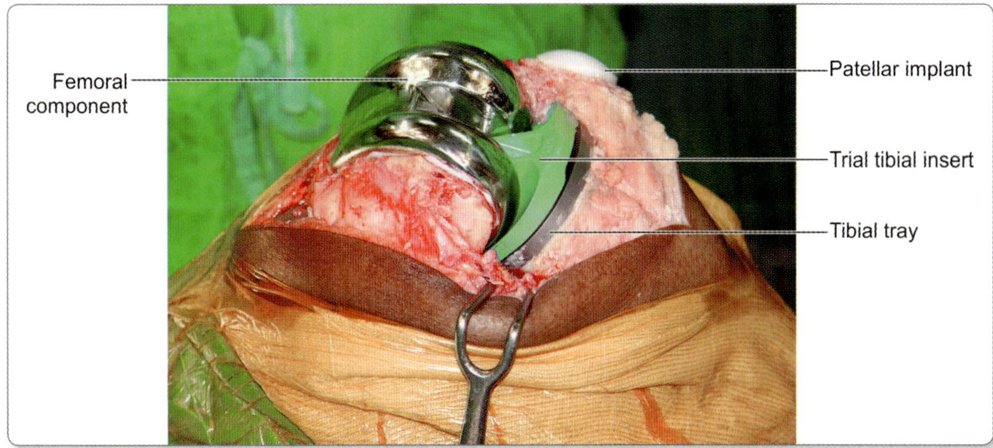

Fig. 2.33 Trial reduction with trial tibial insert to determine the thickness of tibial inserts

sandbag beneath the ankle and apply controlled pressure over the knee to keep it straight. On releasing the pressure from the knee, the flexion deformity should not recoil back. In case of rheumatoid arthritis, small amount of FFD (about 10 degree) is corrected by soft tissue stretching due to exercise later on. Put fresh sheets beneath and above the limb. Put sponges over the knee, apply compression and release the tourniquet. Just before releasing tourniquet, IV antibiotic (1 g Cefotaxime) is given. Blood is started. Achieve hemostasis especially coagulate the lateral inferior genicular artery by electrocautery if it is cut during surgery as described ahead.

Cementing with one packet of bone cement (40 g)—After mixing the 40 g cement as described above, apply the bone cement on the under surfaces of tibial tray, femoral component up to the posterior aspect and patellar implant. Apply the patellar implant, femoral component and tibial tray in sequence as described above. Put the appropriate size and thickness of trial tibial insert in the tibial tray and reduce the joint and extend the knee as described above. The femoral and tibial components are pressurized against each other.

Application of Tibial Insert

Flex the knee fully. Lift the thigh. Remove the trial tibial insert by the help of tibial insert extractor. **Figure 2.34A** shows implanted femoral and tibial components. Apply wet gauze piece over femoral component. Apply big Hohmann on the posterior aspect of upper tibia to dislocate the tibia anteriorly and small curved Hohmann on lateral aspect of upper tibia to retract the patella laterally. Remove the extruded cement by osteotome and mallet or with nibbler. Slightly extend the knee and look for bleeders (i.e. lateral inferior genicular artery) on the lateral aspect of the knee and coagulate it by electrocautery. Again flex the knee fully. Thoroughly wash the tibial tray with pulse lavage (Normal saline mixed with gentamicin). Clean the upper surface of tibial tray with wet gauze piece. Take the appropriate size and thickness of tibial insert (according to the size of tibial tray). Keep it over the tibial tray seated posteriorly and its anterior margin resting on the lip **(Fig. 2.34B)**. Assemble the universal handle with nylon punch and put it over the tibial insert in such a way that the 'FRONT' written surface will face anteriorly. Blow the hammer 2–3 times over the top of the universal handle till the tibial insert is in position. Seating is confirmed by circumferential inspection. Remove the big and small Hohmann and gauze piece from over the femoral component. Reduce the Knee **(Fig. 2.34C)** and extend it. For reduction, one assistant will hold the ankle and other will lift the thigh and the surgeon will press the top of upper tibia downward and posteriorly and simultaneously extend the knee.

Wash the wound with gentamicin mixed normal saline by pulse lavage. Again check the stability of the knee, mediolateral stability in full extension, midflexion and flexion at 90° and anterior drawer test in 90° flexion. Check the patellar tracking by moving the knee from full extension to full flexion **(Fig. 2.34D)**. If patella is not tracking well then lateral release can be done at this stage taking care not to do over release and jeopardizing the blood supply of patella. The lateral release is performed from inside the knee joint with anterior and lateral retraction of patella by cutting the synovium and retinaculum longitudinally, to a variable extent, from the Gerdy tubercle distally to the muscle fibers of the vastus lateralis proximally. Put a sand bag under the knee to keep the knee flexed at 70° to 80° for better approximation of the cut margins of wound and skin flap.

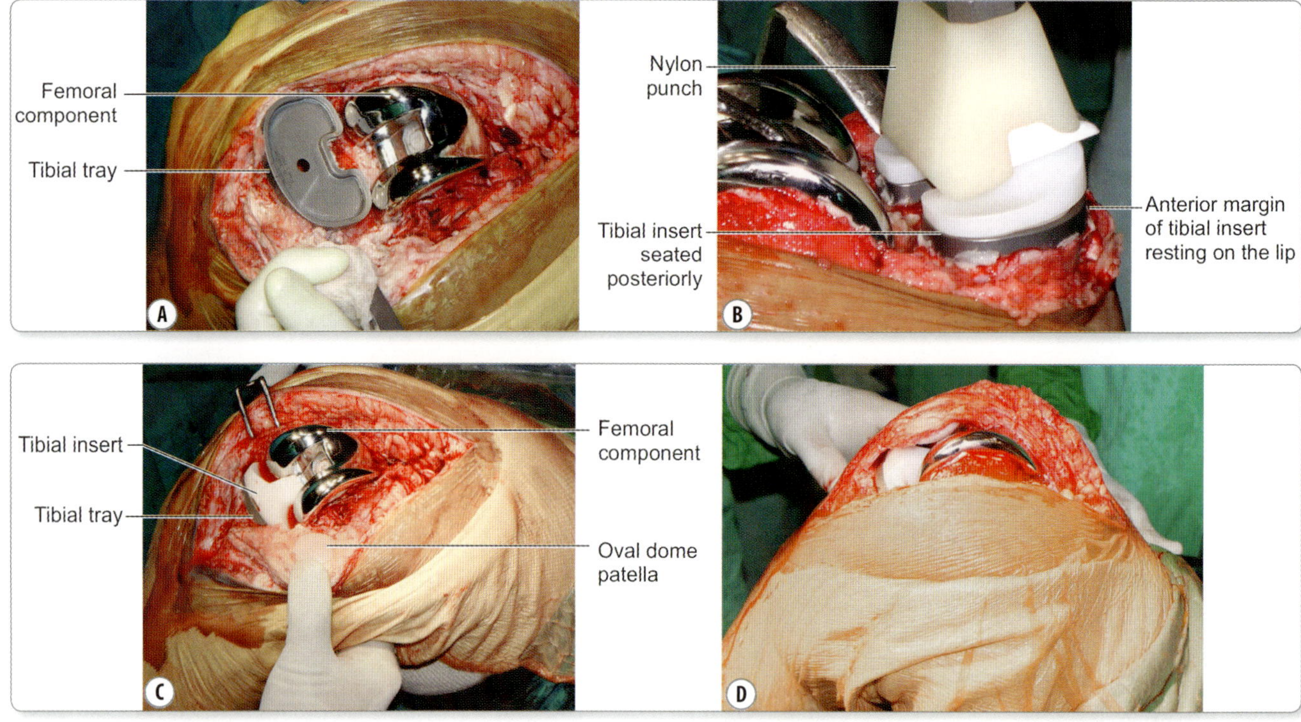

Figs 2.34A to D (A) Implanted femoral and tibial components; (B) Application of tibial insert; (C) Final implantation; (D) Excellent patellar tracking

Wound Closure

Apply two drains No.14, one in lateral and another in medial gutter and brought out through the thigh just above the starting point of incision. Knee extension during application of drain will facilitate the drain insertion. Take No.1 vicryl and stitch the capsule and quadriceps tendon starting from the upper pole of patella by interlocking continuous suture up to the tibial tubercle. The periosteal sleeve will fall back in position. Apply 3–4 interrupted sutures for extra strength. Take another No.1 Vicryl and stitch the quadriceps tendon starting from the upper pole of patella by interlocking continuous suture up to the starting point of incision in the thigh. The knee is put through a range of motion from full extension to full flexion to confirm patellar tracking and the integrity of the capsular closing. Apply interrupted subcutaneous sutures with No.1 vicryl. Remove the Ioban and clean the skin margin with betadine-soaked gauze piece. Close the skin by skin stapler taking care not to invert the margins of skin. Fix the drain with thread. Connect the drains to extension tubes which are connected to drain bottles with negative pressure. Clean the wound with betadine soaked gauze piece and make the area dry with sponge. Apply betadine-soaked gauze piece and cotton pad over the wound. Fix it by elastoplast transversely. Remove the cuff of tourniquet. Apply cotton roll, crepe bandage and knee brace.

Transfer of Patient from OT

Empty the urine bag. Put the drain bottle and urine bag on the sheet kept on the patient. Bring the OT table out of operation theater. Transfer the patient from OT table to wheeled cot. During transfer take care of drain tube and urinary catheter so that they should not be pulled out. Shift the patient in ICU after recording the vitals (e.g. pulse, BP, respiratory rate, etc.)

Postoperative Advice

1. Nil orally for 4 hours.
2. Injection Cefotaxime 1 g IV BD for 3 to 5 days.
3. Injection Amikacin 500 mg IV BD for 3 to 5 days, in cases where BUN and serum creatinine are on higher side, use Augmentin 1.2 g IV BD in place of injection Amikacin. (For 3 days in osteoarthritis cases and 5 days in rheumatoid and diabetic cases)
4. Intravenous (IV) fluid: Ringer's lactate (R/L)—2 units, dextrose normal saline (DNS)— 2 units.

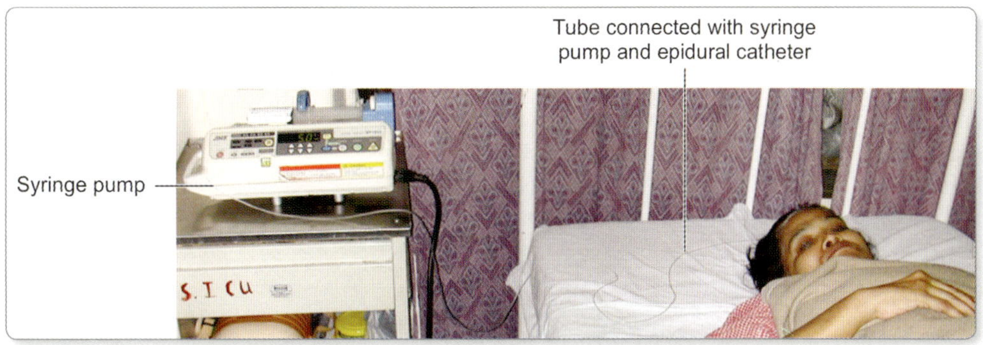

Fig. 2.35 Syringe pump connected with epidural catheter

5. Postoperative analgesia: One of the following methods can be used:
   i. *Continuous epidural analgesia*: Patient is connected to continuous infusion through epidural catheter with 'automatic reservoir pump' or 'syringe pump'. **(Fig. 2.35)**. One of the following combinations can be given:
      - Bupivacaine 0.125%; runs at the rate of 5 mL/hr. For making this solution, take 12.5 mL of 0.5% Bupivacaine in 50 mL syringe and mix with normal saline to make total 50 mL solution.
      - Bupivacaine 0.125% with fentanyl 5 µg/mL; runs at the rate of 5 mL/hr. For making this solution, take 12.5 mL of 0.5% Bupivacaine and 2½ amps. (250 µg) of Fentanyl (2 mL amp. 50 µg/mL) in 50 mL syringe and mix with normal saline to make total 50 mL solution.
      - Bupivacaine 0.125% with Buprenorphine 3 µg/mL; run at the rate of 5 mL/hr. For making this solution, take 12.5 mL of 0.5% Bupivacaine and ½ amp (150 µg) of Buprenorphine (1 mL amp, 300 µg/mL) in 50 mL syringe and mix with normal saline to make total 50 mL solution (most commonly used).
      - Bupivacaine 0.0625% with morphine 0.05 mg/mL, at the rate of 5 mL/hr. For making this solution, take 12.5 mL of 0.5% Bupivacaine and morphine ½ amp (5 µg) in 100 mL syringe and mix with normal saline to make total 100 mL solution.

      Initial bolus dose (5 mL) of prepared solution is given after patient is shifted to surgical ICU, about 45–60 minutes after end of the surgery. Then the solution is run at the rate of 5 mL/hr for 24–48 hours **(Fig. 2.36)**.

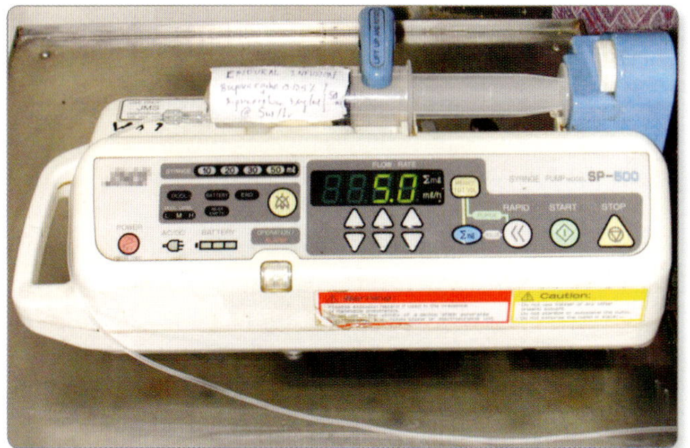

Fig. 2.36 Syringe pump set at 5 mL/hr

   ii. *Intermittent epidural analgesia*: It can be given where infusion is to be avoided in certain patients, syringe pump is not available or those patients showing persistent side-effects like nausea, vomiting, itching or hypotension. One of the combinations can be given:
      - Bupivacaine 0.25%, 6–8 mL 6 hourly through epidural catheter.
      - Bupivacaine 0.25% with injection Tramadol 50 mg 6 mL 8 hourly.
      - Bupivacaine 0.125% with Fentanyl 25 µg, 6–8 mL 6 hourly through epidural catheter. For making this solution, take 2.5 mL of 0.5% Bupivacaine and 0.5 mL Fentanyl in 10 mL syringe and mix with normal saline to make total 10 mL solution.
      - Bupivacaine 0.125% with Buprenorphine 150 µg, 6–8 mL 6 hourly through epidural catheter. For making this solution, take 2.5 mL of 0.5% Bupivacaine and 0.5 mL Buprenorphine in 10 mL syringe and mix with normal saline to make total 10 mL solution.
      - Injection Tramadol 50 to 100 mg (50 mg/mL, 1–2 mL) mix with normal saline total 10 mL 6–8 hourly through epidural catheter.
   iii. *Patient-controlled epidural analgesia*: It can be given with patient-controlled analgesia (PCA) pump, which is very small, lightweight and run on pencil cells. The pump gives continuous background infusion superimposed on patient-controlled boluses. It can be programmed to deliver as specific

dose by patients themselves on an as-needed basis, the minimum interval between doses (lockout period) and maximum dose of drug that can be given in a given period. Patients can be ambulating and do exercise also by carrying electronic PCA pump with them. The pump is connected to epidural catheter and one of the following combinations can be given:
- Bupivacaine 0.0625% with morphine 0.05 mg/mL solution with pump setting of 2–4 mL/hr. continuous infusion, 4–6 mL demand dose and 30 minutes lockout interval (2–4, 4–6, 30).
- Bupivacaine 0.0625% with Fentanyl 5 μg/mL solution with pump setting of 4 mL/hr continuous infusion, 4 mL demand dose and 30 minutes lockout interval (4, 4, 30).
- Bupivacaine 0.125% solution with pump setting of 4 mL/hr. continuous infusion, 4 mL demand dose and 30 minutes lockout interval (4, 4, 30).

iv. *Patient-controlled IV analgesia*: It can be given when epidural catheter is not inserted for any reason or not working properly (i.e. blocked or displaced). Patient-controlled analgesia (PCA) pump is connected to peripheral intravenous line and one of the following combinations can be given:
- Morphine 0.5 mg/mL solution with pump setting of 0 mL continuous infusion, 2 mL demand dose and 15–20 minutes lockout interval (0, 2, 15).
- Fentanyl 5 μg/mL solution with pump setting of 0 mL continuous infusion, 2 mL demand dose and 15–20 minutes lockout interval (0, 2, 15).
- Tramadol 5 mg/mL solution with pump setting of 2 mL/hr continuous infusion, 2 mL demand dose and 30 minutes lockout interval (2, 2, 30).

v. *Intermittent IM/IV analgesia*: One of the following combinations can be given alone or in combination with above routes:
- Injection Diclofenac 75 mg IM or IV formulation (other than IM oily formulation) 75 mg in 100 mL of normal saline, 8 hourly IV or SOS.
- Injection Tramadol 50–100 mg IM or diluted up to 10 mL with normal saline, 6 hourly IV or SOS.

Dose and volume of drug depends on age, weight and height of patient and adequate hepatic-renal function. Patients need monitoring of pulse, BP, respiratory rate, Sedation and any side-effects like nausea, vomiting, itching, hypotension, urinary retention, constipation or excessive motor blockade.

6. Injection Dexona (Dexamethasone, 4 mg)—1 amp IV at 8.00 PM (3rd dose, 12 hours after 2nd dose).
7. Monitor TPRBP (Temperature, pulse, respiratory rate, blood pressure) ½ hourly for 2 hours and then 4 hourly.
8. Monitor Input-output chart.
9. BT (blood transfusion)—2nd unit started.

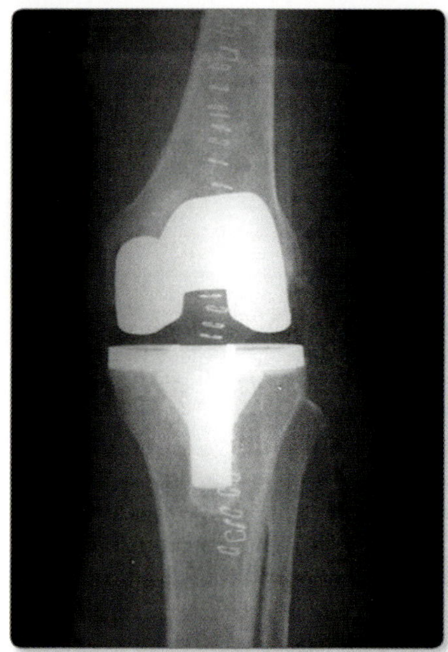

Fig. 2.37 Postoperative AP view

10. Capsule Omeprazole 20 mg after 4 hours and then oral fluids. Light diet at night.
11. Check that suction drain is working properly.
12. Quadriceps exercise, active ankle and toe movements.
13. Bed side portable check X-ray of operated knee-AP view **(Fig. 2.37)**.

1st Postoperative Day

1. Blood investigations—TLC, DLC, Hb%, PCV, blood sugar, LFT (serum billirubin, SGOT, SGPT, serum protein), RFT (BUN, serum creatinine), serum electrolyte. (Neutrophilic leucocytosis is a common postoperative finding.)
2. Continue antibiotics.
3. Injection Enoxaparin sodium (LMWH) 40 mg/0.4 mL SC at 8.00 AM (2nd dose, 24 hours after surgery).
4. Epidural analgesia for pain.
5. Remove knee brace. Physiotherapy—Quadriceps exercise, knee bending exercise, active ankle and toe movements, chest physiotherapy (blowing of football bladder or spirometer after full inspiration). After quadriceps exercise, re-application of knee brace.
6. Normal diet.
7. Use of bedpan.

2nd Postoperative Day

1. Remove epidural catheter (At least 10–12 hours after the last dose of LMWH) and urinary catheter.
2. Injection Enoxaparin sodium (LMWH) 40 mg/0.4 mL SC at 8.00 AM (3rd dose, 48 hours after surgery) atleast 2 hours after the removal of epidural catheter.

3. Continue antibiotics.
4. Removal of suction drain and change of dressing: While removing suction drain, keep negative pressure in the suction bottle and ask the patient to do quadriceps exercise so that whatever collection inside the joint will come out. Clean the incision line and adjacent area with betadine-soaked gauze piece. Apply betadine-soaked gauze piece and cotton pad over the wound. Make the adjacent area dry and apply elastoplast longitudinally without stretching. This will help in knee movement while flexing the knee. Apply knee brace.
5. Patient will stand up with help of walker and if possible start walking **(Fig. 2.38)**.
6. Physiotherapy: Continue quadriceps exercise, knee bending exercise, ankle and toes movement, chest physiotherapy.
7. Tab Combiflam TDS after meals.
8. Tab Proxyvon BD after meals.
9. Cap Omeprazole 20 mg 1 OD.
10. Tab B-complex forte BD.
11. Shift the patient in ward from ICU and transfer the patient from wheeled cot to nonwheeled cot to avoid slipping of cot while patient is coming out from the bed or wheeled cot should be locked and supported with wall. Otherwise patient may fall due to slip of wheeled cot.
12. Use of bedpan.

3 doses of LMWH (Enoxaparin sodium, 40 mg/0.4 mL)—1st dose 24 hours before surgery, 2nd dose 24 hours after surgery and 3rd dose 48 hours after surgery. Thromboprophylaxis is extended SC or oral anticoagulant once daily for 4 weeks in high-risk cases. Early mobilization and use of mechanical methods like thromboembolic deterrent (TED) stockings, Sequential/intermittent pneumatic compressions are helpful in prevention of DVT.

Total 3 doses of Dexona (Dexamethasone)—1st dose 12 hours before surgery, 2nd dose just before surgery and 3rd dose 12 hours after 2nd dose.

One dose of 100 mg Efcorlin (hydrocortisone succinate) IV is given peroperative just before cementing.

3rd to 5th Postoperative Day

1. Continue antibiotics.
2. Continue analgesics.
3. Apply knee brace and patient starts walking with the help of walker.
4. Use of bedpan.
5. Physiotherapy—Quadriceps exercise, ankle and toe movements, chest physiotherapy, knee bending exercise/CPM **(Fig.2.39)**. Special attention is given over quadriceps and knee bending exercises under supervision of physiotherapist. CPM is not required in all cases. It is more beneficial in cases where preoperative movement of knee is limited. Do straight leg raising exercise.

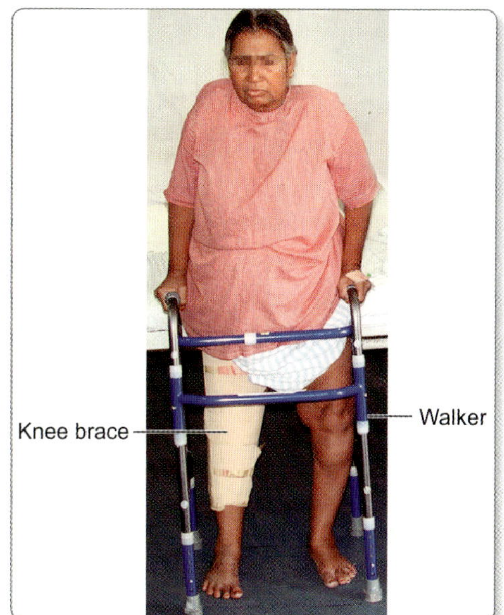

Fig. 2.38 Patient starts walking with help of walker and knee brace from second postoperative day

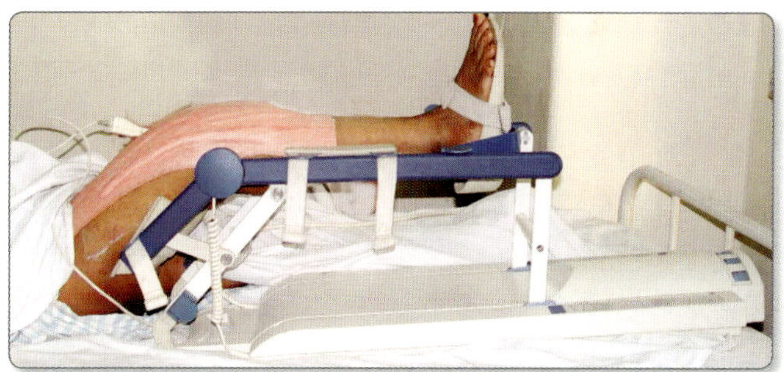
Fig. 2.39 Knee bending exercise with CPM machine

6th to 14th Postoperative Day

1. Stop injectable antibiotics.
2. Start Tab Ceftum/Ciprofloxacin 500 mg BD for 5 days.
3. Tab B-complex forte BD.
4. Analgesic tablets depending upon severity of pain.
5. Physiotherapy—Quadriceps exercise, ankle and toe movements, knee bending exercise/CPM **(Fig. 2.39)**, straight leg raising exercise, chest physiotherapy. Special attention is given over quadriceps and knee bending exercise under supervision of physiotherapist. Patient is asked to put a folded towel or cotton roll beneath the heel and extend the knee **(Fig. 2.40A)**. Patient is also asked to keep a cotton roll under the knee and press it **(Fig 2.40B)**. Patient is asked to sit at the edge of the

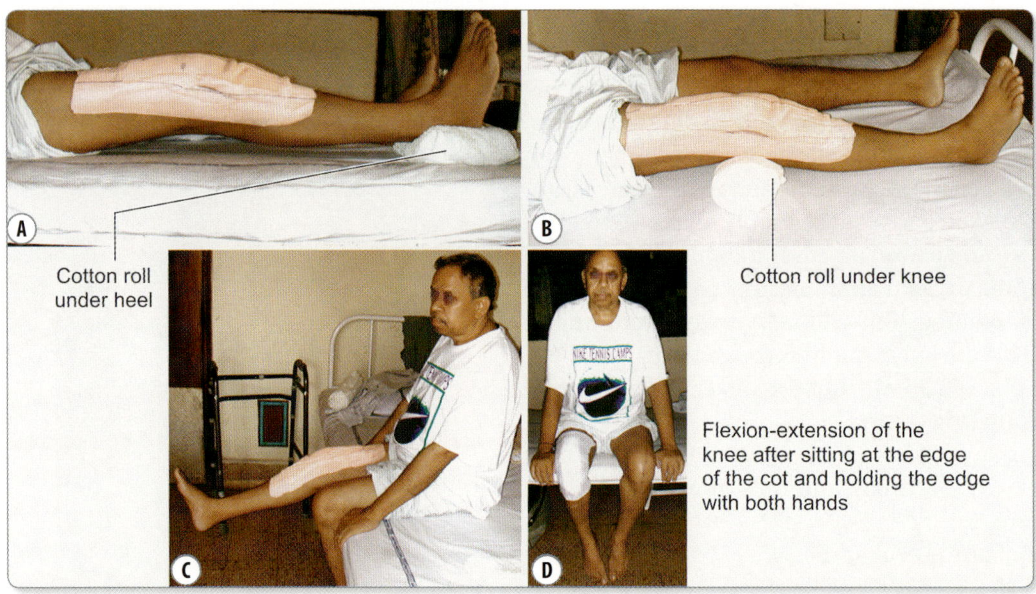

Figs 2.40A to D Quadriceps and knee bending exercises

cot, hold the edge firmly and flex and extend the knee **(Figs 2.40C and D)**. Full extension (i.e. no FFD) and more than 90° flexion should be gained within 2 weeks of surgery. Do straight leg raising exercise.

6. Apply knee brace and walk with help of walker.
7. Stitches are removed preferably in OT under full aseptic precaution on 14th day. After removal of stitches, clean the area with betadine. Apply betadine-soaked gauze piece and then apply dry gauze piece and fix the dressing with Omnifix transversely.
8. Use of western type of toilet/bedpan depending upon patient's mental and physical status.
9. Check X-ray both knees AP and lateral views after removal of stitches **(Figs 2.41A and B)**.

15th–16th Postoperative Day

If everything is well then patient is discharged with following advice:

1. Continue quadriceps exercise, ankle and toe movements, knee bending exercise and straight leg raising exercise.
2. Walk with help of knee brace and walker.
3. No local massage, no heat therapy,
4. Avoid squatting, sitting on floor, cross-legged sitting, jogging and running.
5. Use western type of toilet.
6. Use chair of approximately 20 inches height.
7. Any infection like UTI, dental infection, boils, abscess should be treated vigorously.
8. Control of weight.
9. Follow-up after 1 month.

Follow-up Schedule

One month after surgery then 3 months, 6 months and 1 year.

After 1 month:
Remove knee brace and walker. Do full weight-bearing walking. Start climbing up and down stairs.

After 2 months:
Almost normal activities with some modification in life style.

"After a successful joint replacement, one can expect to become more independent and enjoy activities of daily living with greater ease and comfort."

Assessment during Follow-up

1. Clinical assessment.
2. Radiological assessment.

Clinical Assessment

- Pain
- Range of motion
- Stability—anteroposterior and mediolateral
- FFD
- Extension lag
- Alignment
- Walking
- Climbing up and down stairs

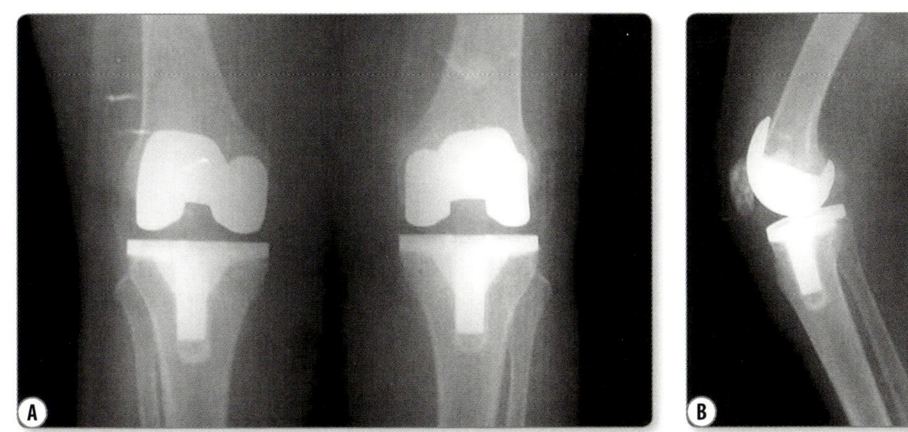

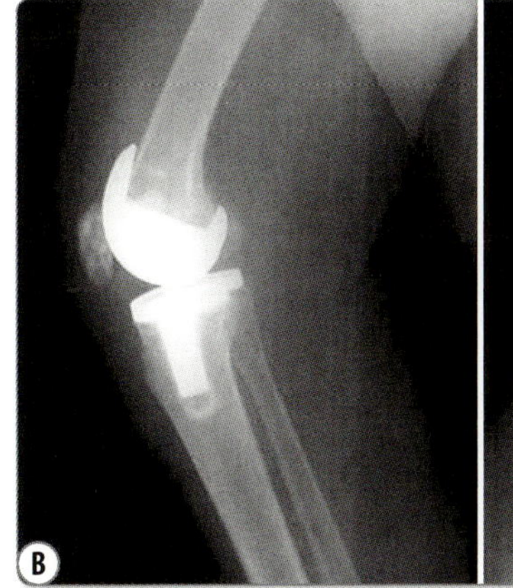

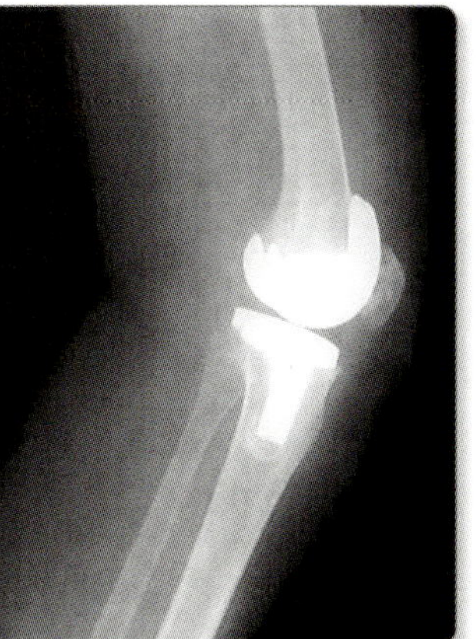

Figs 2.41A and B (A) AP view; (B) Lateral view

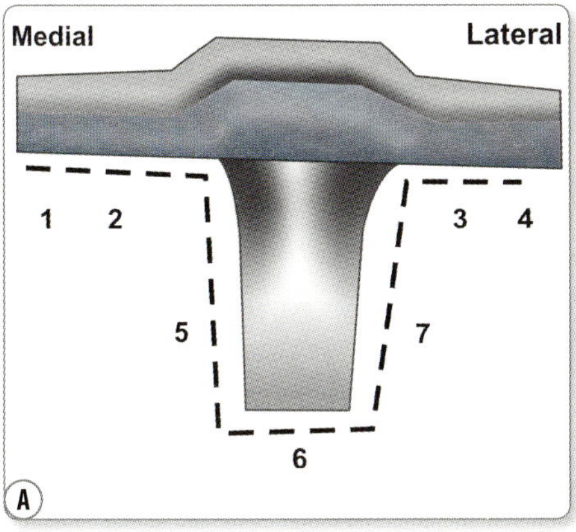

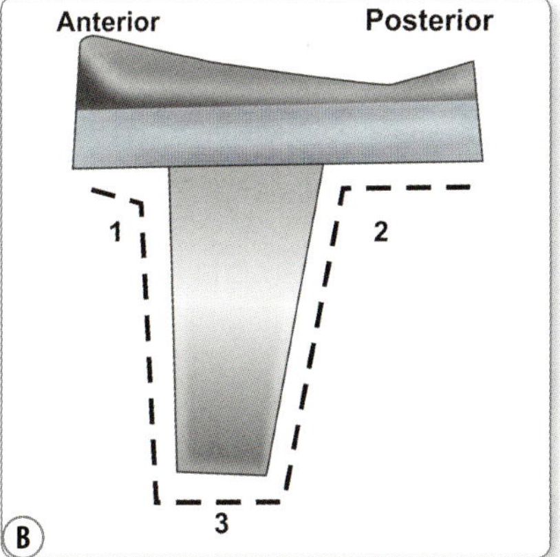

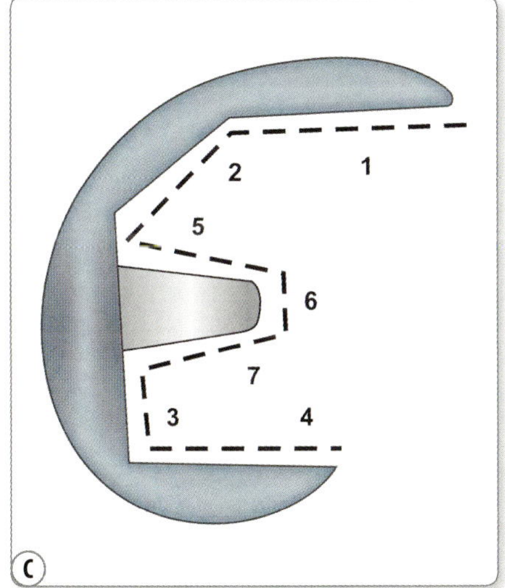

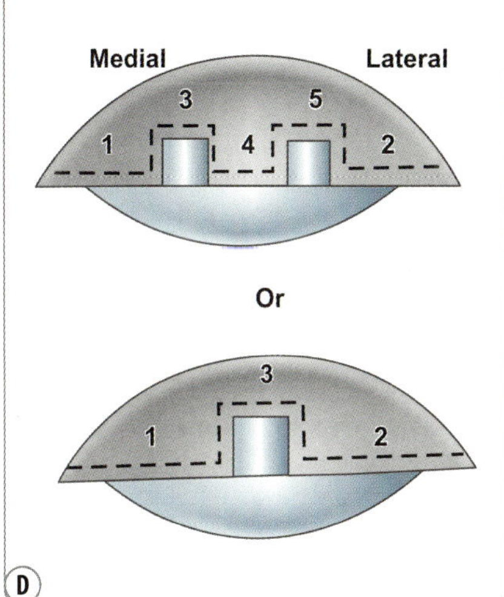

Figs 2.42A to D (A) Zone 1 and 2 for the medial plateau, Zone 3 and 4 for the lateral plateau, Zone 5–7 for the stem fixation ; (B) Zone 1 for anterior part, Zone 2 for posterior part, Zone 3 for the stem fixation; (C) Zone1 and 2 for the anterior flange, Zone 3 and 4 for the posterior area, Zone 5–7 for the central portion; (D) Zone 1 represents medial side, Zone 2 represents lateral side, Zone 3–5 represent the central part of the patellar component

Radiological Assessment (Figs 2.42A to D)

1. AP view to assess the status of tibial component.
2. Anterior-posterior view **(Fig. 2.42B)**.
3. Lateral view to assess the status of femoral and tibial Components **(Fig. 2.42C)**.
4. Patellar skyline view to assess the status of patellar button **(Fig. 2.42D)**.

Difficult Situations and Important Points

3

CHAPTER

Chapter Outline

Total Knee Replacement (TKR) in Difficult Situations

Assess the difficult situations like:

1. FFD >30°
2. Stiff knee (i.e. knee flexion <30°)
3. Large medial or lateral defect (i.e. severe varus >25° or valgus deformity >15°)
4. Post HTO

Plan the surgery properly including templating, keeping many options ready for building up the defect (bone cement, screws and bone cement, bone graft, metallic wedges), tibial tubercle osteotomy, quadriceptoplasty, quadriceps snip, multiple puncture (pie-crusting) in quadriceps tendon (in stiff knee and revision TKR), multiple puncture in iliotibial (IT) band (in fixed valgus deformity), posterior release in femur (in FFD), medialization of tibial tray and possibility of offset stem tibial tray (in post HTO), Extension rod with tibial tray or femoral component. In cases of FFD >30°, preoperative correction of FFD up to 30° or at least 40° must be achieved by vigorous physiotherapy, passive stretching by use of knee brace, traction or serial casting under anesthesia. Postoperative, significant (>15°) flexion contractures can cause persistent pain and altered gait mechanics. In cases of stiff knee (flexion <30°), patient must be informed that regaining flexion will be slow and require considerable time and effort by the patient and the physiotherapist. Even then flexion up to 90° may not be gained in some cases.

Build up the residual defect by:

1. *Bone cement*: If the defect is <5 mm.
2. *Screws and bone cement*: If the defect is between 5 and 10 mm, make two drill holes in defect with 2.5 mm drill bit. The direction of the tip of drill bit is about 10° towards the tibial axis. Measure the depth with depth gauge to determine the length of the screws (usually 18 mm, 20 mm, 22 mm, 24 mm or 26 mm screw length). Tap it with 3.5 mm tap if hard bone. Pass two 3.5 mm cortical screws till they come just below the level of defect **(Fig. 3.1)**. Check the level by putting the trial tibial tray. There is 1–2 mm clearance between head of screws and the tibial

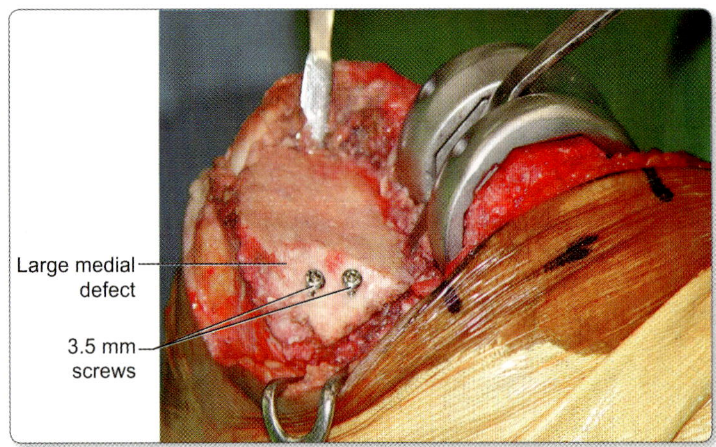

Fig. 3.1 3.5 mm two cortical screws to support the tibial tray and to hold the cement

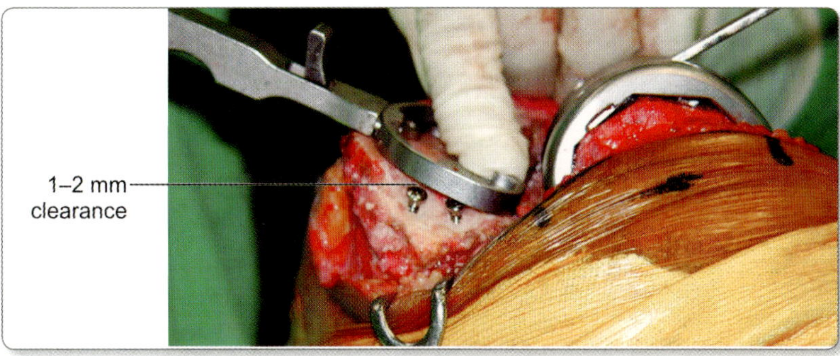

Fig. 3.2 Checking the level of screws in defect by trial tibial tray

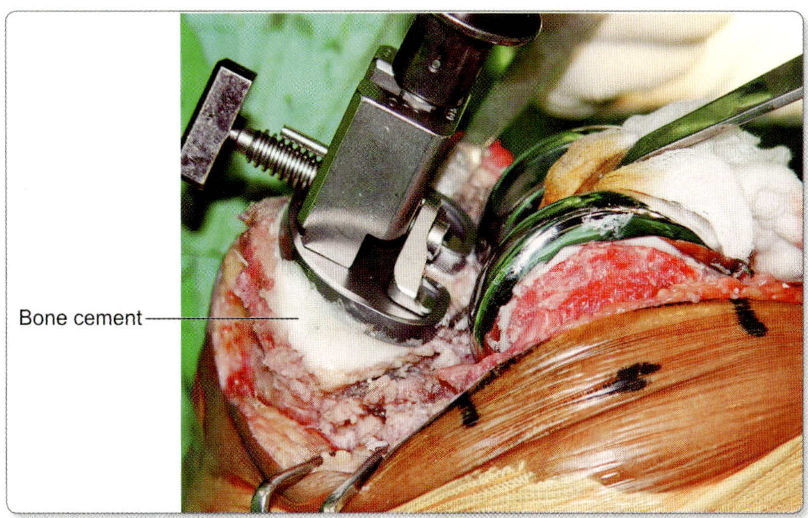

Fig. 3.3 After cementing

tray for bone cement **(Fig. 3.2)**. It will support the tibial tray and hold the cement **(Figs 3.3 and 3.4)**.

3. *Bone graft*: If the defect is >10 mm and patient is younger (<60 years): The bone removed from either posterior part of medial condyle, distal femur, upper tibia or box cut is used as bone graft. The defect of tibial condyle is made box-shaped by backward movement of saw or by high speed drill or microdrive plus for better holding of graft and making the area vascular. The graft is temporarily fixed with one K-wire. Drill through the graft by 2.5 mm drill bit. The direction of the tip of drill bit is about 10° towards the tibial axis. Measure the depth with depth gauge to determine the length of the screws (usually 24 to 30 mm screw length). Countersink, tap with 3.5 mm tap and fix the bone graft by two 3.5 mm cortical screws **(Figs 3.5 and 3.6)**.

In addition, if the tibial defect after resection is less than 50% of the tibial condyle, the peg bone graft without screws may be used. It is usually taken from the intercondylar bone of the femur which is being removed during box cut or resected tibia. Make a hole in the tibial defect by reciprocating saw, burr and/or drill (high speed drill or microdrive plus). Shape the graft in such a manner that it will firmly fit into the hole created in the defect of tibial plateau. Temporarily fix the graft

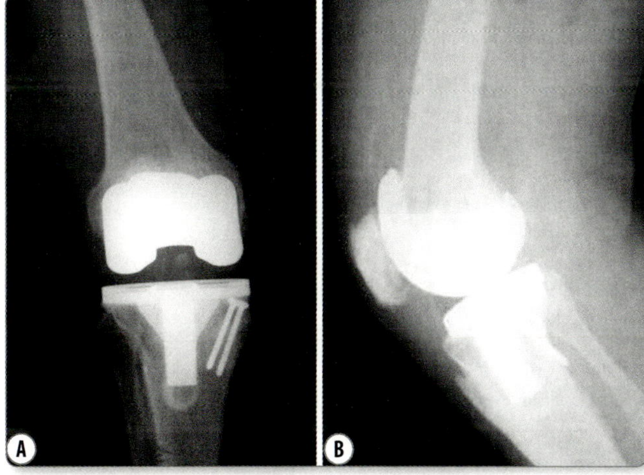

Figs 3.4A and B (A) AP view X-ray; (B) Lateral view X-ray

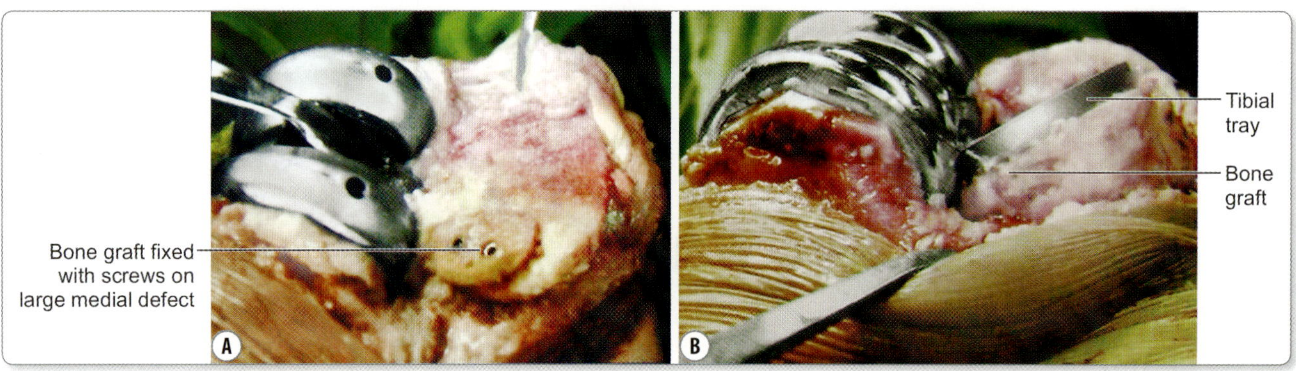

Figs 3.5A and B (A) Bone graft fixed with two 3.5 mm cortical screws on grafted bone; (B) After implantation of tibial tray

transversely with two K-wires taking care not to pass the K-wires in the area of tibial preparation **(Fig. 3.7)**. Re-apply the tibial cutting block and level the graft with saw to resected tibia. If required, augmentation with one or two cortical screws of 3.5 mm may be done. Tibial preparation is done. First fix the tibial tray with bone cement. While cement is setting, remove the K-wires and press the bone cement with fingers near the defect. Hold and pressurize the tibial tray in position till the cement sets.

For central bone defect, do impaction bone grafting.

4. *Metallic wedge*: If the defect is >10 mm and elderly patient (>60 years) **(Fig. 3.8A)**.

Modular plus tibial wedges are used with modular plus tibial tray and 2 enclosed screws **(Figs 3.8C to F)**. The wedges are 10° and 20° hemi and 10° and 15° full in all sizes of tibial tray. There are 10 mm and 15 mm thickness step wedge in all sizes of tibial tray. There is one wedge cutting guide for 10° and 20° hemi wedge and one step cutting guide for 10 mm and 15 mm step **(Fig. 3.8B)**. There are four full wedge cutting guides—10° LL/RM, 10° LM/RL and 15° LL/RM, 15° LM/RL (See details of technique in revision TKR).

Femoral Augmentations

There are posterior augmentation (4 mm and 8 mm) and distal augmentation for right and left (4 mm, 8 mm, 12 mm, 16 mm) (See details of technique in revision TKR).

Posterior Release from Femur

After all bone cuts, lift the femur by bone hook and release posteriorly with curve osteotome and gauze piece by elevating the capsule from the distal femur or proximal tibia in a subperiosteal plane (to avoid injury to popliteal artery or tibial nerve) in case of FFD **(Fig. 3.9)**. Large osteophytes on the posterior aspect of the femur are being removed by using curette.

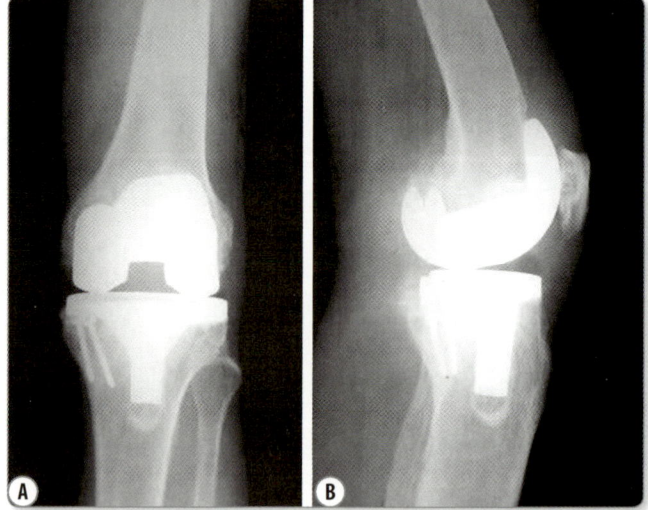

Figs 3.6A and B AP view and lateral view X-ray with bone graft fixed with screws

Extension Rod

In case of large tibial defects **(Figs 3.11 to 3.19)**, old fracture of tibial condyle **(Figs 3.20 and 3.21)**, upper shaft of tibia **(Figs 3.22 to 3.27)** or non-union HTO, extension rod is applied to avoid stress over the condyle of tibia. For application of extension rod with tibial tray, keep the trial tibial tray and punch guide in position after tibial preparation. Remove the drill bushing. Pass the 8 mm drill in tibial canal and ream the tibial canal with gradually increasing diameter reamer till snugly fitting upto the planned length of rod **(Fig. 3.10A)** and then one size higher i.e. for 14 mm rod, ream to 15 mm (Sizes of reamers are 10 mm, 11 mm, 12 mm, 13 mm, 14 mm, 15 mm, 16 mm, 17 mm, 18 mm). Do the trial reduction after application of trial extension rod in Trial tibial tray with peg (For trial reduction with extension rod, the trial tibial tray is separate i.e. with peg). Apply the extension rod of appropriate length and diameter on tibial tray **(Fig. 3.10B)**. For applying the extension rod, hold the appropriate tibial tray with tibial holding clamp. Remove the plastic plug from the lower

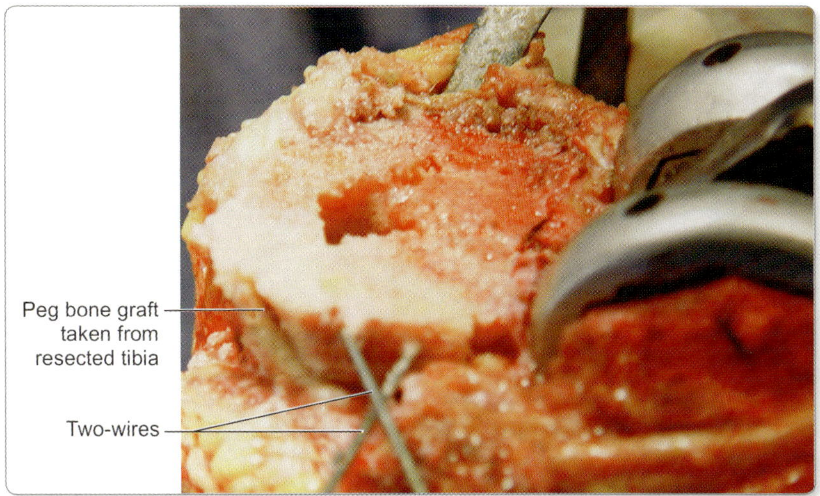

Fig. 3.7 Two K-wires temporarily fixing the graft and passing away from the area of tibial preparation

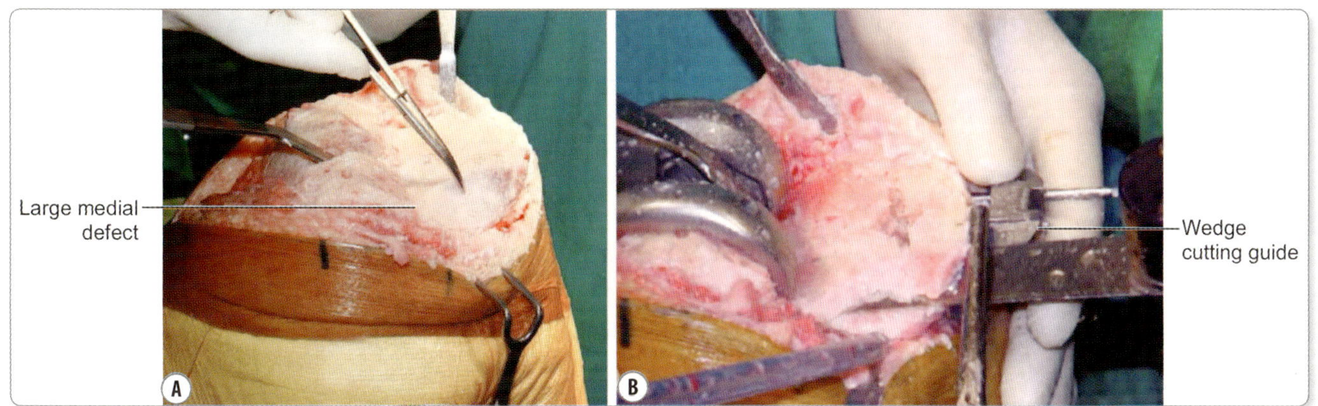

Figs 3.8A and B (A) Large defect >10 mm; (B) Cutting wedge

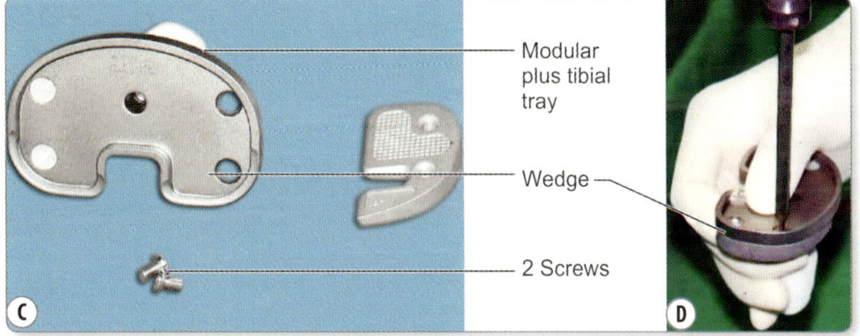

Figs 3.8C and D (C) Modular plus tibial tray, wedge and 2 screws; (D) Fitting of wedge with modular plus tibial tray

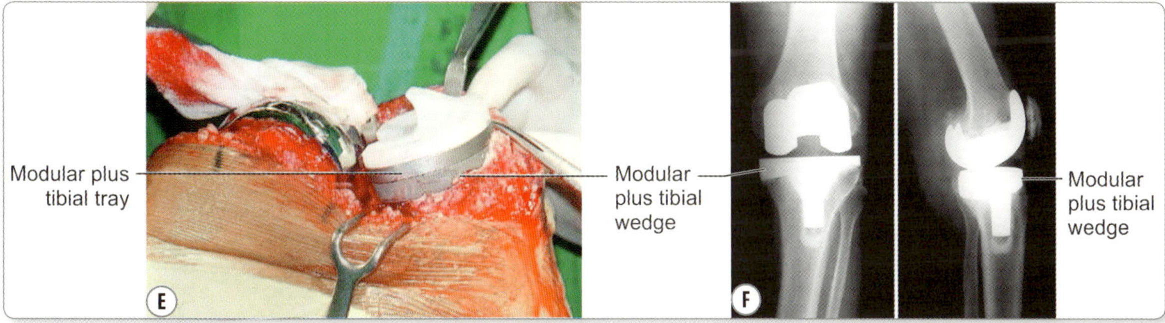

Figs 3.8E and F (E) Modular plus tibial tray with wedge; (F) AP and lateral view X-ray with wedge

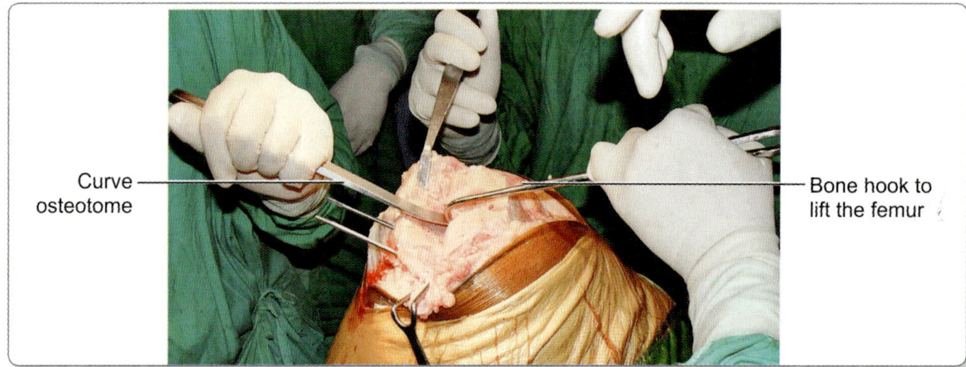

Fig. 3.9 Posterior release of femur

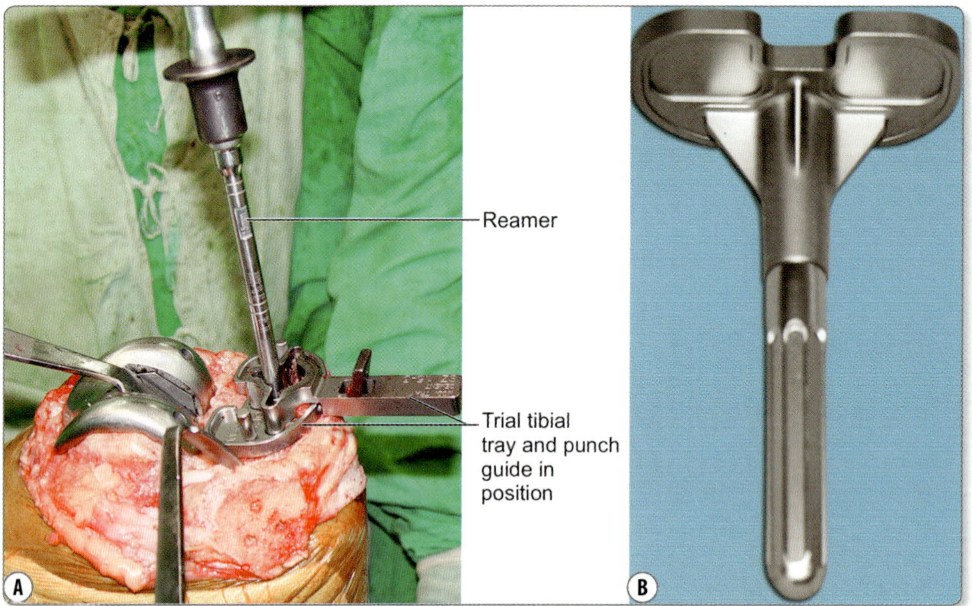

Figs 3.10A and B (A) Reaming upto planned length of rod; (B) Tibial tray fitted with extension rod (Fluted rod)

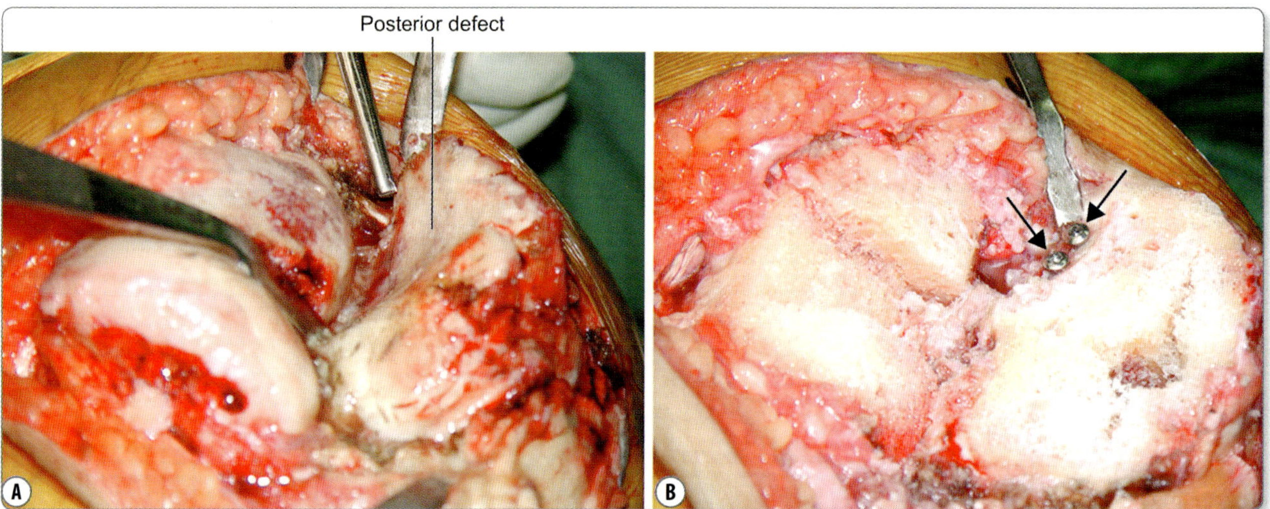

Figs 3.11A and B (A) Large posterior defect of tibia; (B) Built up by 3.5 mm two screws

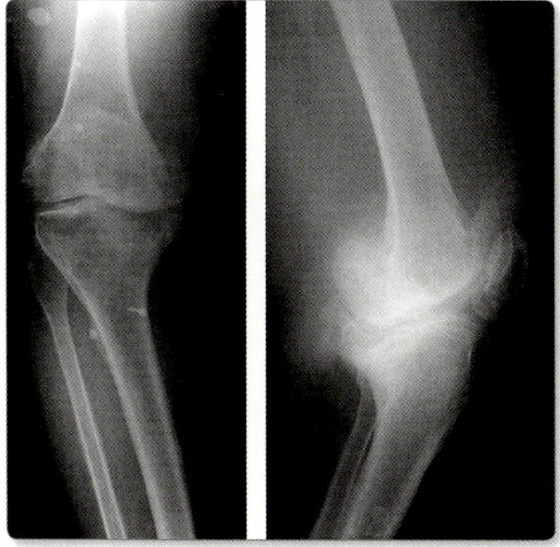

Fig. 3.12 AP and lateral view X-rays showing large posterior defect

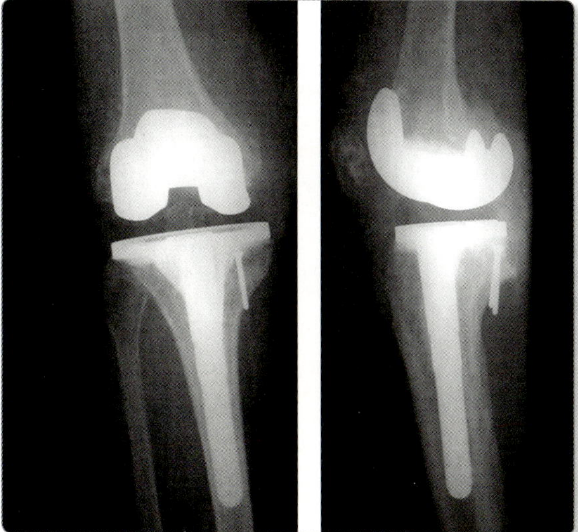

Fig.3.13 In addition to built up by screws, extension rod is applied to avoid stress

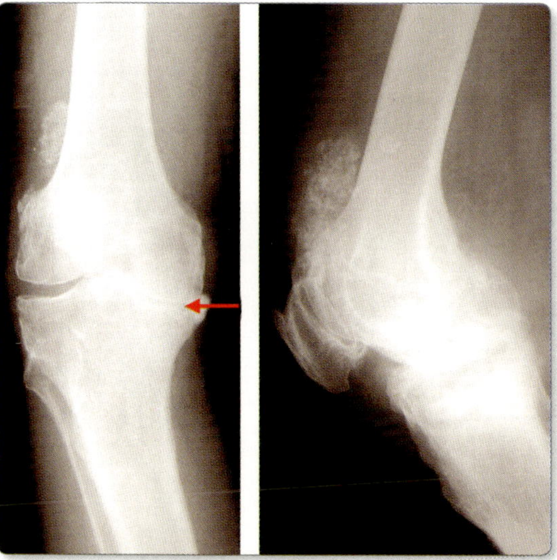

Fig. 3.14 Large medial defect

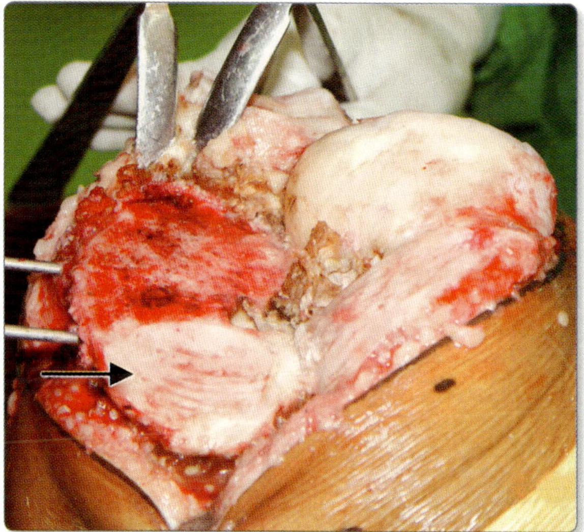

Fig. 3.15 Greater than 10 mm residual medial defect in elderly

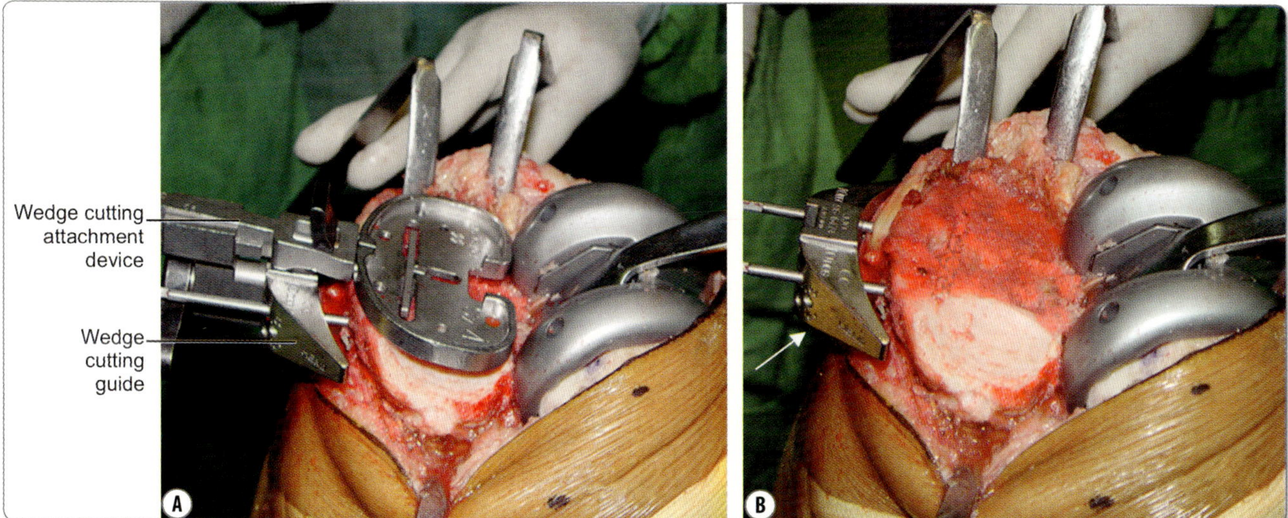

Figs 3.16A and B Positioning of wedge cutting guide

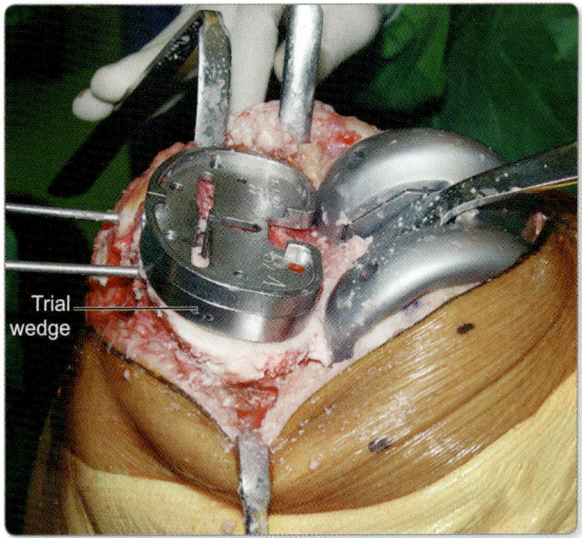

Fig. 3.17 Trial wedge attached with trail tibial tray

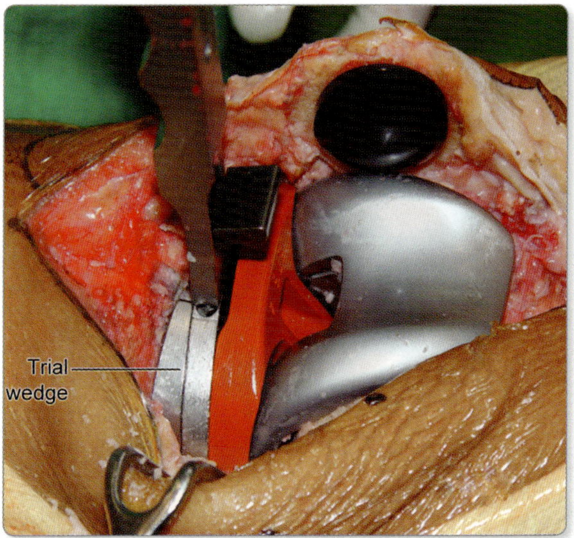

Fig. 3.18 After trial reduction

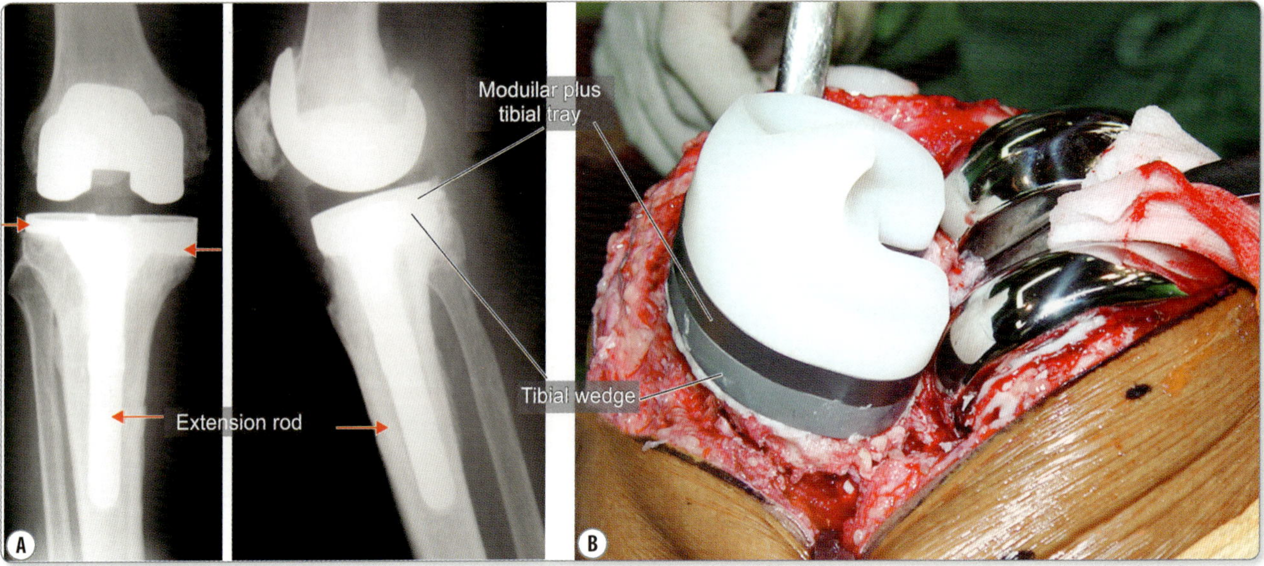

Figs 3.19A and B Modular plus tibial wedge and extension rod fitted with modular plus tibial tray

end of the tibial tray. Extension rod is held with press fit rod wrench and completely tightened with the tibial tray. Similarly ream the femoral canal for femoral rod according to the requirement. Reamers for tibial and femoral rods are same with different marking of tibial rod length and femoral rod length. (Fluted tibial IM rods are available in 3 lengths - 75 mm, 115 mm, 150 mm and diameter 10mm, 12mm, 14mm, 16 mm, 18mm. Fluted Femoral IM rods in 2 lengths—125 mm, 175 mm and diameter 10 mm, 12 mm, 14 mm, 16 mm, 18 mm with 50 and 70 valgus angles, Bolts for fixing IM rod with femoral component—0 mm and 2 mm offset).

It is always a wise decision to use extension rod whenever building up large defects.

Cemented Tibial and Femoral Stem Extension

Recommended in severe osteoporosis **(Figs 3.28 to 3.30)** and whenever building up the large defects **(Figs 3.31A to C)**.

Cemented tibial stems are available in two sizes and two diameters—30 mm, 60 mm length and 13 mm, 15 mm diameters each. Canal preparation is done in the similar way as for fluted rods by same reamer up to desired length and

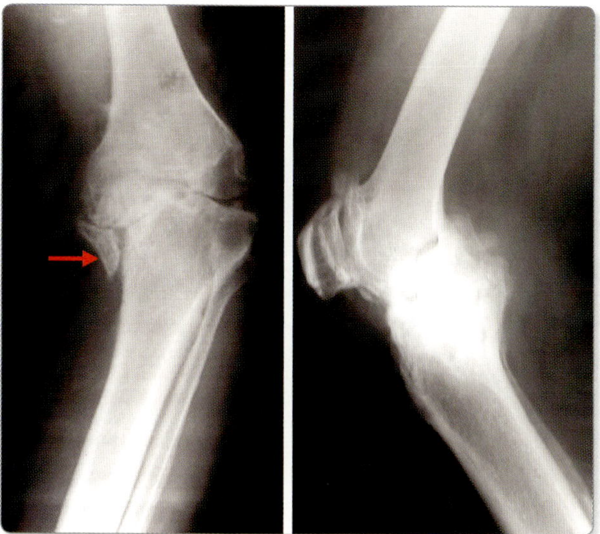

Fig. 3.20 Old fractured medial condyle tibia—AP and lateral view

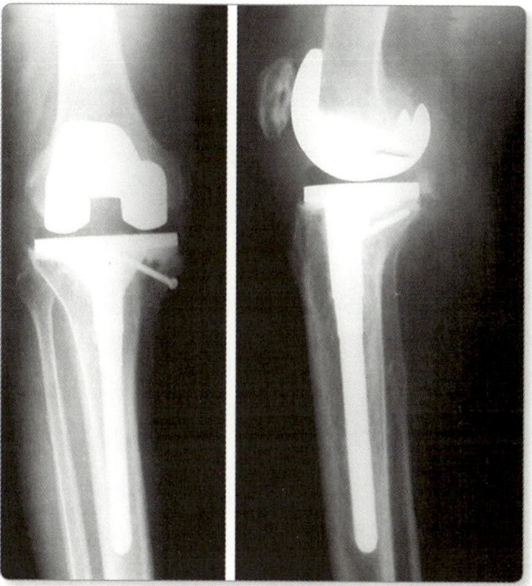

Fig. 3.21 Fixation of fractured of medial condyle with screw and application of extension rod with tibial tray to avoid stress over the fractured medial condyle (AP and Lateral view)

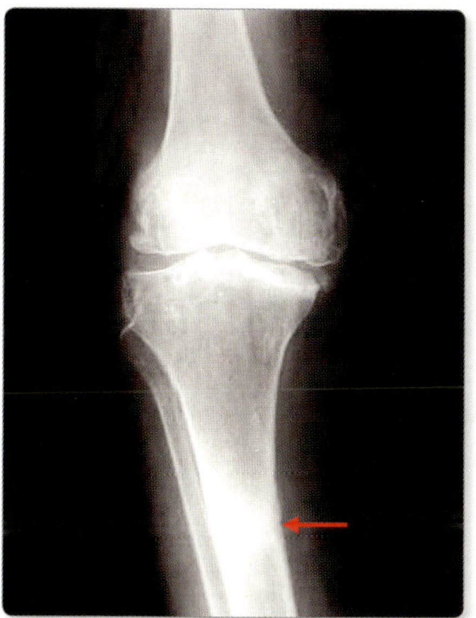

Fig. 3.22 Stress fracture upper tibia with arthritis

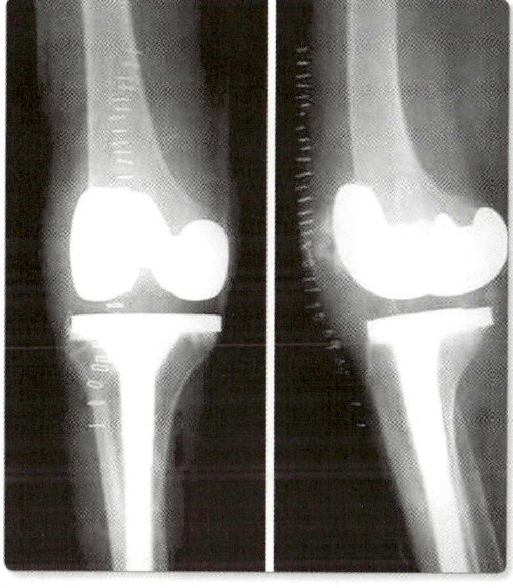

Fig. 3.23 Extension rod with tibial tray to avoid stress over fractured tibia (AP and lateral views)

diameter with trial tibial tray and punch guide in place. Trial reduction is done with trial tibial tray fitted with extension rod. CMW1 bone cement is applied on the selected size tibial tray and stem and applied over the prepared tibia.

Cemented femoral stems (smooth, non-fluted modular stems) are available in two sizes (90 mm and 130 mm lengths), two diameters (13 mm and 15 mm), two angles (5° and 7°) and three stem positions (0 mm, + 2 mm and -2 mm). Femoral canal preparation is done with appropriate diameter femoral stem reamer and desired depth according to marking on the reamer. Stem positioning and trial assembly is done as mentioned in revision TKR ahead. Trial reduction is done with appropriate trial femoral component and stem assembly. Assemble the selected size femoral component and femoral stem. CMW1 bone cement is applied on the femoral component and stem and applied over the distal femur.

Available cemented femoral stems are:

1. 5° and 7° angles each
2. 13 mm and 15 mm +2 mm left/-2 mm right
3. 13 mm and 15 mm +2 mm right/-2 mm left
4. 13 mm and 15 mm 0 mm offset.

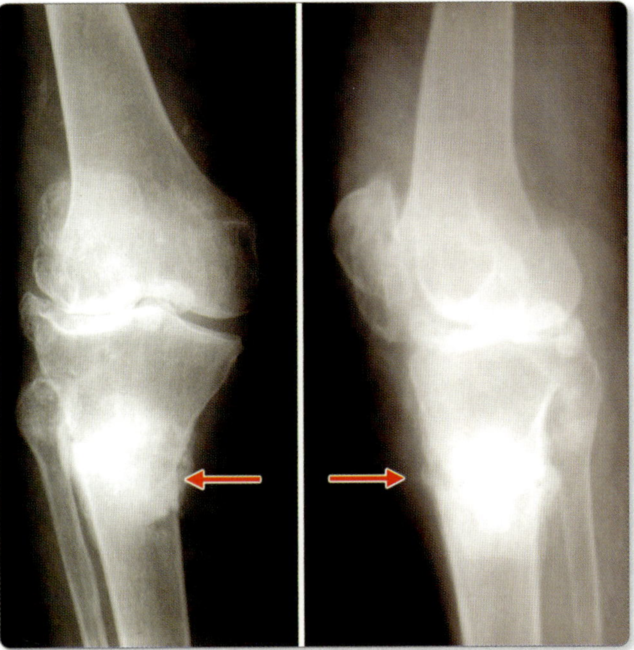

Fig. 3.24 Old fracture upper tibia with arthritis of knee joint

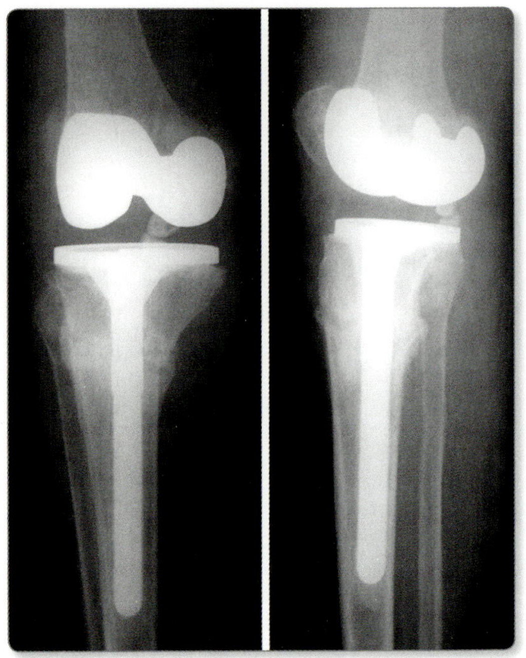

Fig. 3.25 Extension rod with tibial tray to avoid stress over fractured tibia (AP and lateral views)

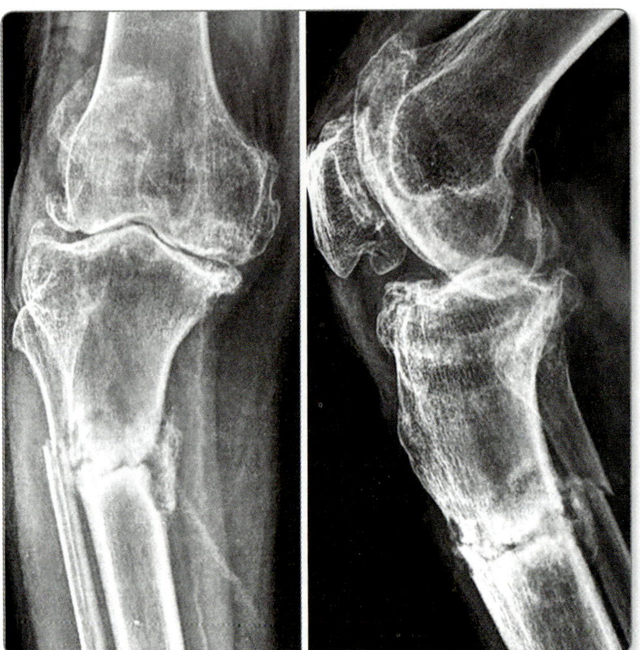

Fig. 3.26 Non-union tibia and fibula with arthritis of knee joint

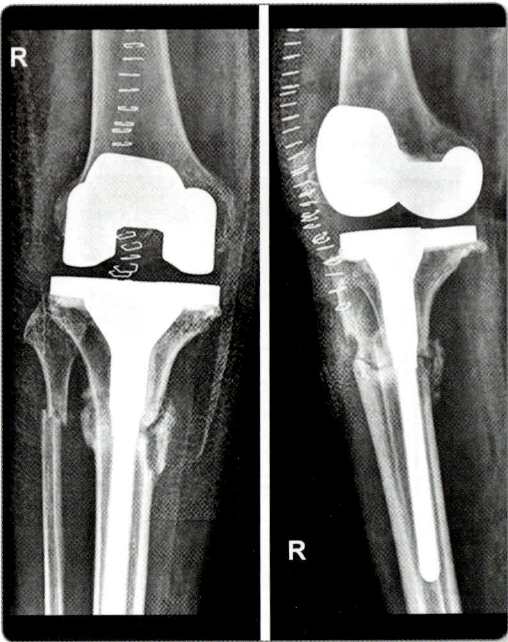

Fig. 3.27 TKR with extension rod

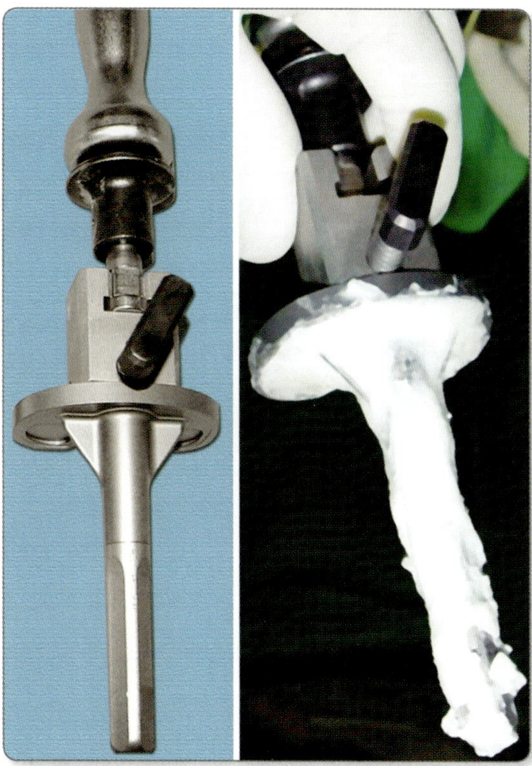

Fig. 3.28 Cemented tibial rod (without and with cement)

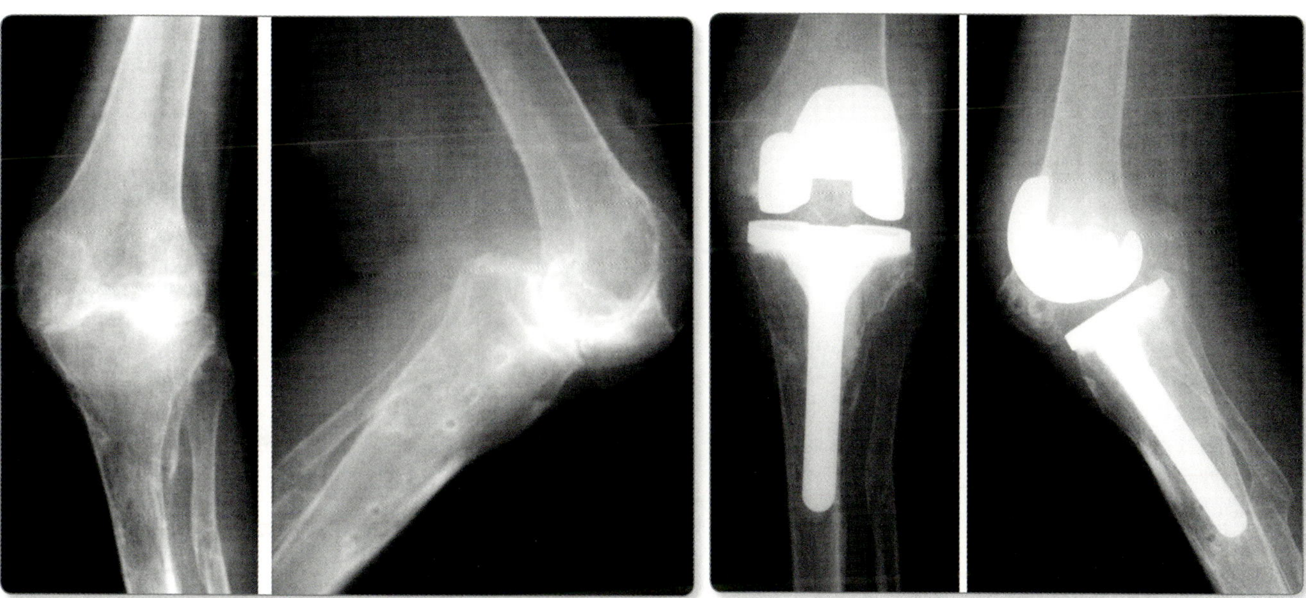

Fig. 3.29 Severe osteoporosis in case of RA

Fig. 3.30 Cemented rod 60 mm with tibial tray

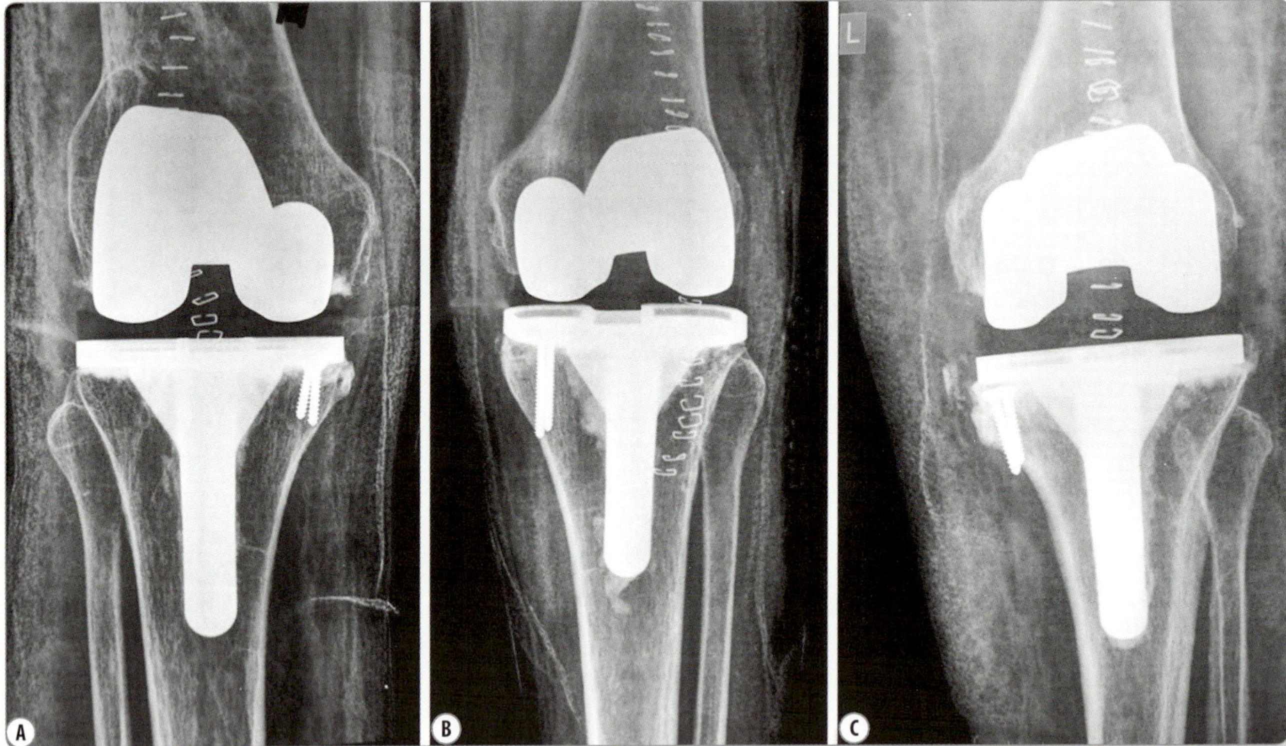

Figs 3.31A to C Buit up the medial defect of tibial condyle by screws and bone cement augmented by 30 mm cemented rod

Post-HTO TKR

Eighty percent of the knees have patella infera after HTO which may contribute to alter biomechanics of patellofemoral joint after TKR. Preoperative templating is helpful in deciding the medialization or use of offset stem. Post HTO TKR is technically more demanding than primary TKR.

Technical Difficulties

Prior Incision

1. Longitudinal midline incision should be used for TKR regardless of incision of previous osteotomy.
2. In case of transverse incision, the longitudinal incision crossing at 90° is ideal, even up to 60° angle is safe.
3. Old healed long previous incision can be incorporated in new incision.
4. If more than one long scars then most lateral scar should be chosen.
5. The intervening bridge between old and new incision should not be less than 2.5 cm.

Soft Tissue Scarring

1. Periosteal exposure of proximal tibia is difficult.
2. Soft tissue dissection is more demanding and preferably done with scalpel or electrocautery rather than periosteal elevator or osteotome.

Patellar Eversion

1. Adherence and scarring of patellar tendon—shortening.
2. Difficult to evert patella.
3. Pin at tibial tubercle.
4. May need quadriceps snip/tibial tubercle osteotomy.
5. Lateral retinacular release.

Patella Infera (Insall-Salvati index)

Insall-Salvati index is defined as the ratio between length of the patellar tendon to the length of the patella in true lateral view X-ray of the knee in at least 30 degree flexion. This ratio is 0.9–1.1 in males and 0.94–1.18 in females (adults) and it is less in post HTO knee **(Figs 3.32A and B)**.

Implant

1. Preferably implants should be removed before TKR.
2. Possibility of subacute infection.

Varus Cut of Tibia

Altered mediolateral slope **(Figs 3.33A and B)**.

Loss of Bone Stock

1. HTO results in reduction in amount of bone stock from proximal tibia.

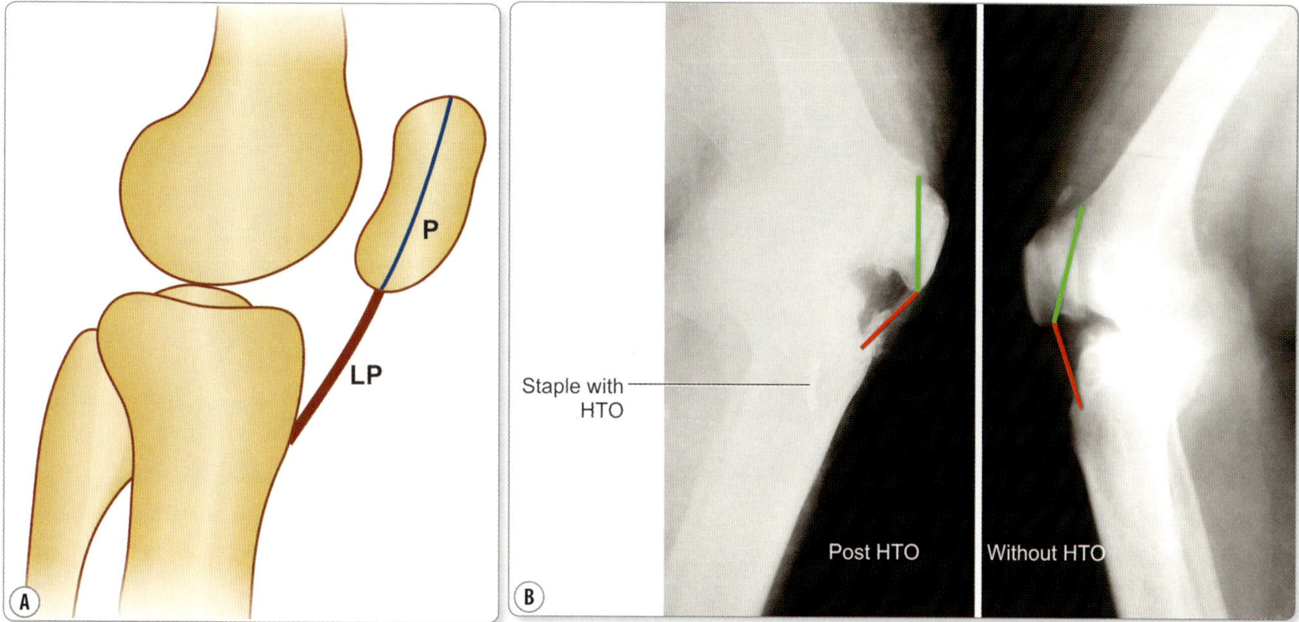

Figs 3.32A and B (A) Diagrammatic picture showing length of patellar tendon and patella; (B) X-ray showing length of patellar tendon and patella

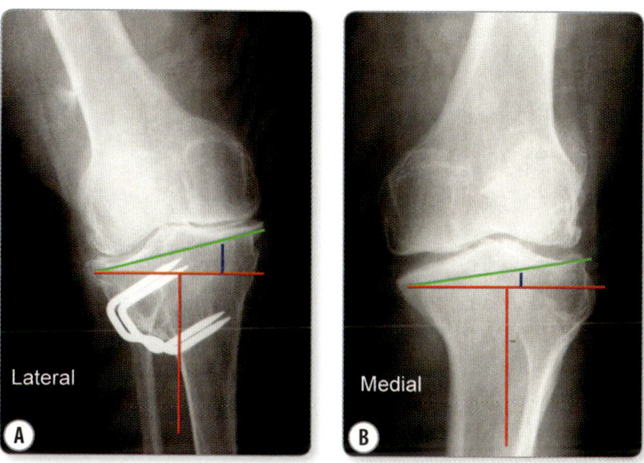

Figs 3.33A and B (A) With HTO, slope on lateral side; (B) Without HTO, slope on medial side

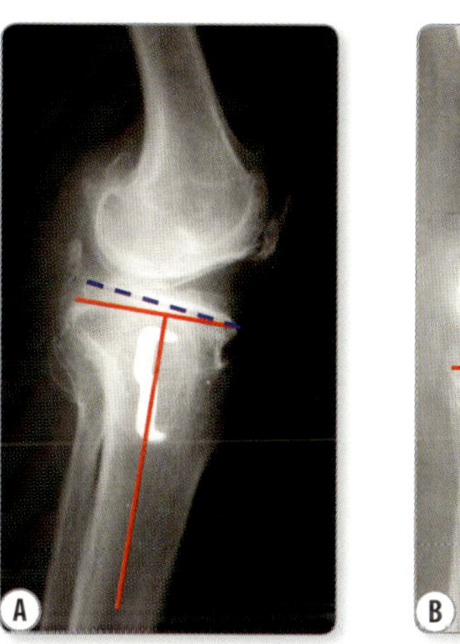

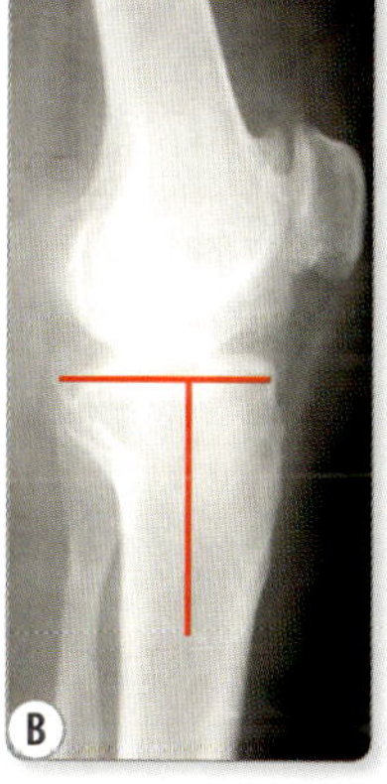

Figs 3.34A and B (A) Tibial cut in Post HTO TKR; (B) Tibal cut in primary TKR

2. In closed HTO, removal of wedge of bone results in deficient lateral tibial plateau for tibial bone cut in TKR.
3. In open wedge osteotomy, wedge of bone elevated results in extra native bone resection from medial tibial plateau during TKR results in implant seated on bone graft.

Anterior Tilting of Tibial Plateau

1. Osteotomy healed with anterior tilting of tibial plateau **(Figs 3.34A and B)**.
2. Considerable amount of bone cut from posterior aspect of tibial plateau.
3. Large space between femoral condyle and tibial plateau in 90° flexion.

Centralizing the Stem

1. Altered geometry of upper tibia.
2. Any offset and malrotation of osteotomy will create mismatch between articular surface of proximal tibia and tibial shaft which results in difficulty to center the implant **(Figs 3.35 and 3.36)**.
3. Medialization of tibial stem but >5 mm medialization of tibial component should be avoided due to high risk of subluxation or dislocation of patella.
4. Possibility of offset stem tibial tray should be kept where there is chance of excessive lateral placement of tibial stem **(Figs 3.37A to F)**. This should be planned in advance after templating.

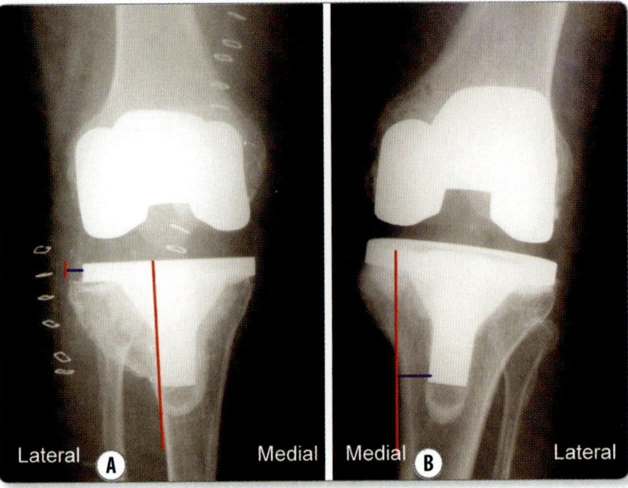

Figs 3.35A and B (A) Post HTO—Lateral placement of tibial stem even after medialization of tibial component; (B) Primary TKR central placement of stem

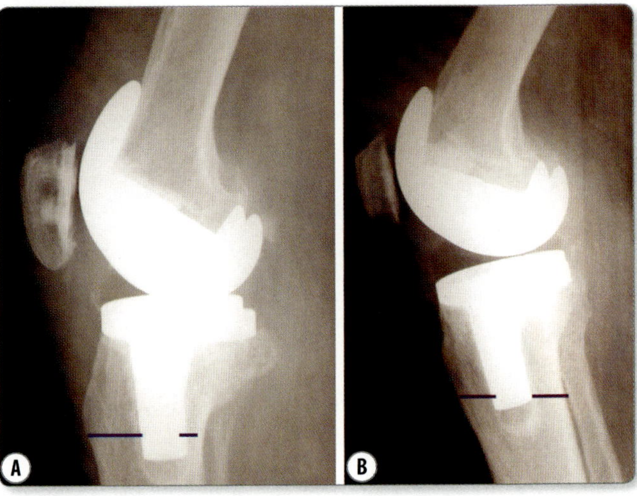

Figs 3.36A and B (A) Post HTO— Posterior placement of tibial stem; (B) Primary TKR central placement of tibial stem

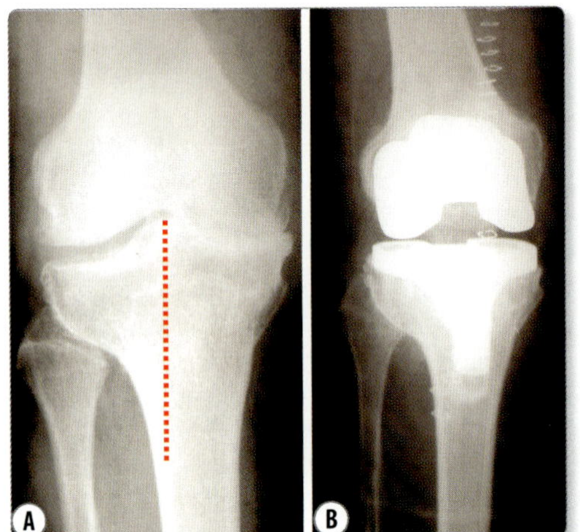

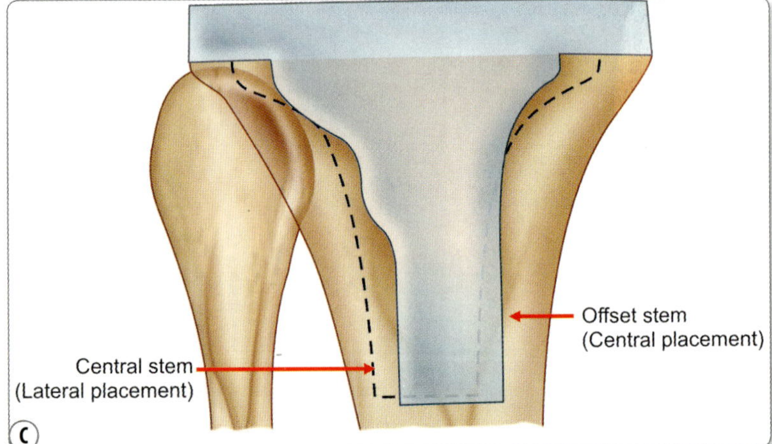

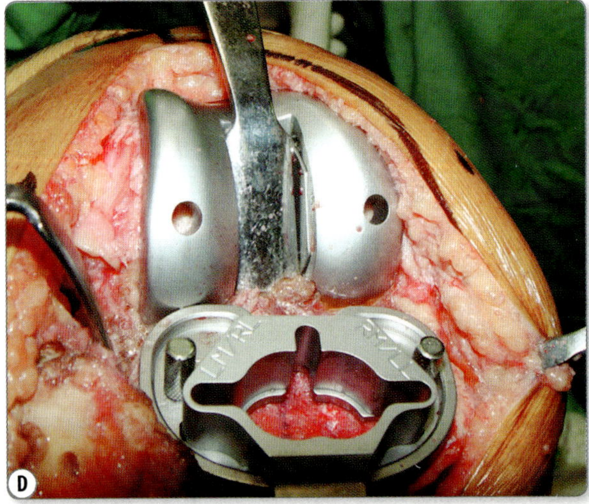

Figs 3.37A to D (A) Post HTO; (B) Offset stem; (C) Diagrammatic picture of central and offset stem in tibial flare following HTO; (D) Tibial preparation for offset stem

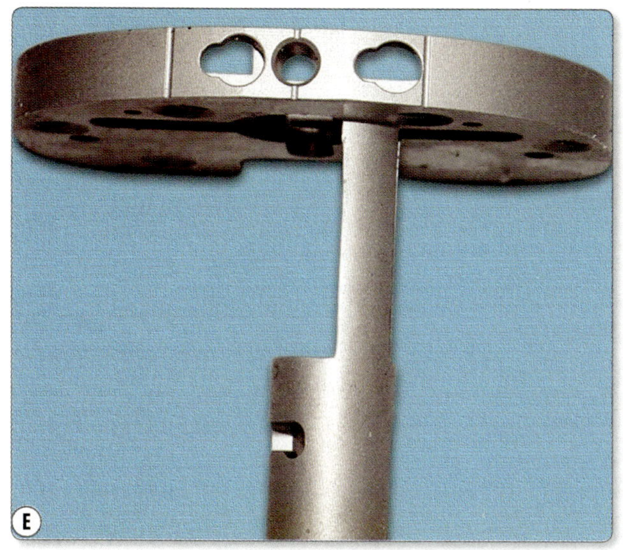
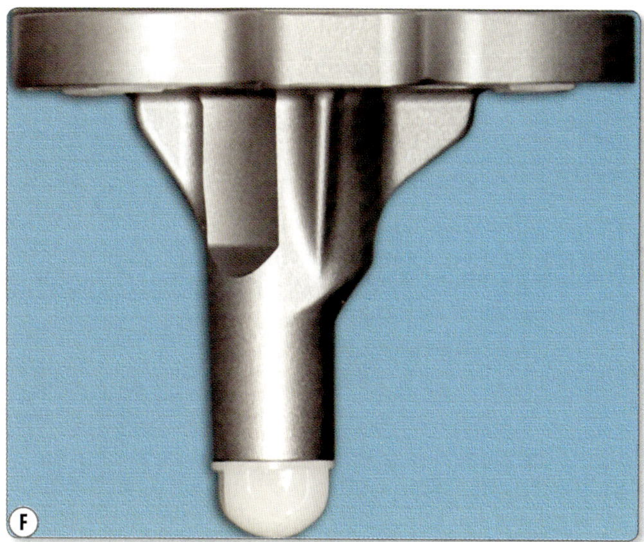

Figs 3.37E and F (E) Trial tibial tray with peg for offset stem (anterior aspect); (F) Offset stem modular plus tibial tray (posterior aspect)

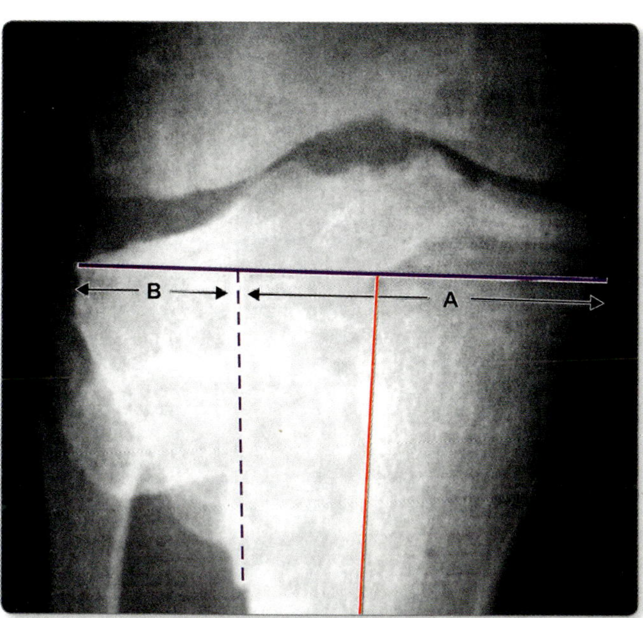

Fig. 3.38 Post-HTO with lateral flare

5. Tibial flare index: Draw a vertical line from the lateral tibial cortex up to the joint surface. Draw a horizontal line across the maximum width of the upper tibia.

$$\frac{\text{Lateral flare to medial tibial margin–A}}{\text{Lateral flare to lateral tibial margin–B}}$$

If the index is <2.5, anticipate difficulty in tibial tray placement and require a tibial tray with offset stem **(Fig. 3.38)**.

Non-union

1. Rare.
2. Long tibial stem is required.

Culture swab should be taken from osteotomy site to rule out possible subacute infection during TKR in cases of post HTO.

Important Points

Do Not Undermine the Skin

During midline skin incision, raise the skin flaps deep to the fascial layer to avoid skin necrosis.

Sequential Soft Tissue Release

Preliminary essential soft tissue release is being done on anteromedial and medial aspect of upper tibia in the beginning. Second time soft tissue release can be done while putting the spacer block between cut ends of femur and tibia if there is tightness in either medial or lateral side. Third time soft tissue releasc (posteromedial and posterior part of upper tibia) can be done when trial is being done with trial femoral and tibial component if there is tightness. Soft tissue release on the posterior surface of femoral condyle is being done in case of FFD.

Adequate soft tissue balance preserves bone stock and reduces cement bone interface stress which prevents early failure. A properly performed soft tissue release, which achieves balance between medial and lateral ligamentous structure and posterior capsule can provide stability to knee even in severe deformities.

1. *Soft tissue balance in varus deformity*: Stagewise soft tissue balance in varus deformity
   i. Generous dissection just below medial joint line.
   ii. Elevation of deep medial collateral ligament.
   iii. Removal of all osteophytes from entire margin of medial femoral condyle, medial and posteromedial margin of tibia.
   iv. Capsular release sub-periosteally from antero-medial and posteromedial margin of tibia.
   v. Release of semimembranosus from postero-medial aspect of joint.
   vi. Release of superficial medial collateral ligament.
   vii. Complete release of superficial medial collateral ligament and pes in severe cases.

   After each release, varus/valgus stability is examined. Care to be taken not to do over release. Under release of varus knee will be tight on medial side in extension. Over release will open on medial side.
2. *Soft tissue balance in valgus deformity*: Valgus deformity consists of bone loss from lateral condyle and lateral plateau tibia, lateral soft tissue contractures of IT band, lateral collateral ligament (LCL), popliteus tendon, posterolateral capsule and hamstrings. Medial collateral ligament (MCL) and capsule are elongated.

   Stage-wise soft tissue release in valgus knee:
   i. Removal of femoral and tibial osteophytes.
   ii. Iliotibial (IT) band (multiple puncture, i.e. pie-crusting of iliotibial band from inside out. Pie-crusting technique involves palpation of tight soft tissues followed by their selective release with multiple stabs of a BP blade No. 11).
   iii. Posterolateral capsule.
   iv. Popliteus.
   v. LCL (Lateral collateral ligament).
   vi. Gastrocnemius.
3. *Soft tissue release in flexion contracture of knee*:
   i. PCL detached from inter-condylar notch of femur.
   ii. Sub-periosteal release of posterior capsule from medial and lateral femoral condyle.
   iii. In severe cases, gastrocnemius release.

In varus deformity, the soft tissues on medial side are contracted which require stage-wise release **(Figs 3.39A and D)**. In valgus deformity, the soft tissues on lateral side are contracted which require stage-wise release **(Figs 3.39B and E)**. In subluxated knee, both medial and lateral collateral ligaments are elongated. So do only essential soft tissue release **(Figs 3.39C and F)**. Thicker plastic insert is usually required in cases of subluxated knee.

Balancing Flexion and Extension Gaps

Where there is preoperative deformity and contracture, imbalance of flexion and extension gaps may be present.

1. *Residual tightness in extension only*: When there is restriction in extension but not in flexion, additional bone is removed from the distal femur. This affects the extension gap but not the flexion gap. When contracture persists following appropriate retinacular release, removal of posterior osteophytes and scar tissues, depending on severity, removal of an additional 2–4 mm of distal femur is indicated. For this, the Steinmann pins are re-applied to their original position in the anterior femur and the distal cutting block returned to the pins using the holes designated +2. The distal cut is accordingly revised. Chamfer cuts are subsequently revised by open chamfer to maintain the correct configuration but A/P cuts are not revised. This affects ligamentous tension but not in flexion.
2. *Residual tightness in flexion and extension both*: A thinner tibial insert or additional tibial resection is indicated, as either will affect flexion and extension gaps. When resection is selected, 2 mm of proximal tibia is removed. For this, the Steinmann pins are re-applied to their drill holes in the anterior tibial cortex and the tibial cutting block returned to the pins using the holes designated +2. The cut is accordingly revised.
3. *Residual tightness in flexion only*: Residual posterior osteophytes, soft tissue and loose bodies may be factor and must be addressed. In the rare cases where tension persists following appropriate correction, 5° of additional posterior slope may be indicated. For this, the pins are re-applied to their holes in the anterior cortex of tibia and the 5° tibial cutting block positioned using the holes designated square. Final slope should not exceed 7°. Alternatively, tightness in flexion may be corrected by downsizing the femoral component, but there should not be anterior notching. The pins are re-applied to the distal femoral surface, the designated cutting block positioned and the cuts revised. As an additional posterior condyle is resected, flexion gap is increased. Alternatively, anteroposterior adjustment of the rod of tibial alignment device also allows the amount of posterior slope to be adjusted apart from the designed slope in the proximal tibial cutting jig. By moving the rod anteriorly about 5 mm at the ankle, 1° of posterior slope is increased at the proximal tibial jig.

Posterior Tibial Slope

Usually take 3° posterior sloped tibial cutting block for tibial cut but there are three circumstances in which posterior slope should not be applied. One is the severe flexion contracture. Every degree of posterior slope is building in a degree of flexion contracture. Therefore, posterior slope is not applied to relieve a severe flexion

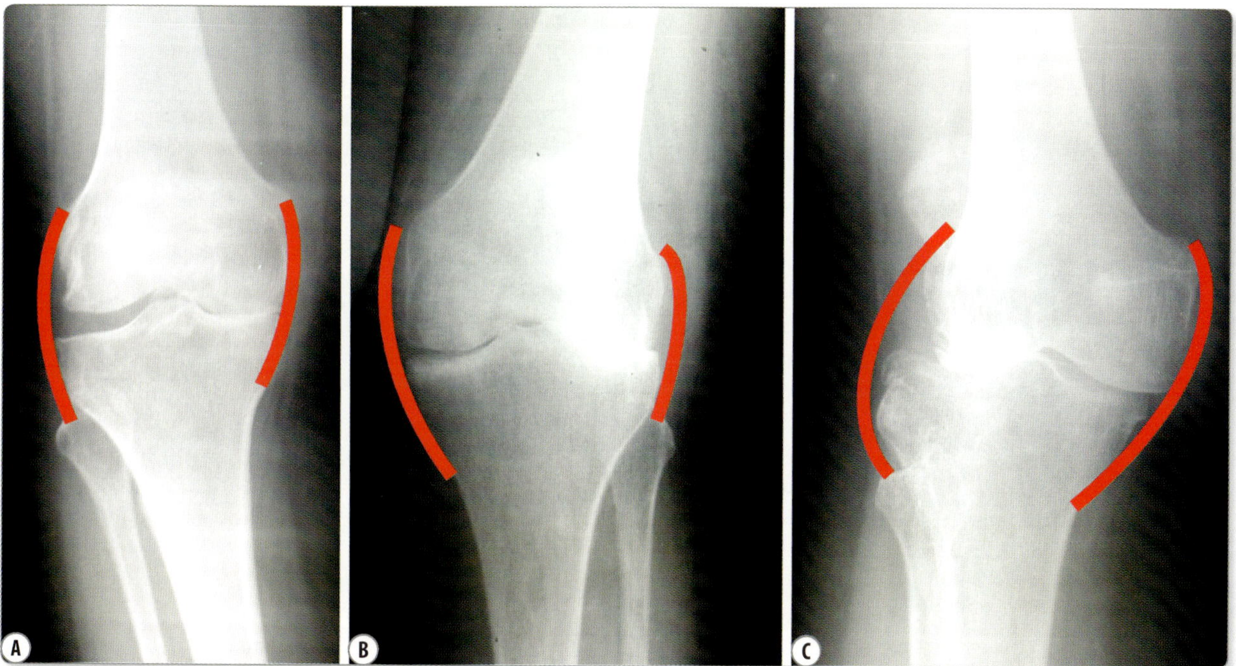

Figs 3.39A to C (A) Varus knee (contracted medially); (B) Valgus knee (contracted laterally); (C) Subluxated knee (elongated both medially and laterally)

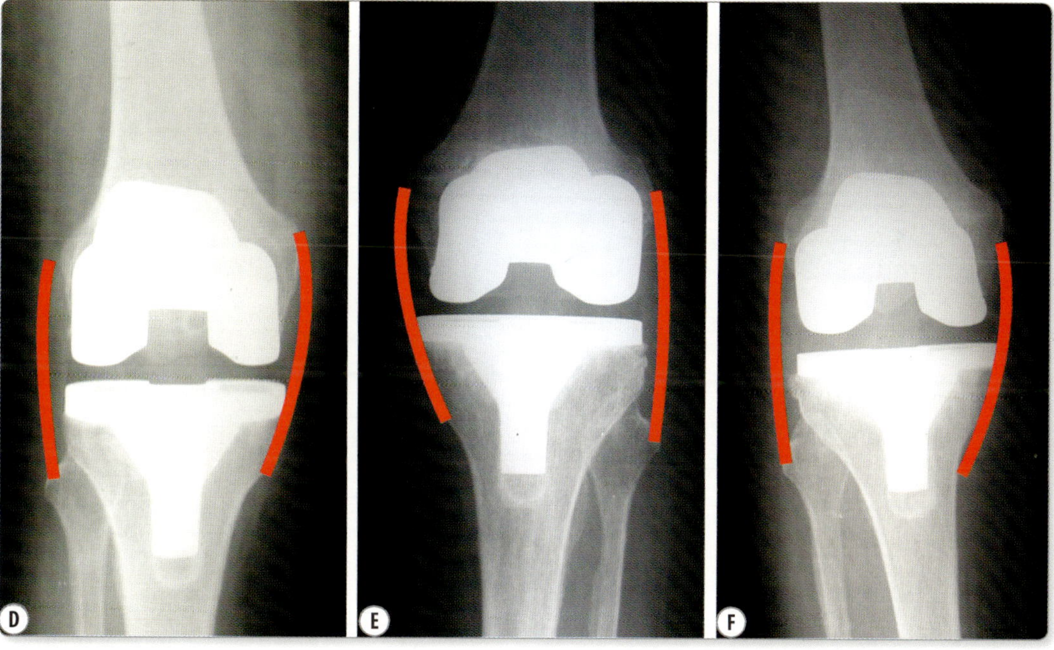

Figs 3.39 D to F Properly performed soft tissue release achieves adequate soft tissue balance after TKR in varus, valgus and subluxated knees

contracture. Second is the distorted tibial joint line. Post-osteotomy is the most frequent situation in which the tibial joint line slopes up instead of normally down. In that case, it is easier to balance the knee by not giving posterior slope. The third situation is with posterior stabilized component in which most system does not allow hyperextension of the articulating surfaces beyond 8–10°. Excessive posterior slope will increase the potential for tibial post impinging against the femoral housing in extension.

3° External Rotation

Upper surface of tibia has 3° varus slope **(Fig. 3.40)**. So ideally the tibial cut should be done at 87° to the mechanical axis of tibia **(Fig. 3.41)**. But tibial cutting at 87° is very difficult as one may cut more tibia. So chance of error in cutting tibia at 87° is very high. It has been demonstrated that tibial component placed in more than 5° of varus tend to fail by subsiding into more varus **(Figs 3.44 and 3.45)**. To avoid this error, we cut the tibia at 90° to the mechanical axis of tibia and this 3° varus slope of tibia is compensated by 3° externally rotating the AP cutting block of femur and cutting more posterior part of medial condyle of femur and creating rectangular space at 90° flexion of tibia (i.e. rectangular flexion gap) **(Fig. 3.42)**. If 3° external rotation of AP cutting block is not done then the space between femur and tibia at 90° flexion will be trapezoidal (i.e. trapezoidal flexion gap) which will lead to tight medial collateral ligament and lax lateral collateral ligament on flexion of knee at 90° **(Fig. 3.43)**.

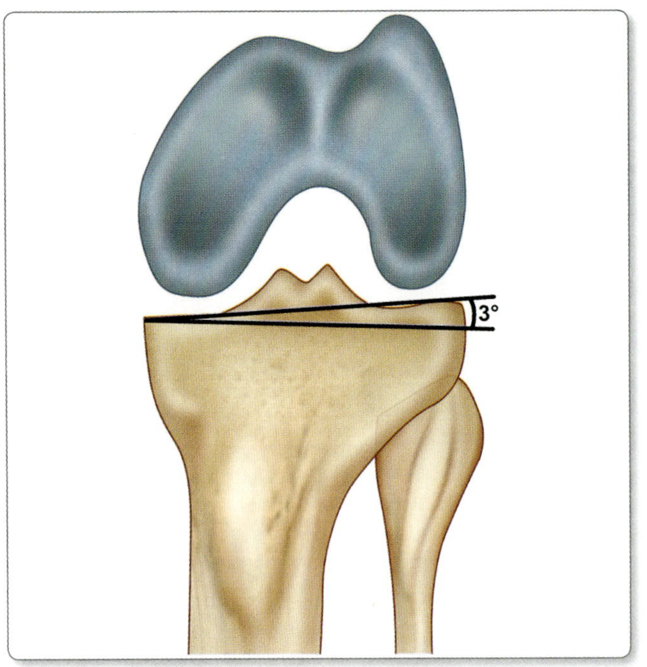

Fig. 3.40 Diagrammatic picture showing 3 degree varus slope of upper surface of tibia

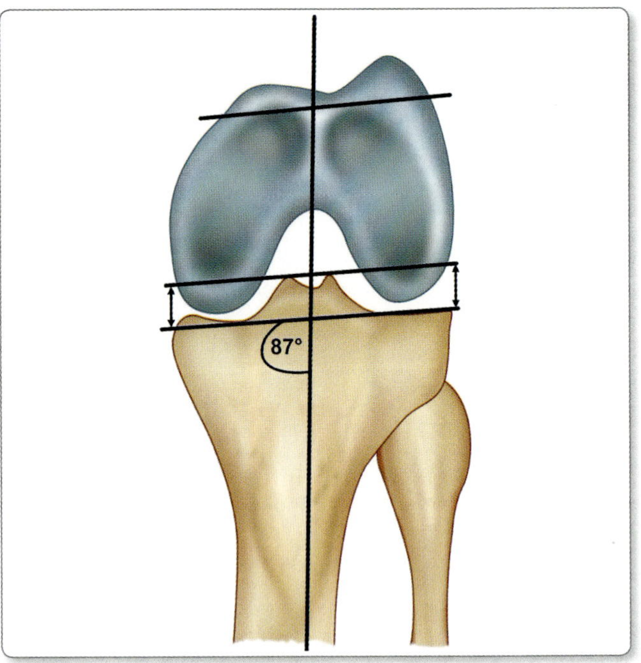

Fig. 3.41 Diagrammatic picture showing rectangular flexion gap if the tibial cut is done at 87° to the mechanical axis of tibia and posterior cut in neutral rotation but cutting the tibia at 87° is difficult and error in cutting is very high

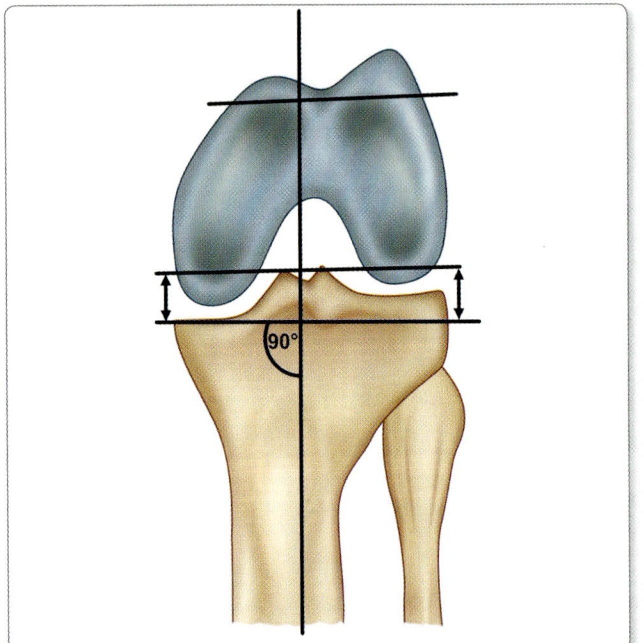

Fig. 3.42 Diagrammatic picture showing rectangular flexion gap if the tibial cut is at 90° to the mechanical axis of tibia and posterior cut in 3° external rotation

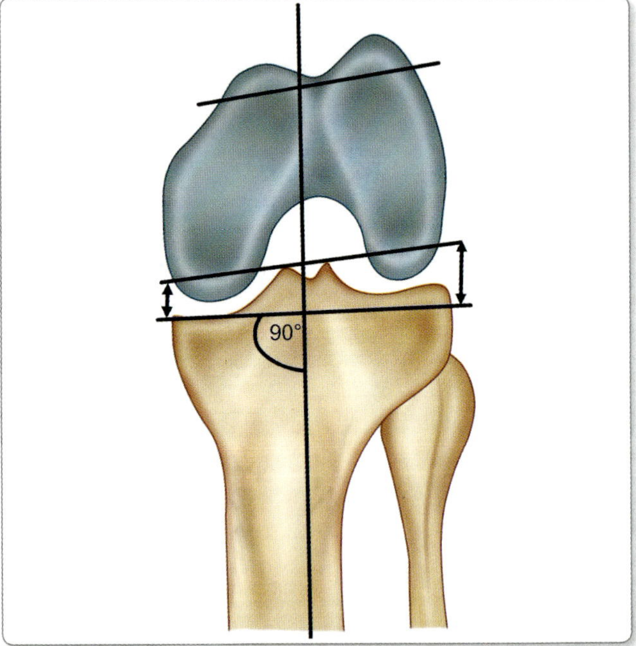

Fig. 3.43 Diagrammatic picture showing trapezoidal flexion gap if the tibial cut is done at 90° to the mechanical axis of tibia and posterior cut is not done in 3° external rotation (tight medial collateral ligament and lax lateral collateral ligament on flexion of knee at 90°)

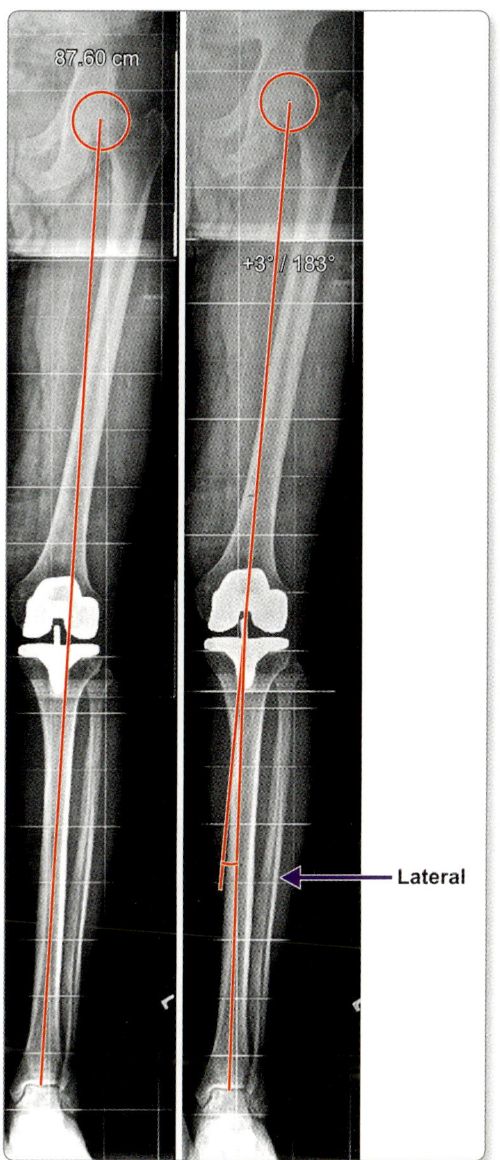

Fig. 3.44 Left knee—3° valgus (perpendicular cut of tibia) normal alignment

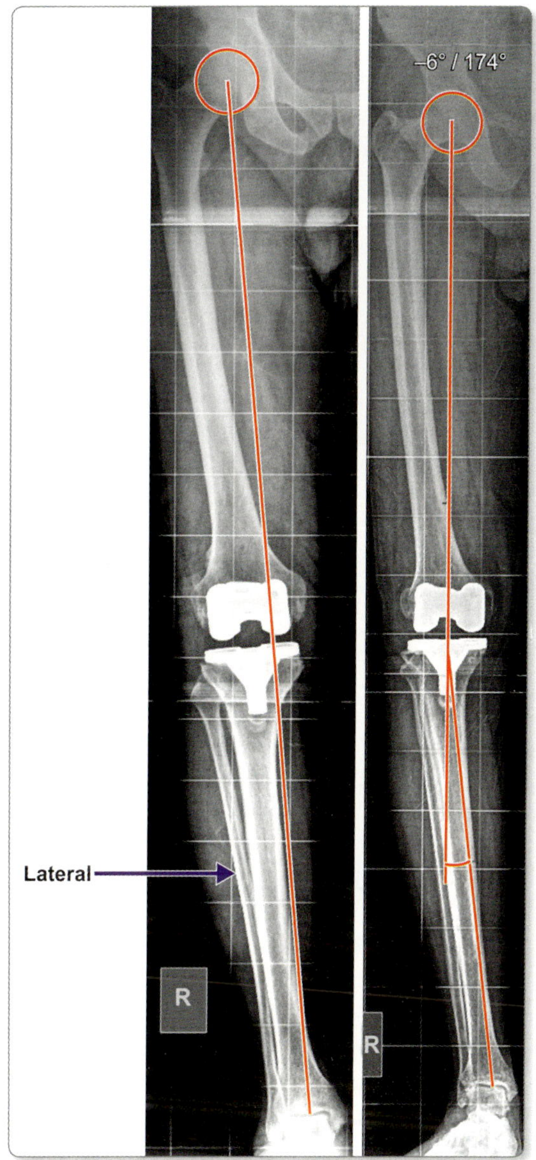

Fig. 3.45 Right knee—6° varus (varus cut of tibia—tends to fail) malalignment

Downsizing Versus Upsizing the Femoral Component

When the femur measures between two sizes, a decision needs to be made whether to "up-size" or "down-size" the femoral component. If the decision is made to downsize, the drill guide is set to lower size, and a lower size A/P cutting block is used. The anterior cut remains constant and more bone will be resected from the posterior condyles. If the decision is made to upsize, the drill guide needs to be set to higher size, and a higher size A/P cutting block is used. The anterior cut will remain constant, but less bone is removed from the posterior condyles. In both cases, the under or over resection of the posterior condyles will affect the flexion gap, and therefore, care must be taken to ensure that the flexion/extension gap is correctly balanced. Undersizing of the femoral component will create looseness in flexion and possible notching of the femoral cortex. Oversizing will create tightness in flexion and increased excursion of the quadriceps mechanism.

Important Points for TKR in FFD >20 Degree

1. Try to minimize the FFD preoperative by vigorous physiotherapy, passive stretching by use of knee brace and if required by traction and serial casting.
2. Resect the femur 11 mm in place of 9 mm. This will slightly increase the extension gap.

3. Remove posterior osteophytes as much as possible but take care of vessels lying nearby.
4. Do posterior release.
5. Lastly if not correcting the FFD, then resect tibia 2 mm more. This will slightly increase both flexion and extension gap.
6. Dedicated physiotherapy and use of knee brace postoperatively.

Avoid Elevating or Lowering Joint Line

Elevated joint line (>8 mm) leads to motion problems

1. Midflexion instability.
2. Patellofemoral tracking problems—increased stress over the patellofemoral joint.
3. Patella baja.

Lowered joint line leads to:

1. Lack of full extension.
2. Flexion instability.

Patellofemoral Alignment

Q angle: It is the angle between axis of extensor mechanism (ASIS to center of patella) and axis of patellar tendon (center of patella to tibial tuberosity). The normal Q angle is 7 degree for better patellar tracking **(Figs 3.46 and 3.47)**. Any increase in the Q angle will lead to increased lateral subluxation forces on the patella relative to the trochlear groove which can lead to pain and mechanical symptoms, accelerated wear, and even dislocation. It is critical to avoid techniques that lead to increased Q angle. Common errors include:

1. Internal rotation of the femoral component
2. Medialization of the femoral component
3. Internal rotation of the tibial tray
4. Placing the patellar implant laterally on the patella.

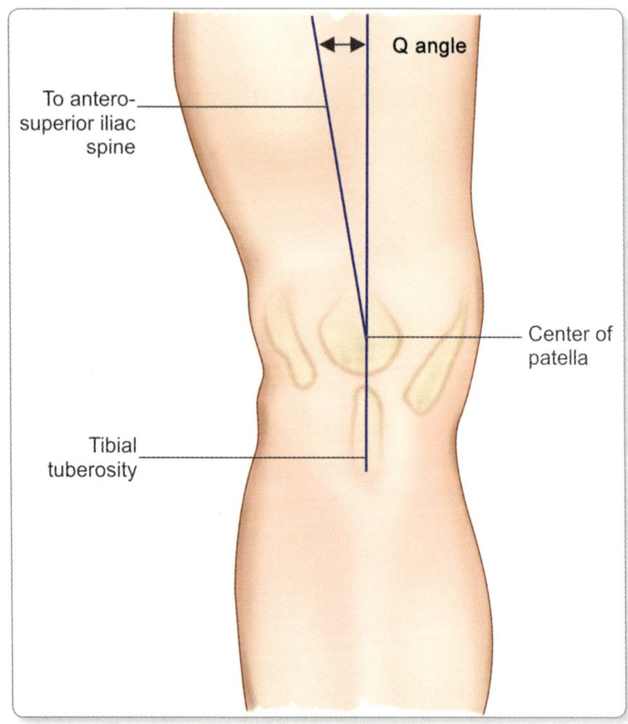

Fig. 3.46 Q angle

Check Variations

After exposure of the knee, look for variation in tibial condyle, femoral condyle and patella which, sometimes, may not be appreciated on preoperative X-ray of the knee. Deficiency in either condyle or patella may require proper adjustment of the guide, cutting block and the implants. For example, in deficient posterior part of either condyle or femur, the skid of femoral sizing guide will not sit against the deficient posterior condyle or sit in excessive rotation and hence the guide is adjusted in such a way that it lies perpendicular to the mechanical axis of the tibia. So the appreciation of variation is helpful to avoid the errors in cutting **(Fig. 3.48)**.

Two Packets Cement (CMW 1–40 g and 20 g)

Advantages:

1. Surgeon is more comfortable as there is no hurry for early setting of cement.
2. Two packets of cement are sufficient for bigger size knee while one packet may be less.

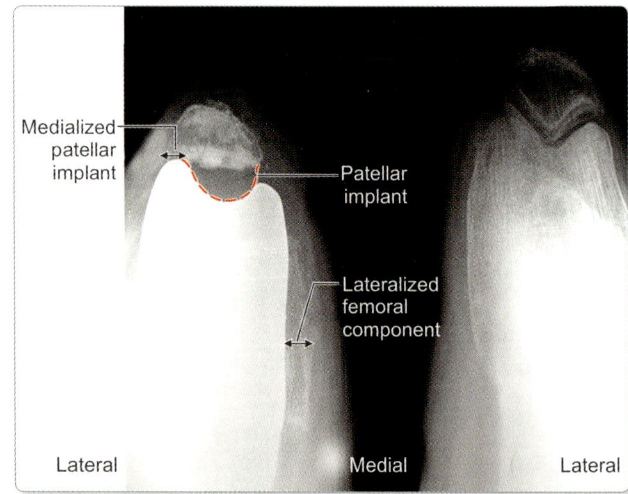

Fig. 3.47 Skyline view showing excellent patellar tracking when femoral component is lateralized and patellar implant is medialized (compare from nonoperated knee)

3. With two packets cement, the tibial component is pressurized against fixed femoral component hence there is no chance of tilting of component while pressurization. With one packet cement while pressurizing the femoral and tibial component against each other simultaneously, there may be tilt of component in cases of osteoporosed bone and rheumatoid arthritis cases.

One Packet Cement (CMW 1–40 g)

After gaining experience, one can do the cementing with one packet of 40 g bone cement especially in cases of osteoarthritis with good bone stock. The femoral and tibial components are pressurized against each other. The bone cement should be brought out from the refrigerator just before starting the cementing to avoid early setting.

Miscellaneous Points

1. Equal size tibial tray and femoral component are used but one size up or down tibial and femoral component can be used, e.g. size 2.5 tibial tray can be used with size 2 or size 3 femoral component and vise versa.
2. Lateralize the femoral component and medialize the patella for better patellar tracking.
3. Switch off the fan while cementing. This will avoid the change of cement setting time.
4. Don't talk while mixing the cement and implanting the components. This will avoid the distraction of mind and possibility of error.
5. Do not invert the skin while suturing it. This will avoid the non-healing of wound and bad scar.
6. Don't use tourniquet in cases whose preoperative X-rays show vessel calcification.
7. Must have minimum **two different sets** of saw system, e.g. pneumatic, electric or battery operated to avoid inconvenience if one system fails during surgery.

Precautions to Prevent Peroperative Complications

1. Always have a look over the insertion of patellar ligament while everting and retracting the patella to avoid avulsion. If patellar ligament is tight, fix it with a pin.
2. Avoid notching of anterior cortex of femur. Must check before cutting that AP and chamfer cutting block is placed properly and not upside down.
3. Always check with visualization guide before each cut.
4. Be careful while box cutting in smaller femur.
5. In short statured patient, keep 1.5 size implants also and size 5 in tall patient. Common sizes are 2, 2.5, 3 and 4.
6. In Indian patients, the anteroposterior diameter of lower end of femur is less than the mediolateral diameter and hence may affect the sizing of tibial and femoral components. Anteroposterior diameter of lower end of femur determines the size of femoral component.
7. In smaller femur, be careful while passing pins in AP and chamfer cutting guide and box cutting guide. It is better to drill with 2.5 mm drill before passing the pins to avoid avulsion of lateral or medial epicondyles.

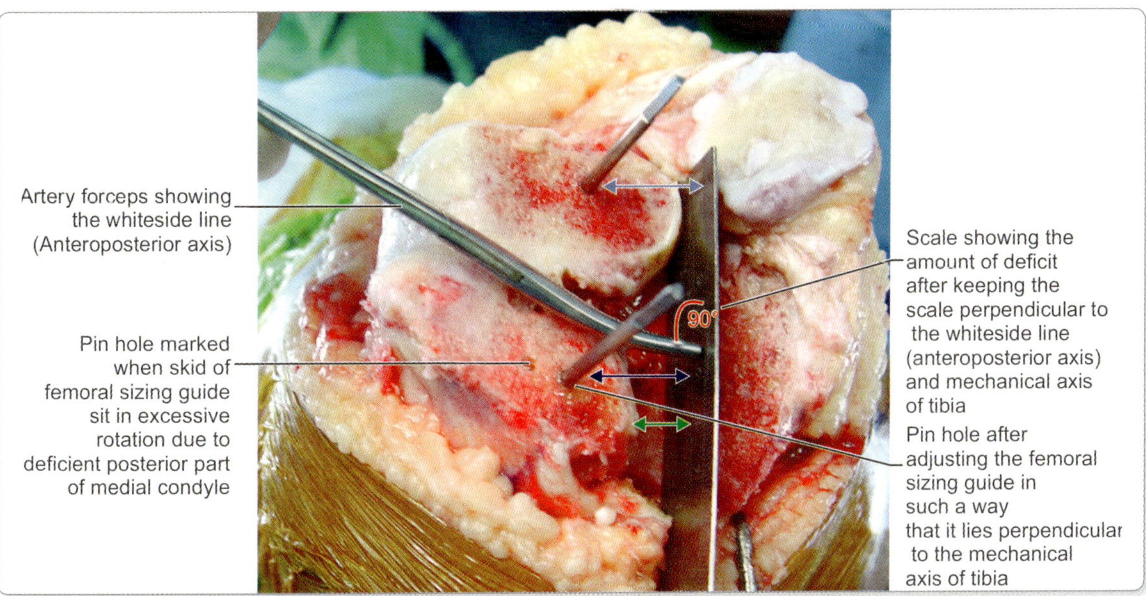

Fig. 3.48 Deficient posterior part of medial condyle (green line) where proper adjustment of femoral sizing guide avoids excessive removal of bone from deficient medial condyle

8. Box cut must be proper and adequate. First cut with saw then with osteotome to avoid splinter of femoral condyles. Fine tuning should be done by bone file and nibbler before putting the trial femoral component box assembly. The trial femoral component box assembly should be applied first with pressure of palm then with femoral punch and gentle hammer to avoid splintering of femoral condyles.
9. Use saw and osteotome for widening during upper tibial preparation before broaching to avoid shattering of upper tibia.
10. While cementing and pressurization of the components, keeping the knee in extension, apply controlled force to avoid supracondylar fracture especially in osteoporosed bone and rheumatoid arthritis cases.
11. While cementing, take care that appropriate size and side of femoral component is being applied without posterior tilt and the tibial tray in proper orientation.

Avoid Silly Mistakes

Never put wrong femoral component (i.e. putting right femoral component on left femur or vice versa). This silly mistake can be avoided by:

1. Be sure that the decided knee is being operated.
2. Keep the femoral component of the same side only.
3. The operating surgeon must see the packet of femoral component before opening and make sure that the same side femoral component is being opened.
4. Do not be in hurry while performing such type of special surgery where mistakes and errors are not acceptable.

Contraindications of TKR

1. Acute infection in joint or elsewhere in body.
2. Neuropathic arthropathy.
3. Severe deformity which is away from knee joint due to old fracture, bowing of bones.
4. Nonfunctioning muscles acting on joint.
5. Painless ankylosis.
6. Very poor bone stock.
7. Non-compliant patients.
8. Low socioeconomic conditions.

Ideal Indicated Patient for Successful TKR

1. Demand of the patient.
2. Understanding risk-benefit ratio.
3. Shared decision making.
4. Acceptance of postoperative follow-up protocol.

Complications

1. Thromboembolism
2. Infection
3. Patellofemoral complications: Patellofemoral instability, patellar fracture, patellar component failure, patellar component loosening, patellar clunk syndrome and extension mechanism tendon rupture.
4. Neurovascular complications: Arterial compromise (rare), peroneal nerve palsy.
5. Periprosthetic fractures.
6. Polyethylene wear.
7. Arthrofibrosis.
8. Aseptic loosening.
9. Flexion instability: This is a sense of instability without giving way, recurrent knee effusions, multiple areas of soft tissue tenderness about the knee and substantial anterior tibial translation at 90 degrees of flexion. The revision operation focused on balancing the flexion and extension gaps while taking care to fill the enlarged flexion gap. This may occur due to error in tibial cut, malrotation of femur, excessive ligament release, MCL rupture, flexion-extension mismatch in flexion contracture, thin poly syndrome and Next size syndrome.
10. Joint jack phenomenon: Correction of varus/valgus deformity via soft tissue balancing is the accepted technique in knee arthroplasty surgery. However, in rare instances, excessive ligamentotaxis can result in overly stretched periarticular structures leading to pain and impaired function. This has been called the "joint jack phenomenon." A very thick polyethylene insert will result in a painful knee and leg length discrepancy. Solution is to use a salvage hinge knee arthroplasty to achieve joint space reduction, restore equal leg lengths, and avoid global instability.

Implants and Cement Required for Primary TKR (Fig. 3.49)

1. Cruciate substituting femoral component—right and left
   (M/L—Mediolateral, AP—Anteroposterior)
   Size—1.5 (57 mm M/L, 53 mm AP)
   2 (60 mm M/L, 56 mm AP)
   2.5 (63 mm M/L, 59 mm AP)
   3 (66 mm M/L, 61 mm AP)
   4 (71 mm M/L, 65 mm AP)
   5 (73 mm M/L, 69 mm AP)

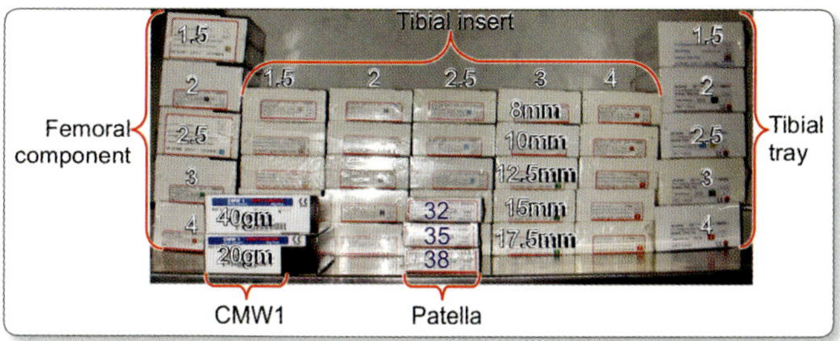

Fig. 3.49 Stock of implants and bone cement usually required during primary TKR

2. Modular tibial tray, (modular plus tibial tray if wedge has to be used and offset stem modular plus tibial tray in post HTO tibial flare, RM/LL and LM/RL)
   RM/LL—Right medial/Left lateral
   LM/RL—Left medial/Right lateral
   Size—1.5 (61 mm M/L, 41 mm AP)
   2 (64 mm M/L, 43 mm AP)
   2.5 (67 mm M/L, 45 mm AP)
   3 (71 mm M/L, 47 mm AP)
   4 (76 mm M/L, 51 mm AP)
   5 (83 mm M/L, 55 mm AP).
3. Stabilized tibial insert
   Size— 1.5, 2, 2.5, 3, 4, 5
   Thickness: 8 mm, 10 mm, 12.5 mm, 15 mm, 17.5 mm
4. Oval dome patella
   Size—32 mm (8 mm thick), 35 mm (8.5 mm thick), 38 mm (9 mm thick) and 41 mm (11.5 mm thick).
5. CMW1 gentamicin—40 g and 20 g.

Knee Implants

Femoral component and tibial tray are made up of Co-Cr-Mo alloy. The femoral components are available in right and left configuration. The components have a grit blasted finish of entire fixation surfaces to provide for enhanced cement fixation.

The tibial insert and patellar implant are made up of ultrahigh molecular weight polyethylene (UHMWPE). A new cobalt-chrome (CoCr) tibial tray and moderately cross-linked tibial insert have been added to the PFC sigma modular knee system. The cobalt-chrome alloy modular tibial tray is having the 12 locking mechanism and moderately cross-linked polyethylene further reduces the potential for polyethylene wear. Improvements in the locking mechanism of modular tibial components minimize the relative motion and thus reduces all forms of backside wear.

Summary of TKR (Steps in Sequence)

1. Midline skin incision and medial para patellar approach.
2. Sequential soft tissue release.
3. Removal of osteophytes, infrapatellar fat pad, medial meniscus, lateral meniscus, ACL, PCL, supracondylar synovectomy and release of patellofemoral plicae.
4. Tibial cut perpendicular to tibial axis (0 mm on more involved condyle or 8 mm or maximum 10 mm on less involved condyle) with usually 3° posterior sloped tibial cutting blocks.
5. Femoral cuts (7° valgus, 9 mm thickness, 3° external rotation)—6 cuts
   i Distal cut.
   ii. Anterior cut.
   iii. Posterior cut.
   iv. Anterior chamfer cut.
   v. Posterior chamfer cut.
   vi. Box cut (in lateralized position).
6. Rectangular and equal flexion—extension gap.
7. Resurfacing of patella and drilling for 3-pegs of patellar implant in superiorly and medialized position.
8. Tibial preparation in 3 degree external rotation (appropriate size drilling, widening with saw and osteotome, broaching).
9. Wash with gentamicin mixed normal saline by pulse lavage.
10. Cementing of patella, femoral component and tibial tray in sequence.
11. Apply appropriate size and thickness of tibial insert, reduce and extend the knee.
12. Apply two drains and suture the wound in layers.

Instruments Required for TKR (Figs 3.50 to 3.54)

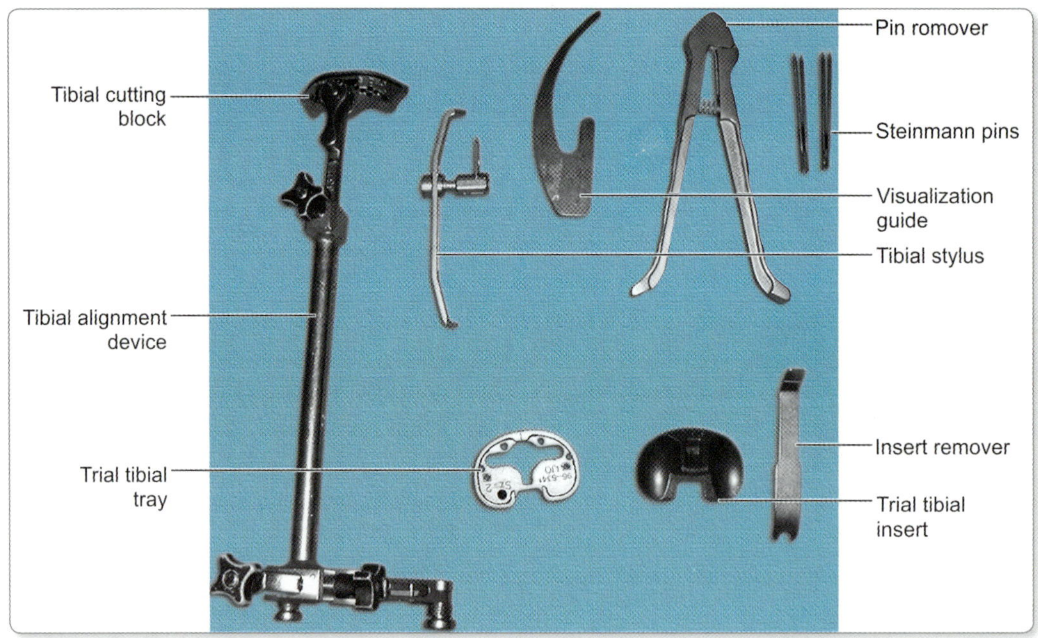

Fig. 3.50 Instruments required for tibial cutting and sizing, insert and insert remover

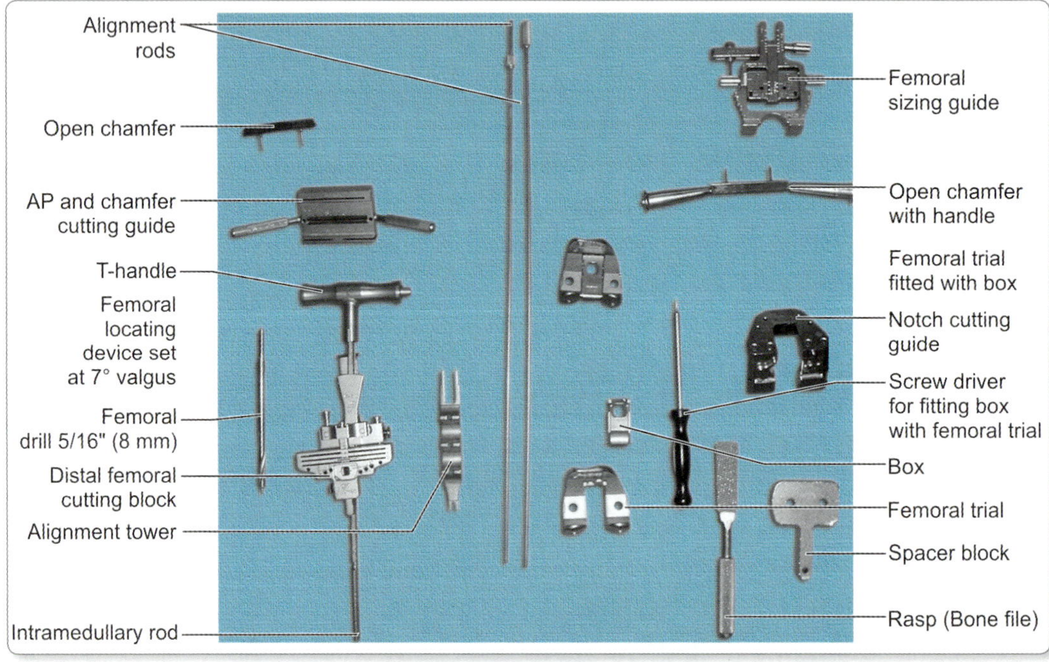

Fig. 3.51 Instruments required for femoral cutting

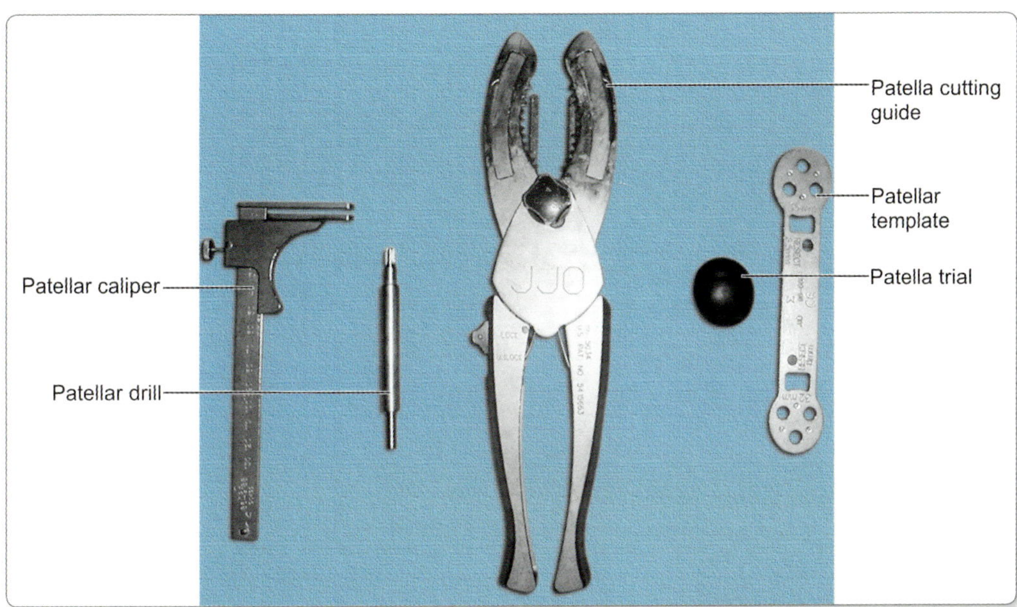

Fig. 3.52 Instruments required for patellar resurfacing

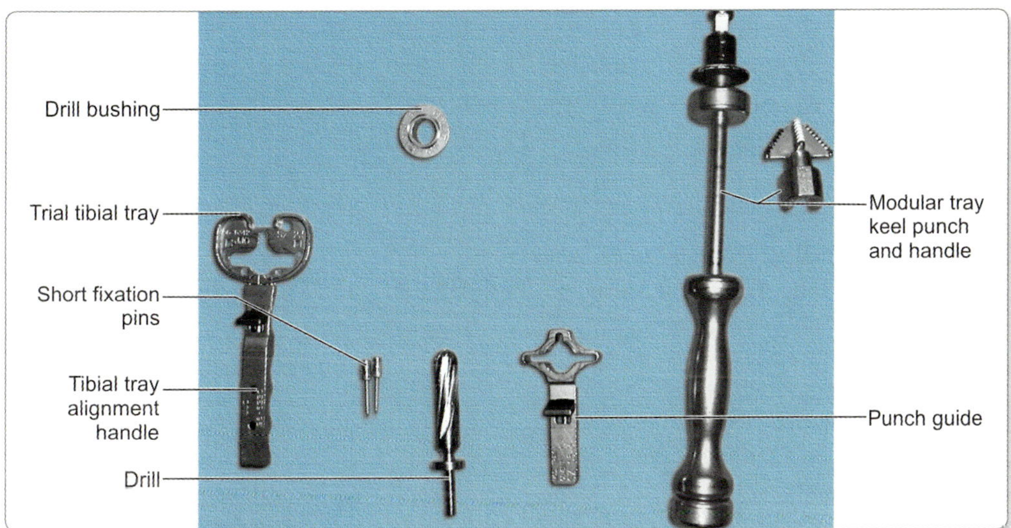

Fig. 3.53 Instruments required for tibial preparation

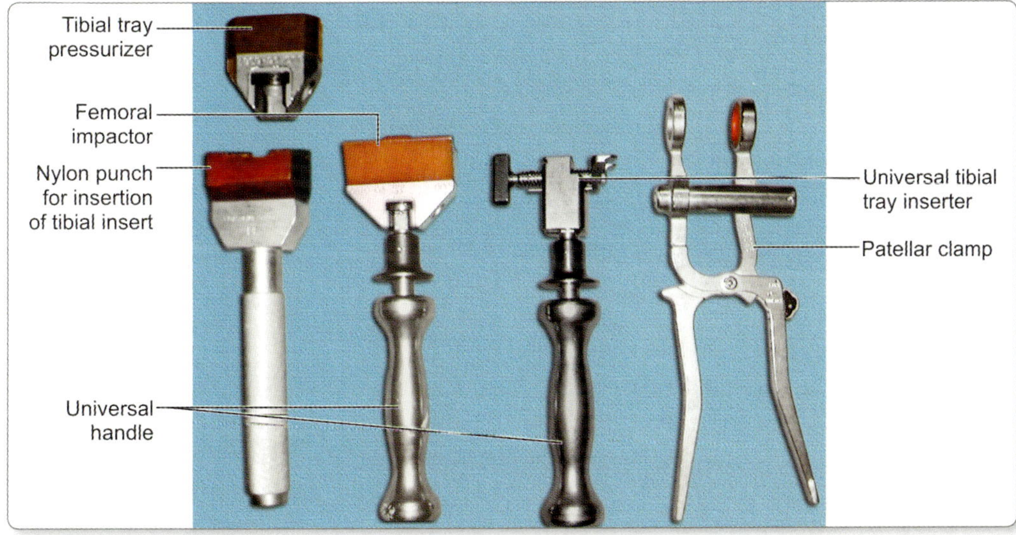

Fig. 3.54 Instruments required for cementing and insertion of tibial insert

Rotating Platform High Flexed TKR

4 CHAPTER

CHAPTER OUTLINE

- Fixed Bearing Versus Mobile Bearing TKR (RPF)
- Instruments Required for RPF TKR
- Fundamental of TKR

Fixed Bearing Versus Mobile Bearing TKR (RPF)

Rotating platform high flexion (RPF) TKR differs from fixed bearing TKR on the following technical points:

1. *Tibial cut*: It is done with **0° tibial cutting block** and tibial stylus set at **10 mm on less affected condyle.** Cutting is done in the same way as described for fixed bearing TKR. Put the MBT (mobile bearing tibial) tray trial over the upper surface of resected tibia and determine the size of the tibial tray. It should rest on the cortex. It should not overhang, otherwise it will cause friction to the collateral ligaments and it should not be undersized otherwise it will sink.
2. *Femoral cuts*: Distal, anterior, posterior, and chamfer cuts are same and cut with the same guides and oscillating saw blade (1.25 mm thick saw blade, No. 519.115) as described for fixed bearing TKR.

After the distal cut, place the base block with insert tightness shim of appropriate thickness over the cut surface of tibia and extend the knee and check the extension gap. After the anterior, posterior and chamfer cuts, check the flexion gap with base block, the insert tightness shim along with flexion adapter shim at 90° of flexion.

Notch cutting and extra 2 to 4 mm posterior cut of femoral condyles is done with different notch cutting guide (**RPF femoral cutting guide**). It has smaller notch. 2 mm to 4 mm extraposterior cut supposed to provide high flexion of knee.

For cutting the notch and extra posterior cut, apply the RPF femoral cutting guide on the prepared femur (i.e. after cutting the distal, anterior, posterior and chamfer cuts) in such a way that the lateral flange of the guide coincide with lateral margin of the femur and check the cutting line for the posterior cut. Fix it by four Steinmann pins, 1st in superolateral hole, 2nd in inferomedial, 3rd in superomedial and 4th in inferolateral (i.e. contralateral) to avoid rotation or tilt of cutting guide. Cut the notch first with reciprocating or oscillating saw (0.9 mm thick saw blade, No. 519.107) then with osteotome. Do fine tuning with bone file and small nibbler. Notch cut must be adequate. Perform the extraposterior cut with the oscillating saw (0.9 mm thick saw blade, No. 519.107) through the slot attached with RPF femoral cutting guide. Remove the Steinmann pins by pin puller. Remove the femoral notch cutting guide.

Apply the appropriate size femoral trial and see that it is flushed well. Apply medium Hohmann on the posterior aspect of upper tibia and dislocate it anteriorly. Apply one small Hohmann on lateral aspect to retract the everted patella and one on medial aspect to retract the medial collateral ligament. Apply the tibial tray alignment handle with appropriate size MBT tray trial and put it on the resected tibial surface. Apply the lock off evaluation bullet into the cut-out of the MBT tray trial. Put 10 mm thick appropriate size RPF tibial insert trial (according to the size of femoral trial) onto the MBT tray trial. Remove the Hohmann. Reduce the knee and extend it. For reduction, one assistant will hold the ankle and other will lift the thigh. The surgeon will hold the alignment handle with MBT tray trial with trial insert and push it posteriorly and downward and simultaneously extend the knee. The tray trial will take its position according to kinematics of the knee **(trial reduction in nonrotation mode)**. Some adjustment of tibial tray can be done by using the alignment handle to rotate the tray and tibial insert into congruency with the femoral trial with knee in full extension. The rotation of the tibial tray is usually centered on the junction between the medial and central one-third of the tibial tubercle. Check the mediolateral stability both in extension and flexion. Determine the thickness of the tibial insert which allow mediolateral and anteroposterior stability and full extension of the knee. Check the overall alignment in anteroposterior and mediolateral plane. Mark by electrocautery over the anterior aspect of upper tibia in center and on medial according to the marks on the center of tibial tray alignment handle and tray trial respectively. The amount of rotation of tibial insert can be checked by replacing the lock off evaluation bullet with pinned evaluation bullet into the cut-out of the MBT tray trial and tap down lightly to secure the tray to the proximal tibia. Apply the tibial insert trial and do the movement and check the movements of tibial insert **(trial reduction in free-rotation mode)**. Excessive malrotation of the tibial tray relative to the femoral component can result in insert overhang and impingement with soft tissues.

1. **Patellar resurfacing** is same as fixed bearing TKR. Apply the patellar implant and check the patellar tracking. Remove the patellar implant.
2. **Tibial preparation** is different. There are separate drill and broach for MBT tray. Flex the knee fully. Assistant will lift the thigh. Remove the tibial insert trial by bone hook after applying it in the hole on the top of tibial insert trial. Remove the MBT tray trial and evaluation bullet. Apply the medium Hohmann on the posterior aspect of upper tibia to dislocate it anteriorly and small Hohmann on lateral aspect to retract the everted patella and on medial aspect to retract the medial collateral ligament. Connect the tibial tray alignment handle with MBT tray trial and put over the resected surface of upper tibia as per electrocautery marks after assessing the overall tibial coverage. Fix the tray trial with two fixation pins inserted through the recessed holes. Remove the tibial alignment handle. Seat the MBT drill bushing into the tibial tray trial by lightly taping the top of the drill bushing. Assemble the drill stop onto the MBT drill and position at the selected tray size. Advance the drill through the drill bushing into the cancellous bone until it hits the drill stop. Remove the drill. Assemble the punch bushing impactor/extractor with MBT keel punch bushing. Hold the handle of punch bushing impactor/extractor and insert the MBT keel punch bushing into the MBT tibial tray trial. Lightly tap with hammer over the top of punch bushing impactor/extractor till the superior surface of punch bushing is flushed with superior surface of the tibial tray trial. Remove the punch bushing impactor/extractor. Use oscillating saw and osteotome to widen the keel slot in sclerotic bone of upper tibia to avoid shattering during broaching. Assemble the universal handle to the appropriately sized MBT keel punch and insert it into the MBT punch bushing by hammering over the top of universal handle till the shoulder of punch is in even contact with the MBT punch bushing. Disconnect the universal handle, leaving the MBT keel punch in place. Remove the two fixation pins. Apply the appropriate size and thickness of RPF trial tibial insert according to size of femoral trial. Apply the trial patellar implant. Reduce the knee and extend it fully. For reduction, one assistant will hold the ankle and other will lift the thigh. The surgeon will hold the trial insert anteriorly to avoid rotation and press the top of upper tibia downward and posteriorly and simultaneously extend the knee. Check the overall alignment, stability, movement and patellar tracking. If there is any instability, exchange the tibial insert trial with the next greater thickness and repeat reduction. Select the insert that gives the greatest stability in flexion and extension and allowing full extension.

Flex the knee. Lift the thigh. Remove the insert by bone hook. Apply medium Hohmann on the posterior aspect of upper tibia and small Hohmann on lateral and medial aspect. Assemble the universal handle to the MBT keel punch and remove it by slap hammer. Assemble the punch bushing impactor/extractor with keel punch bushing and remove it. Remove the MBT tray trial. Remove the trial femoral component. Make multiple drill holes with 2.5 mm drill bit in the hard area of bone. Wash the femoral canal with 100 mL normal saline and block the canal with bone graft by the bone of extraposterior cuts, chamfer cuts or box cut. Thoroughly cleanse with gentamicin mixed normal saline by pulse lavage.

Cementing

Cementing of patella and femoral component is similar to fixed bearing knee. Apply medium Hohmann on the posterior aspect of upper tibia to dislocate it anteriorly and small Homanns on medial and lateral aspect to retract the collateral ligaments and soft tissues. For cementing the MBT tray, apply the bone cement over the upper surface of tibia and under surface of the MBT tray. Insert the tibial tray fully in prepared tibia with manual pressure to avoid malrotation. Put a swab over the tibial tray in order to protect the bearing surface. Place the MBT tray impactor over the swab on tibial tray and deliver several mallet blows to the top of the universal handle. Remove the extruded bone cement by curette. Apply the MBT trial post into the central stem of MBT tray and apply the RPF tibial insert trial **according to the size of the femoral componenet**. Reduce the knee and extend it. Keep the sand bag under the heel and maintain even pressure across bone/tibial implant interface. Avoid hyperextension which may cause posterior lift-off. Assistant will keep the ankle dorsiflexed. Maintain the position till cement sets. Release the tourniquet. Achieve the hemostasis specially coagulate the lateral inferior genicular artery by electrocautery.

Application of Tibial Insert

Flex the knee. Remove the tibial insert trial and MBT trial post. Apply medium Hohmann (Big Hohmann may be jammed in the notch as the notch of femoral component is smaller) on the posterior aspect of upper tibia and small Hohmann on the lateral and medial aspect of upper tibia. Remove the extruded cement with small osteotome and mallet or nibbler. Cleanse with gentamicin mixed normal saline by pulse lavage. Apply the appropriate size **(according to size of femoral component)** and thickness of RPF tibial insert. Remove the Homanns and reduce the knee as described. Check the stability, movement and patellar tracking. Close the wound under two suction drains as described for fixed bearing TKR.

Note: In fixed bearing TKR, the size of tibial insert is according to the size of tibial tray while in RPF TKR, it is according to the size of femoral component.

Technically well-performed TKR and good **postoperative physiotherapy** give excellent results whether using fixed bearing or mobile bearing (RPF) **(Figs 4.1 to 4.4)**. In RPF design, there is extraposterior bone cut, hence be careful in small femur (size 1.5 and 2), osteoporosed bone and rheumatoid arthritis. RPF TKR is indicated when the preoperative knee movement is 0–120° and varus/valgus deformity is less than 20°. RPF TKR is avoided in cases of gross instability, large bone defect, quadriceps wasting and stiff knee.

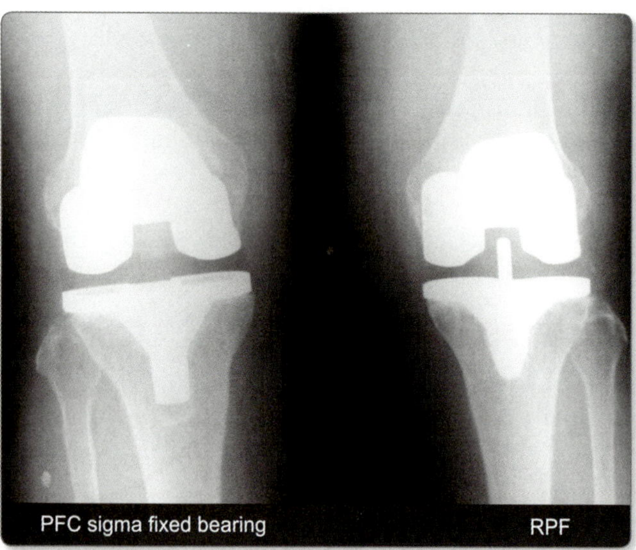

Fig. 4.1 AP view

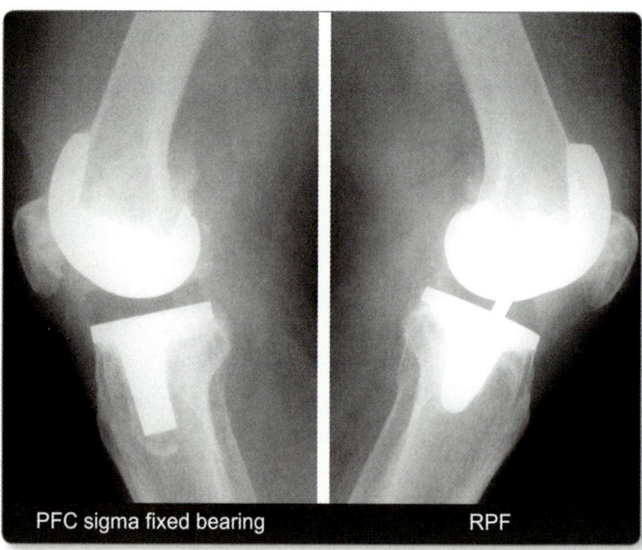

Fig. 4.2 Lateral view

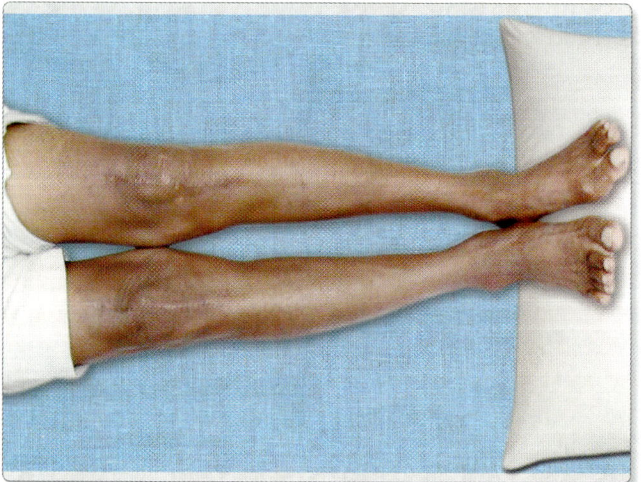

Fig. 4.3 Full extension

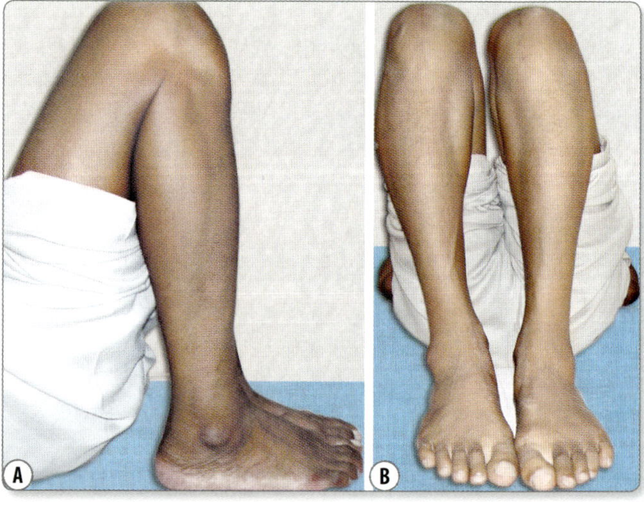

Figs 4.4A and B (A) Right knee—PFC sigma fixed bearing; (B) Left knee—RPF in same patient with full range of movement (full flexion and extension in both knees)

Instruments Required for RPF TKR

Instruments required for RPF TKR are given in **Figure 4.5**.

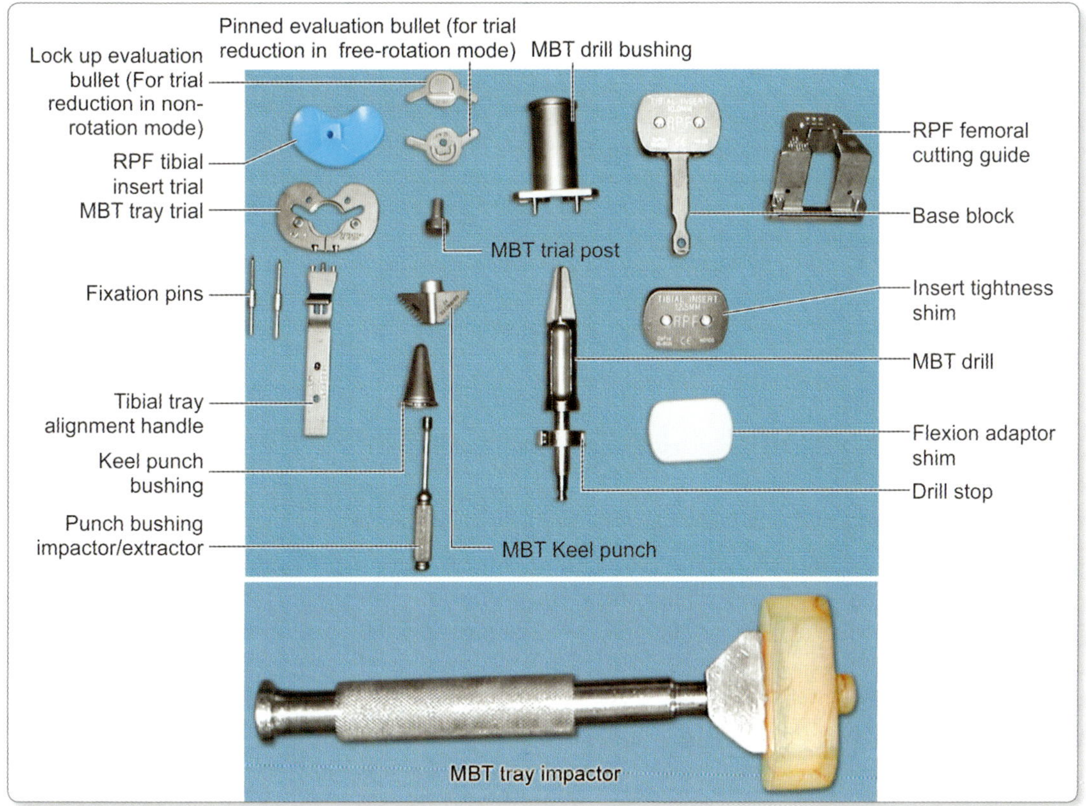

Fig. 4.5 Different instruments required for RPF and TKR

Fundamentals of TKR

Restoration of—3 Points

1. Femorotibial alignment.
2. Patellofemoral alignment.
3. Ligament balancing.

Achievement of Above Goals by—3 points

1. Cuts.
2. Sequential soft tissue release.
3. Component insertion.

Tibial Cut—3 points

1. Perpendicular to the mechanical axis of tibia.
2. 10 mm thickness measured on less involved condyle.
3. 3° posterior slope for fixed bearing and 0° for RPF.

Femoral Cuts—3 points

1. Distal cut in 7° valgus, 9 mm thickness.
2. Anterior, posterior and chamfer cuts in 3° external rotation (2–4 mm extraposterior cut for RPF).
3. Box cut in lateralized position.

Patellar Cut—3 points

1. Measurement of thickness.
2. Retain patella minimum 14 mm.
3. Drilling in superiorly and medialized position.

Tibial Preparation—3 points

1. 3° external rotation.
2. Drilling and widening.
3. Broaching.

Cementing of Components—3 points

1. Patellar implant in superiorly and medialized.
2. Femoral component in 7° valgus, 3° external rotation and lateralized.
3. Tibial tray in 3° external rotation.

Tibial Insert—3 points

1. Proper thickness.
2. Size according to size of tibial tray for fixed bearing.
3. Size according to size of femoral component for mobile bearing (RPF).

Final Achievement of Goals—3 points

1. Restotaion of normal alignment of limb.
2. Normalize range of motion.
3. Painless stable joint.

Always Avoid—3 points

1. Medialization and internal rotation of femoral component.
2. Internal rotation and varus positioning of tibial tray.
3. Lateralization of patellar implant.

Complications and Revision TKR

5

CHAPTER

CHAPTER OUTLINE

Periprosthetic Fracture

Femoral and patellar fractures are more common than tibial fractures.

Supracondylar Fracture Femur (Lewis and Rorabeck)

It is of three types—This classification depends upon fracture displacement and prosthesis stability.

1. Type I—Undisplaced with well-fixed prosthesis.
2. Type II—Displaced (>5 mm mediolateral displacement or >5° angulation anteroposteriorly or both) with well fixed prosthesis.
3. Type III—Displaced or undisplaced with loose prosthesis, polyethylene wear, instability.

The aim of treatment is to achieve fracture union within 6 months, with minimal displacement (<5 mm translation, <5° mediolateral and <10° anteroposterior angulation, <10° rotation, <1 cm shortening) with range of motion at least 90–100°.

Type I fracture may be treated conservatively by traction and functional cast bracing.

Type II fracture requires open reduction and internal fixation by LCP, DCS and 95° barrel plate, condylar blade plate, buttress plate. Other options are closed reduction and internal fixation by flexible nailing, retrograde interlocking nail, antegrade interlocking nail or external fixator. Open reduction and internal fixation by DCS and 95° barrel plate with bone grafting is a good option **(Figs 5.1 to 5.3)**. Lateral approach is used leaving minimum 7 cm distance between the anterior scar and lateral incision to avoid skin bridge necrosis. Presently, locking compression plate (LCP) is the best option for periprosthetic fracture **(Figs 5.4 to 5.6)**. If the fracture line is away from the femoral condyles, it can be fixed by broad LCDCP or DCP with bone grafting **(Fig. 5.7)** or LCP.

Type III fractures are treated by revision TKR using long stemmed components or custom made distal femur replacing components. Bone grafting and prevention of extrusion of cement into the fracture site are essential for successful outcome. Preferably, plan for two-stage procedure. First achieve the fracture union then revision TKR which makes the surgery easier.

Tibial Fractures (Figs 5.8A and B)

These are very rare and classified into four types (Felix et al.) depending on the major anatomic pattern and three sub-categories based on stability of the implant and whether

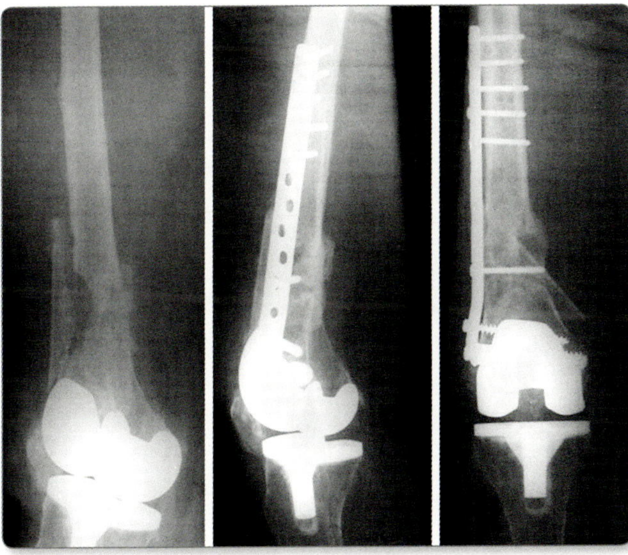

Fig. 5.1 Type II comminuted supracondylar fracture femur fixed with DCS and 95° barrel plate with bone grafting

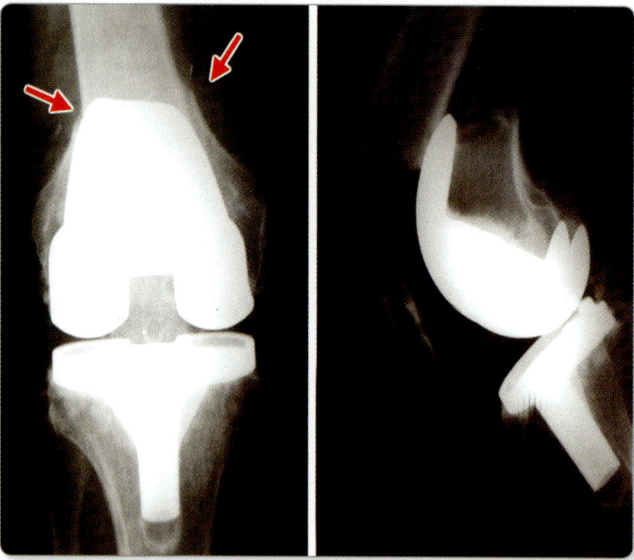

Fig. 5.2 Type II supracondylar fracture femur—AP and lateral views

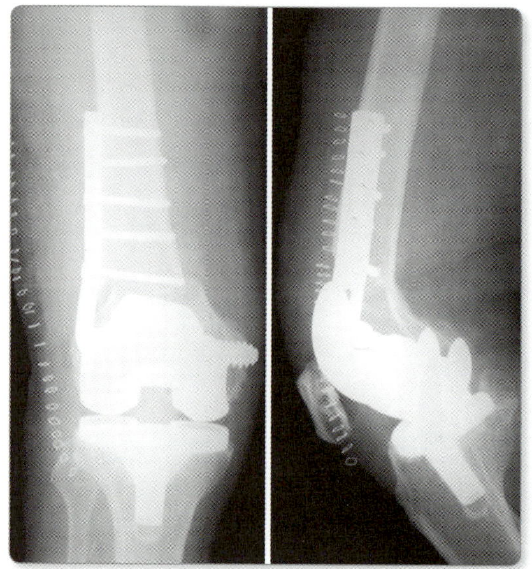

Fig. 5.3 Fixation with DCS and 95° barrel plate with bone grafting

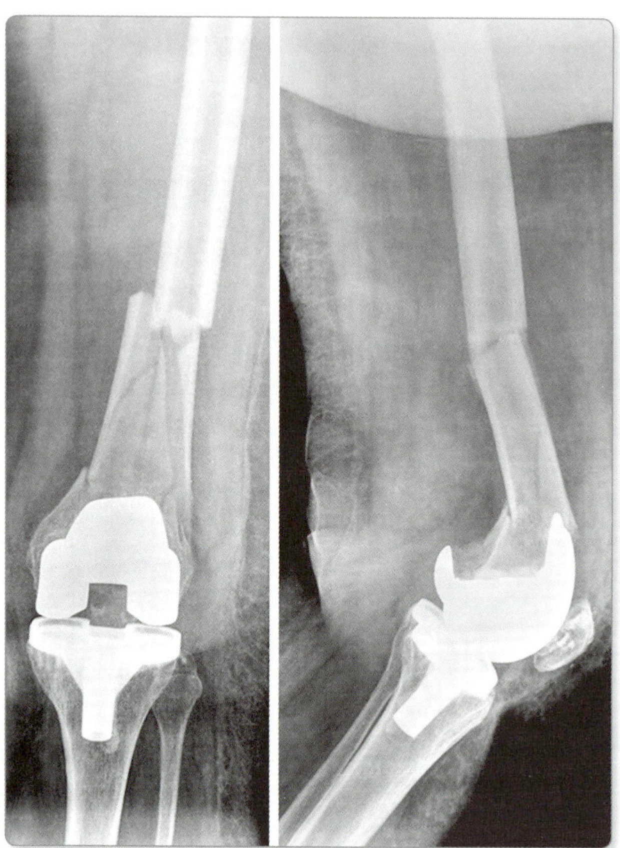

Fig. 5.4 Type II Comminuted supracondylar periprosthetic fracture femur

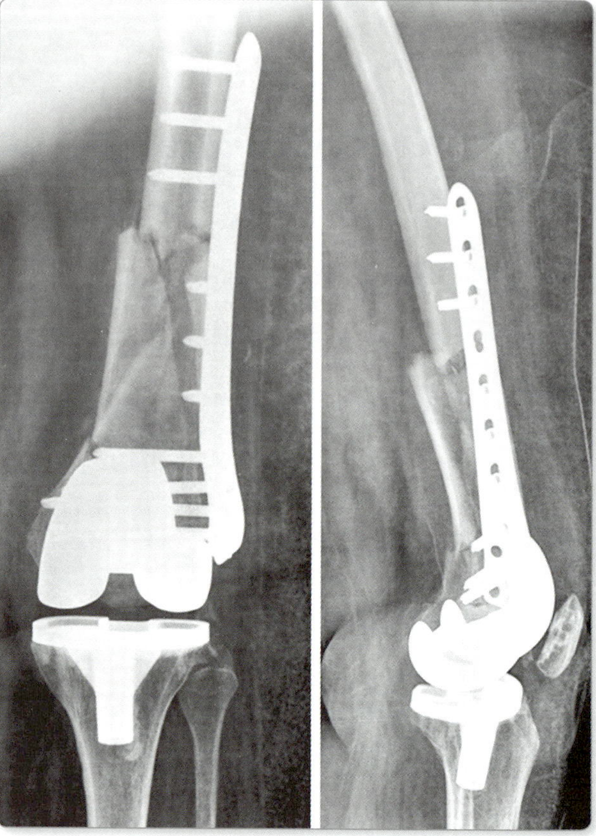

Fig. 5.5 Fixation with LCP

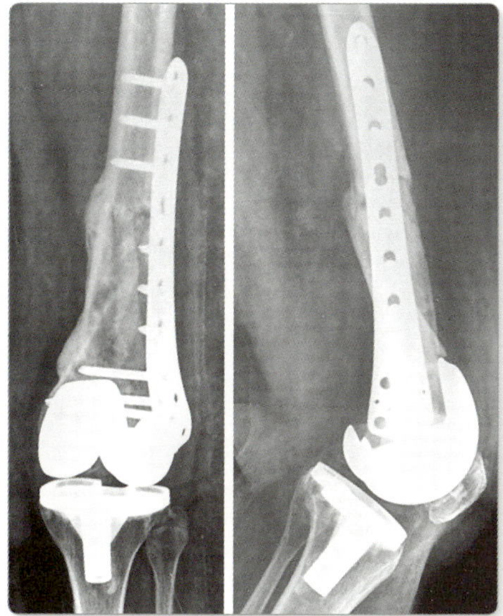

Fig. 5.6 After union of fracture at 3 months

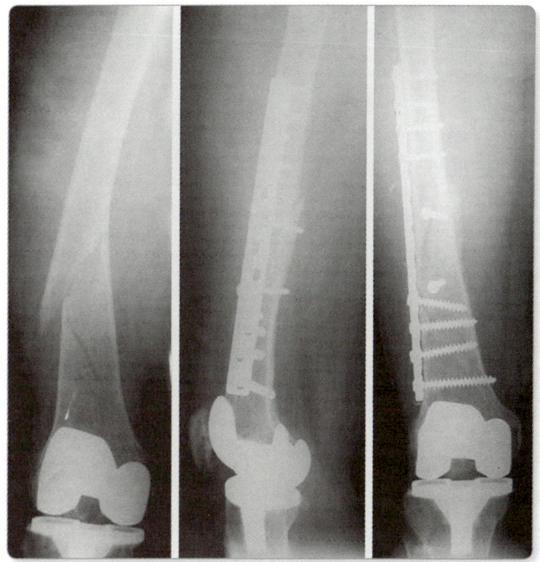

Fig. 5.7 X-rays showing fracture of lower shaft femur extending to supracondylar region and fixation with broad LCDCP with bone grafting

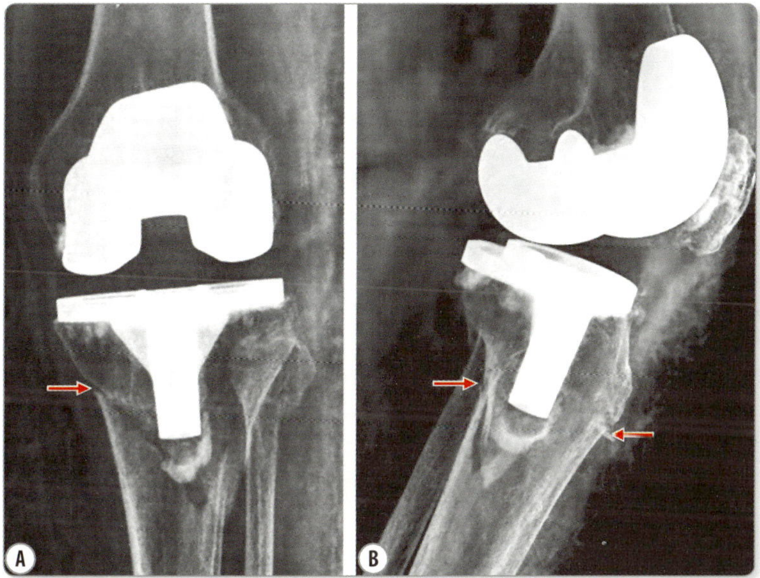

Figs 5.8A and B Periprosthetic fracture tibia

the fracture occurred intraoperatively or postoperatively **(Figs 5.9A to D)**.

1. Type I—Tibial plateau fracture.
2. Type II—Fracture adjacent to stem.
3. Type III—Fracture distal to stem.
4. Type IV—Fracture tibial tubercle.

Subcategories:

A. Well-fixed prosthesis.
B. Loose prosthesis.
C. Intraoperative:
   i. Stable, undisplaced.
   ii. Unstable, displaced.

Type III B:

i. Proximal fracture.
ii. Distal fracture.

Type IV:

i. Displaced (unstable).
ii. Stable.

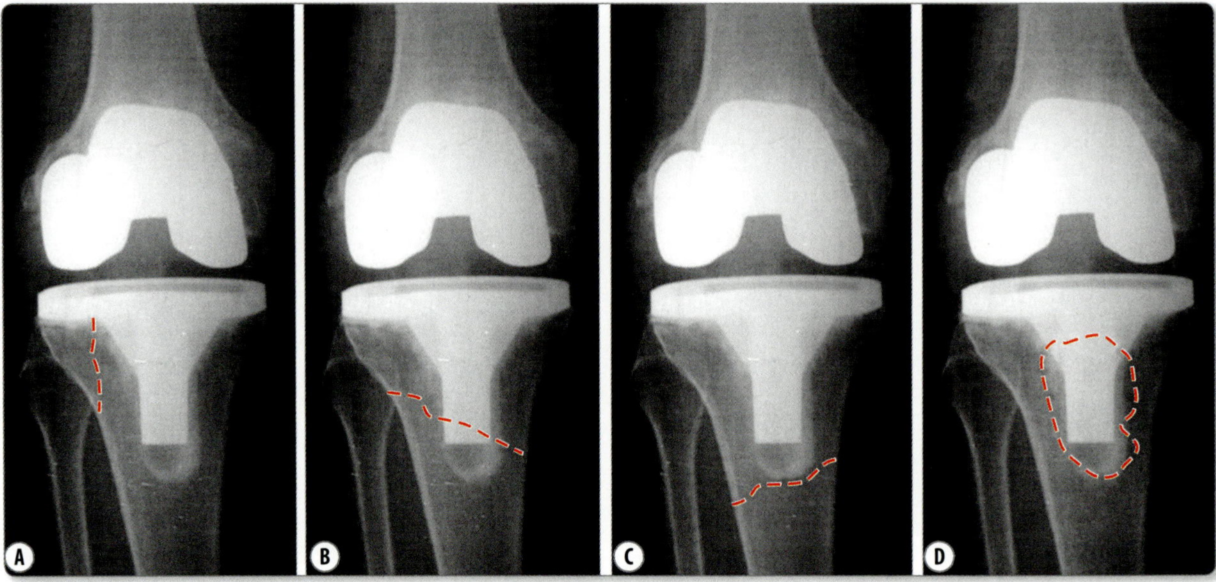

Figs 5.9A to D Diagrammatic pictures showing periprosthetic tibial fracture

Treatment Plan of Tibial Fractures based on Classification

1. Type I, II, III A and C (i) Conservative—POP cast and non weight-bearing walking.
2. Type I, II, III B—Revision TKR with stem. Type I B requires long stem components, bone graft/Augments, III B: (i) Proximal fracture requires revision TKR with long stem and (ii) Distal fracture requires two stage procedures: Stage I—osteosynthesis, and stage II—revision TKR.
3. Type I, II, III C (ii)—Long stemmed components. In Type III C (ii), try close reduction and casting, if fails then use modular TKR with long stem to bypass fracture or ORIF
4. Type IV—
   i. Open reduction and internal fixation.
   ii. Extension immobilizer brace.

Patella Fractures

It is of four types (Goldberg):

1. *Type I*: Fractures not involving cement/implant composite or quadriceps mechanism.
2. *Type II*: Fractures involving cement/implant composite (prosthetic loosening) and/or quadriceps mechanism.
3. *Type III*: Inferior pole fractures
   IIIA: With patellar ligament disruption
   IIIB: Without patellar ligament disruption.
4. *Type IV*: Fracture-dislocations.

Treatment Plan of Patella Fractures based on Classification

Type I and IIIB—Conservative—Cylinder cast or knee brace for 4 to 6 weeks with partial weight bearing walking with crutches.

Type II, IIIA and IV—ORIF (TBW) with revision of prosthetic patella.

Fragment excision may be done for small fragments that do not compromise implant stability or patellar tracking. Patellectomy may be required in cases of extensive comminution or devascularization with osteonecrosis.

Infection

It is disaster for TKR. Diabetic and rheumatoid arthritic patients are more prone to infection. Other high risk groups are patients with steroid intake, obese, previous infection, previous major surgery of knee joint and age more than 75 years. It is suspected by pain, swelling, redness, indurations **(Fig. 5.10)**, raised local temperature, tenderness, stiffness, fever, neutrophilic leukocytosis, raised ESR, CRP positive and confirmed by aspiration from joint, Gram staining, pus culture-sensitivity and cytochemical analysis of synovial fluid (i.e. estimation of cell count, glucose and protein) or presence of discharging sinus **(Fig. 5.11)**.

ESR of 30 mm/hr or higher and a CRP level of 10 mg/L or higher are considered to be suggestive of infection unless until proved otherwise. In cases where both ESR and CRP are normal, chance of infection is low. According to a

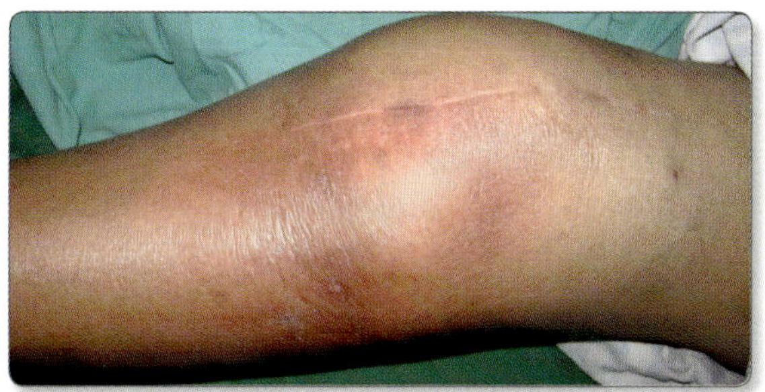

Fig. 5.10 Infected TKR showing swelling, redness, indurations over knee

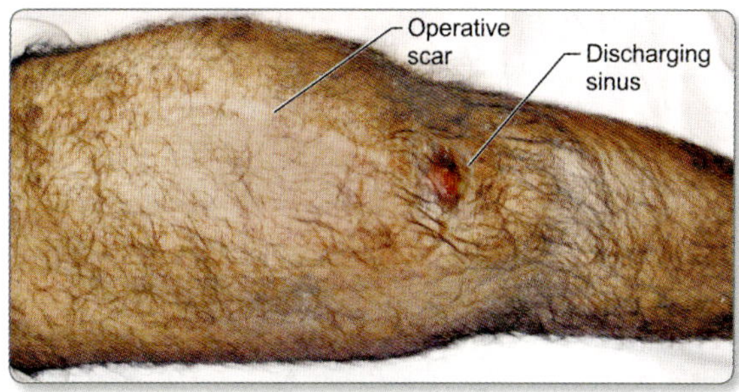

Fig. 5.11 Infected TKR showing discharging sinus

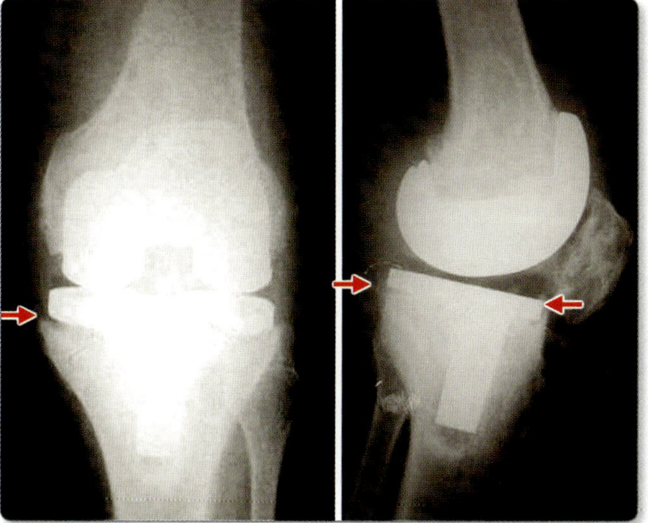

Fig. 5.12 Periprosthetic osteolysis

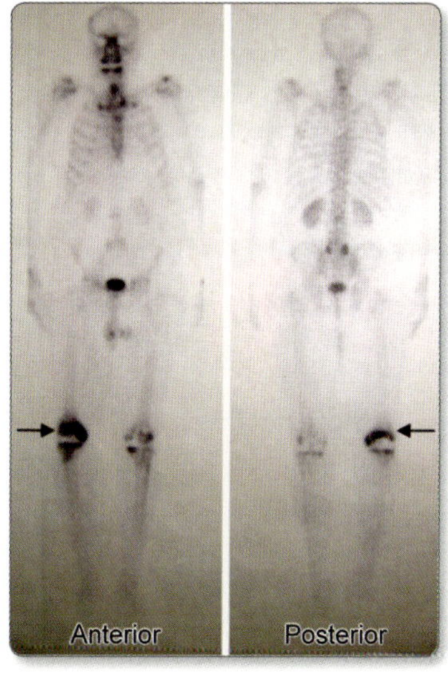

Fig. 5.13 Bone scan showing increased tracer uptake in the right knee suggestive of infection

recent study, C-reactive protein levels in synovial fluid are potentially strong markers for periprosthetic joint infection. A white cell count more than 25,000 cells per millimeter with more than 75% polymorphonuclear leukocytes in synovial fluid aspirate is suggestive of infection. Low glucose and elevated protein levels in synovial fluid aspirate as compared to plasma levels is also suggestive of infection. A Gram stain of synovial fluid aspirate may show the organism in 25% of cases. Periprosthetic osteolysis is the most frequent radiographic finding of infected TKR **(Fig. 5.12)**. Bone scan with technetium-99m, gallium-67 and indium-labeled WBCs and antibodies are most useful in cases with unclear diagnosis **(Fig. 5.13)**. Polymerase chain reaction (PCR) can also be used to diagnose infection but there is high rate of false positives and the potential for amplification of noninfectious agents. In PCR, the synovial fluid aspirates are analyzed for the presence of bacterial deoxyribonucleic acid indicative of infection. Histopathology of periprosthetic tissue obtained by arthroscopy or arthrotomy reveals acute inflammatory response with polymorphonuclear leukocytes in patients with infected TKR. The presence of 5 PMN's per high power field in five sections is suggestive of infection.

Pathophysiology of periprosthetic joint infection includes following steps:

1. Adherence of bacteria to implant.
2. Biofilm formation.
3. Intracellular internalization.

Adherence of bacteria to the implant is the first step in pathogenesis of periprosthetic joint. There are two phases of bacterial adhesion to the surface of the implant—reversible (nonspecific) and irreversible (specific). The reversible adhesion depends on nonspecific physical and chemical characteristics of the bacteria, biomaterial and surrounding joint fluid while the irreversible adhesion depends on more specific structures and receptors.

Biofilm is a complex structure comprised of microorganisms enveloped in macromolecules of glycocalyx and other protective structures. Attachment of bacteria to a surface involves cell-to-cell adhesion between microorganisms and the artificial surface.

According to the concept of intracellular internalization, the staphylococci invade and live inside the host cells (in bone) and become resistant to antibiotics and immune system responses. "Small colony variant" strains are particularly skilled in invading and living inside the host cells. These strains have mutations that impair the electron transport pathway.

The most common organism in periprosthetic joint infection is *Staphylococcus aureus*. Occasionally, there are Gram-negative bacteria, fungi and polymicrobial.

According to the proposed criteria by the Musculoskeletal Infection Society (MSIS), periprosthetic joint infection exists when:

1. There is a sinus tract communicating with the prosthesis, or
2. A pathogen is isolated by culture from at least two separate tissue or fluid samples obtained from the affected prosthetic joint, or
3. Four of the following six criteria exist:
   i. Elevated serum erythrocyte sedimentation rate (ESR) and serum C-reactive protein (CRP) concentration.
   ii. Elevated synovial white blood cell (WBC) count.
   iii. Elevated synovial neutrophil percentage (PNM%).
   iv. Presence of purulence in the affected joint.
   v. Isolation of a microorganism in one culture of periprosthetic tissue or fluid.
   vi. Greater than 5 neutrophils per high power field in five high power fields observed from histologic analysis of periprosthetic tissue at X400 magnification.

Periprosthetic joint infection may also be present if fewer than four of these criteria are met and clinical suspicion is high.

Deep prosthetic infections following TKR are of 3 types:

1. Early infection—less than 2 months of surgery.
2. Intermediate infection—between 2 months to 2 years of surgery.
3. Late infections—after 2 years of surgery.

Early infections may be associated with local wound complications such as delayed healing, skin slough or hematoma formation. Intermediate infections may occur either due to periprosthetic contamination or hematogenous spread. Late infections are more common than early infections and are usually due to hematogenous spread of microorganism from a distant site. Prosthetic retaining procedures are more likely to be successful in early infections while late infections require prosthetic removal and exchange.

Once infection is confirmed, the joint should be opened at the earliest. Persistent serous discharge for more than 5 to 7 days is an indication for surgical exploration and debridement. Early rather than late intervention in these cases may prevent deep infection. Anesthesia, positioning, dressing and draping are similar to TKR. Apply the tourniquet in proximal thigh. Elevate the limb for 5 minutes and raise the tourniquet pressure up to 400 mm Hg. Open the joint by same incision and medial parapatellar approach.

Take multiple swabs for culture and sensitivity test at the time of reoperation. It is recommended that 3 to 5 samples from various locations around the prosthesis be taken to increase the likelihood of obtaining positive culture. The broad spectrum IV antibiotics, e.g. Cefotaxime 1 g IV BD and Amikacin 500 mg IV BD preferably by central line (neck line) should be started only after taking the swabs for culture sensitivity test and exchanged with definitive antibiotics according to culture sensitivity report. Apply one pin over the insertion of patellar tendon at tibial tubercle to avoid avulsion. Apply one curved small Hohmann on the lateral aspect of tibial condyle to evert the patella and one small Hohmann on medial aspect of tibial condyle to retract the medial collateral ligament. Everting of the patella is difficult due to lot of fibrosis. Remove the fibrous tissues from infrapatellar and suprapatellar regions which are helpful in everting the patella. Reestablish the medial and lateral gutters by removing the redundant synovial tissue and scar from the medial and lateral gutters. Assistant will lift the thigh and apply one big Hohmann on the posterior aspect of upper tibia to dislocate the tibia anteriorly. Remove the plastic insert by plastic insert remover (Fig. 5.14). Sometimes, the notch of plastic insert is deformed by plastic insert remover. Then use osteotome and hammer for insert removal. Take another swab from the undersurface of the tibial insert for culture and sensitivity test.

After full exposure of the knee, clean thoroughly first by betadine solution mixed with hydrogen peroxide then by pulse lavage with copious amount of normal saline mixed with gentamicin. Remove the infected granulation tissues and fibrous tissue membranes. Check the loosening of femoral, tibial and patellar components. If these are not loose, release the tourniquet and check that the tissues are freshly bleeding. Apply the trial tibial insert. Remove the Hohmann and reduce the joint and extend it. Check the mediaolateral stability of the knee both in extension, midflexion and 90° flexion and select the proper thickness of new tibial insert. Again flex the knee. Remove the trial insert.

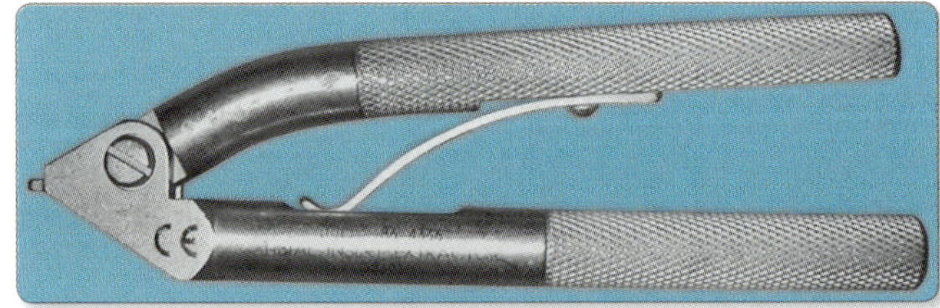

Fig. 5.14 Plastic insert remover

Apply the big Hohmann on the posterior aspect of the upper tibia and small Hohmann on medial and lateral aspect of upper tibia. Apply the new tibial insert of appropriate size and thickness. Remove the Hohmann and reduce the joint. Close the wound under two suction drains one in medial and another in lateral gutters. After 48 hours, remove the suction drains under full aseptic precaution. Change the antibiotics according to pus culture and sensitivity report and continue IV antibiotic for 3 weeks then oral antibiotics for further period of 3 weeks. Usually the infection is controlled.

If the components are loose or there is recurrence of infection, remove the femoral, tibial and patellar components and plan for two stage revision TKR. Oscillating saw with a thin and flexible blade, osteotomes, punch and hammer are used for gradual removal of tibial tray, femoral and patellar components. The osteotome is directed at the prosthesis-cement interface. Stacked osteotomes technique is used for removal of the components **(Fig. 5.15)**. Pass one thin osteotome at prosthesis-cement interface and then pass another thick osteotome between prosthesis and the first osteotome. Avoid leverage of the implant against bone to prevent bone collapse. Gigli saw is used for separation of the components from bone to avoid bone loss and iatrogenic fracture of condyles. While using Gigli saw, it should point up, i.e. away from bone **(Fig. 5.16)**.

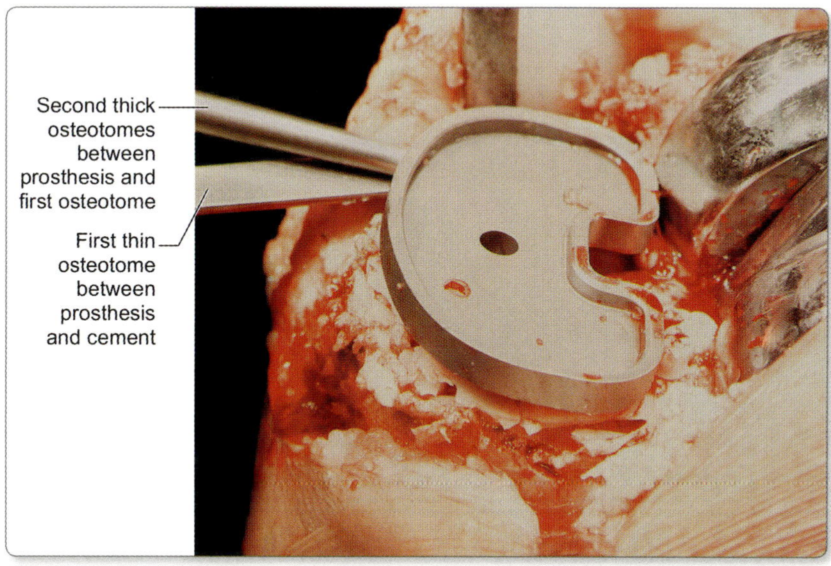

Fig. 5.15 Stacked osteotome technique for removal of component

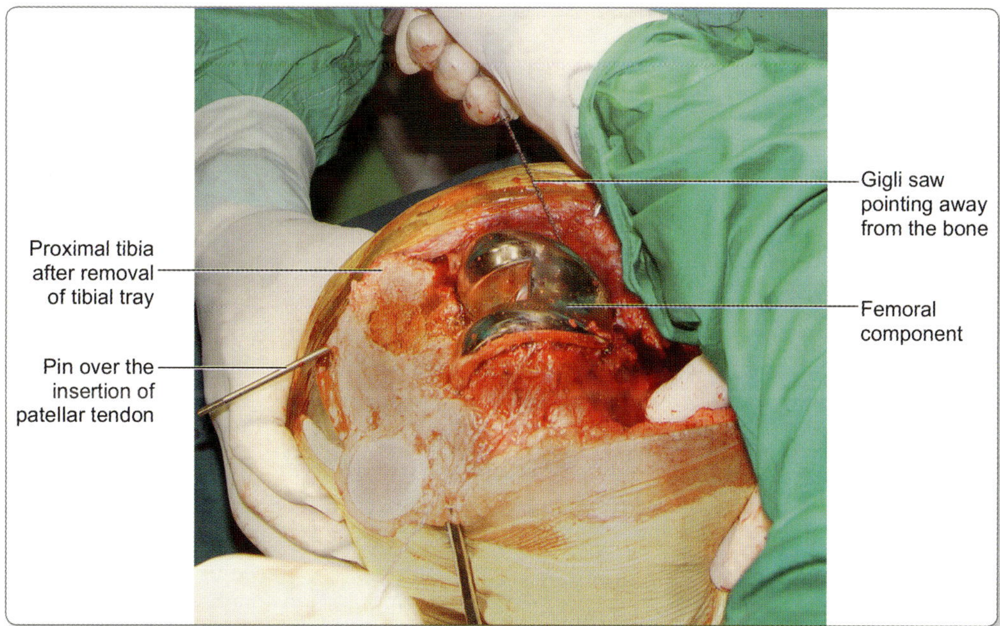

Fig. 5.16 Separating the femoral component from femoral condyles by Gigli saw

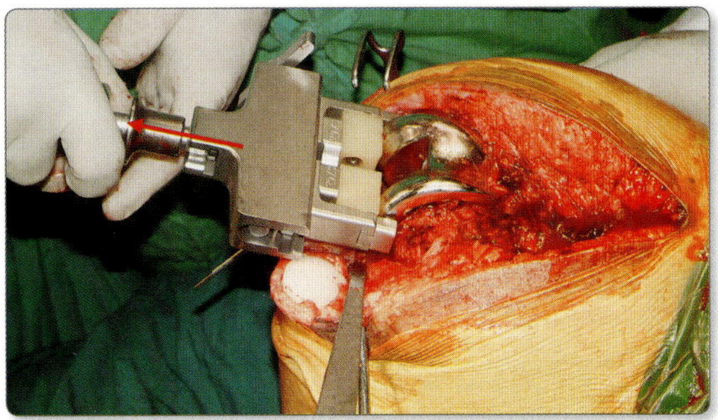

Fig. 5.17 Extraction device with slap hammer applying longitudinal force

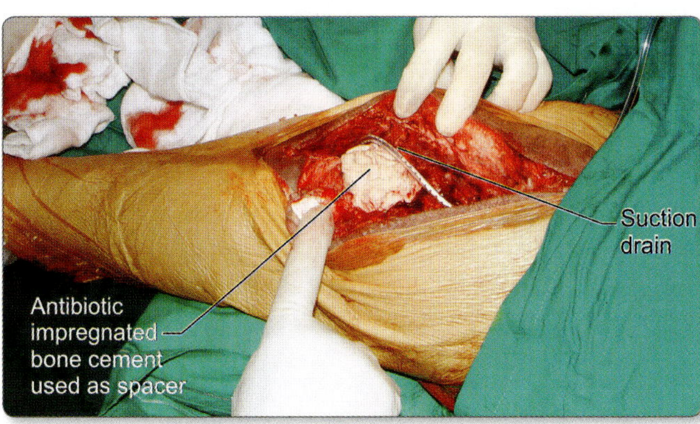

Fig. 5.18 Bone cement used as spacer (Static spacer)

After complete disruption of the fixation surfaces, the femoral component is removed with extraction device that uses a slap hammer which delivers longitudinal force to the component **(Fig. 5.17)**. Gently remove bone cement. Ultrasonic cement removal system is useful in removing the cement from tibial canal (chapter 10).

Thoroughly clean the wound first by betadine solution mixed with hydrogen peroxide then by pulse lavage with copious amount of normal saline mixed with gentamicin. Remove the all infected granulation tissues and fibrous tissue membranes. Mix bone cement (CMW1 40 g of two packets) with 1 g/40 g of vancomycin and 3.6 g/40 g of tobramycin. If tobramycin in powder form is not available, then mix 2 g/40 g vancomycin with 2 packets of 40 g gentamicin impregnated bone cement (CMW1 gentamicin). However, there are few reported literatures regarding risk of nephrotoxic effect. A wide variety of antibiotic concentration ratios are used internationally but in general no more than 8 g per 40 g of cement should be utilized to minimize systemic side-effects. Put one Surgicel and Abgel posteriorly in the gap between the distal femur and proximal tibia to protect the posterior soft tissues. When the bone cement is almost half set (i.e. in the doughy stage), apply it between the distal femur and proximal tibia as a spacer (Static spacer) **(Fig. 5.18)**.

In place of this, the commercially available Spacer-K (Dynamic spacer) can be applied **(Fig. 5.19)**. It is available in three sizes - small, medium and large. The size is selected which is nearest to the size of the removed implant. It is fixed with antibiotic impregnated bone cement. Apply femoral part first and wait for the polymerization of the cement then apply the tibial part. Reduce the joint and perform some flexion-extension movements to allow the self-centering of the tibial component in relation to the femoral component.

Alternatively dynamic articulating spacer can be applied. For this, proper size and thickness of new plastic insert can be applied with thick layer of antibiotic impregnated bone cement (to ensure high local antibiotic concentration) in the doughy stage (to prevent bonding with bone facilitating easier removal at the time of revision) directly over the cut surface of tibia (without tibial tray). However, the plastic insert of RPF will not stick with bone cement and hence directly cannot be applied. The same femoral component, after removal of bone cement and autoclaving, is re-implanted with antibiotic impregnated bone cement in the doughy stage for maintaining the space which is required during revision TKR **(Fig. 5.20)**. In case of infected RPF total knee, same femoral component and tibial tray are re-implanted after removal of cement and autoclaving. Apply the new plastic insert of appropriate size and thickness. The advantages of dynamic articulating spacer are preserving stability and mobility, providing high local antibiotic concentration and preventing the soft tissue contractures.

Apply two suction drains and close the wound. Apply knee brace. Drains are removed after 48 hours. IV antibiotic is given according to pus culture and sensitivity test for 6 weeks and then oral antibiotic for a further period of 6 weeks. Wait for 3 months and if there is no sign of infection, negative synovial fluid cultures on repeat aspiration and less than 5 PMN's per high power field in intraoperative frozen section specimens, then revision TKR is done.

If infection persists even after 3 months or recur after revision TKR, plan for arthrodesis. Limb reconstruction system (LRS) is a better option for arthrodesis.

It may be difficult for the surgeon and patient to decide on a knee arthrodesis because preserving motion with a revision total knee arthroplasty is an attractive option. But destroyed bone or soft tissues may make implantation of another prosthesis very difficult following the staged treatment of an infected total knee arthroplasty. In this setting, arthrodesis following a knee arthroplasty that was complicated by infection is associated with a low risk of reinfection and provides a stable, pain-free limb. However, the energy required to walk with a knee fusion is 25% to 30% higher than that required for normal walking. As multiple

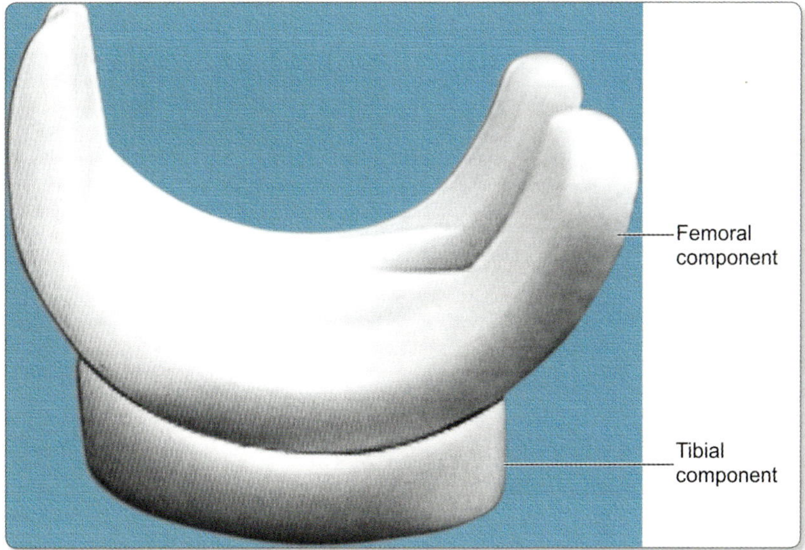

Fig. 5.19 Spacer-K (Dynamic spacer)

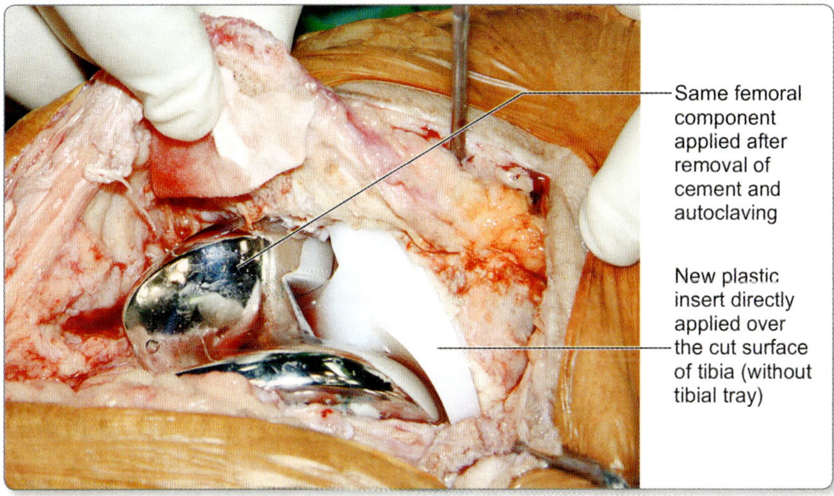

Fig. 5.20 Same femoral component after autoclaving and new plastic insert used as spacer in fixed bearing total knee (Dynamic articulating spacer)

revisions with chronic infection, severe bone loss, and intractable pain may lead to above knee amputation and the energy required to walk with an above-the-knee amputation is 25% greater than that required with a knee fusion. Rand and Stulberg have proposed using the following indications for arthrodesis following a failed total knee replacement:

1. High functional demand.
2. Disease involving a single joint.
3. Relatively young age.
4. Deficient extensor mechanism.
5. Poor soft tissue coverage.
6. Immunocompromised condition.
7. The presence of a highly virulent microorganism causing infection that requires highly toxic antimicrobial therapy.

Knee Arthrodesis with Limb Reconstruction System in Cases of Infected TKR

Introduction

Arthrodesis of the knee is the method that most readily controls septic processes and results in a nonpainful, stable knee joint. However, the disadvantages of this technique are shortening of the limb and a loss of joint function. Femorotibial arthrodesis with the LRS provides all the advantages of monolateral external fixation while allowing compression at the point of arthrodesis, achieving perfect coaptation, and providing extraordinary rigidity to the mounting. It is applied on the anterior aspect of thigh and leg to stabilize the knee arthrodesis.

Limb reconstruction system consists of an assembly of clamps which can slide on a rigid rail and can be connected by compression-distraction unit.

Items Used—(Manufactured by SH Pitkar)

1. 400 mm Rail-1.
2. End clamps-2, (End clamp is having 5 screw seats with compression-distraction unit mounting at one end).
3. Central clamps-2, (Central clamp is longer and having 5 screw seats with compression-distraction unit mountings at both ends. The screw seats are at the same level in both end and central clamps).
4. 6/5 mm tapered, Schanz screws preferably HA (Hydroxy-apatite) coated for enhanced fixation and improved stability at the pin-bone interface—10 (170 mm × 40 mm – 3, 150 mm × 40 mm – 2, 150 mm × 50 mm – 2, 150 mm × 30 mm – 3). The thread length is selected such that about 5 mm of thread will remain outside the entry cortex and about 2 mm will project beyond the second cortex.
5. CD unit (compression-distraction unit, 40 mm)—1.
6. 6 mm Allen Wrench—1.

Items Required

1. 9" long drill bit 4.5 mm—1.
2. 4.8 mm drill guides—10 (5 long Drill guides for the femur and 5 medium drill guides for the tibia).
3. 6 mm screw guides—10 (5 long screw guides for the femur and 5 medium screw guides for the tibia).
4. Clamp templates—4.
5. Pointed scissors—1.
6. BP blade No. 11—1.
7. T-wrench—1.

Procedure

A radiolucent table is used and the image intensifier is placed at right angle to the table on the opposite side of operative limb. Keep a folded sheet or sand bag beneath the greater trochanter to keep the limb in neutral rotation. The skin of whole limb is prepared from umbilicus to toes. Tourniquet is applied in the upper third of thigh as high as possible. Use of tourniquet is optional. Draping is done as in TKR. Open the joint by same incision and medial parapatellar approach. Spacer or implants are removed and thorough debridement is done as described earlier. The bone ends of femur and tibia are approximated and temporarily fixed with two cross K-wires. Insert two suction drains No. 14, one in medial and one in lateral gutters. The wound is closed by interrupted sutures. The assistant will hold the limb in neutral position. Take one 400 mm rail and assemble 4 clamp templates on the rail with their locking screws loosened to allow free movement. The precise positions of clamps and screws are planned. The clamp templates face medially and the rail laterally **(Fig. 5.21)**. Apply 4.8 mm drill guide and 6 mm screw guide one in each other in 1st, 3rd and 5th screw seats on proximal and distal templates and 3rd and 5th screw seats in first middle template and 1st and 3rd screw seats in second middle template counting the screw seats from proximal to distal. Tighten the locking screws of templates with drill and screw guides. Keep the central part of rail over the center of the knee and adjust the templates in such a way that 1st screw seat of the proximal template is on the anterior aspect of middle thigh in the line of femur and the 5th screw seat of distal template over the anterior aspect of middle leg in the line of just medial to the anterior border of tibia. This is checked by feeling with 1.8 mm trocar point K-wire and image intensifier. Make a mark over the thigh with the drill guide of 1st screw seat of proximal template.

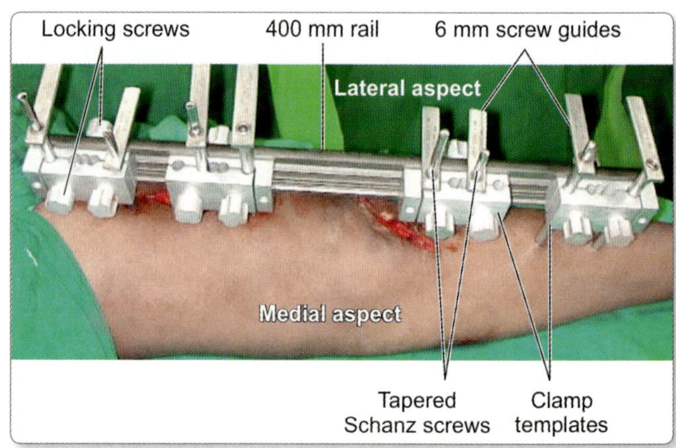

Fig. 5.21 400 mm Rail with clamp templates, screw guides and tapered Schanz screws

Make a small nick on the skin of thigh by BP blade No.11 over the drill guide mark. Separate the soft tissues through the skin nick by pointed scissors till periosteum to create a soft tissue tunnel. For this, put the closed tip of pointed scissors till it touches the bone. Open the tip of scissors and pull it out. Repeat this act 3–4 times in both longitudinal and transverse directions. Press the sleeves deep to the bone to protect the soft tissues during drilling and passing Schanz screws. Pass the long 4.5 mm drill bit through the drill guide up to the bone and center it by moving mediolaterally and by feeling. Check under image intensifier that there is no overlapping of the tip of drill bit and the cortex. Once the drill bit is in the center of bone, drill it till the opposite cortex. Remove the drill bit and 4.8 mm drill guide. Take one tapered Schanz screw (170 mm × 40 mm) preferably HA (hydroxyapatite) coated and load over T-wrench. Pass it in the drill hole through the 6 mm screw guide to protect the soft tissues. Drill through the 5th screw seat of distal template over the center of tibia just

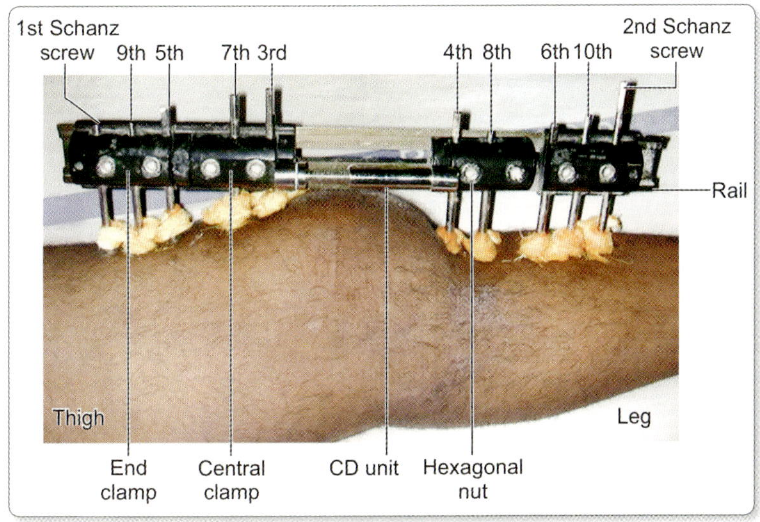

Fig. 5.22 View from medial side, sequence of applying Schanz screws

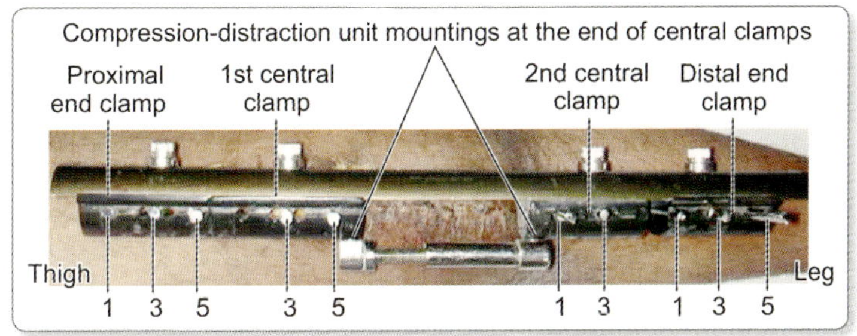

Fig. 5.23 Screw seats (1, 3 and 5) counted from left to right or proximal to distal

medial to the anterior border of tibia in the similar way as done for femur and apply the 150 mm × 30 mm tapered Schanz screw. Now adjust the level of two central templates one proximal and another distal to knee. Drill through 3rd and 5th screw seat in first central template and 1st and 3rd screw seat in second central template in the same way as done for 1st drill screw seat in femur and apply the tapered Schanz screws (150 mm × 40 mm and 150 mm × 50 mm). The 1st screw seat in second central template is just distal to tibial tubercle. Similarly drill through 3rd and 5th screw seats of the proximal template and 1st and 3rd screw seats of the distal template and apply the tapered Schanz screws (for proximal template, two 170 mm × 40 mm and for distal template two 150 mm × 30 mm sizes tapered Schanz screws).

Loosen the locking screws of all four templates holding the screw guides and remove the templates along with rail. Check the position of Schanz screws in lateral view under Image Intensifier because once the Schanz screw goes more; it cannot be brought back due to tapering design. The threading of Schanz screws should hold both cortices and project 2 mm beyond the second cortex. Remove the clamp templates from the rail. Apply two central clamps in the center and two end clamps over the two ends of the rail. Pass the Schanz screws of the limb in corresponding screw seats of the clamps in such a way that clamps face the medial aspect and rail on lateral aspect of the limb. Keep the rail one finger breadth above the skin at the level of knee. Tighten the hexagonal bolt holding the schanz screws and clamp locking screws holding the rail by 6 mm Allen wrench. Apply the 40 mm CD unit facing medially between two nearest compression-distraction unit mountings of the two central clamps **(Figs 5.22 and 5.23)**. Loosen the clamp locking screws of 2nd central and distal end clamp. Remove the two cross K-wires used for temporary fixation of femoral and tibial ends. Turn the CD unit clockwise with 6 mm Allen wrench for compression at the ends of the femur and tibia **(Fig. 5.24)**. After compression, tighten the both clamp locking screws of 2nd central and distal end clamp **(Fig. 5.25)**. Pin site and operative site dressings are done. Suction drains are removed after 48 hours.

1 mm compression (one thread clockwise rotation of CD unit by Allen wrench) is done weekly till the union occurs

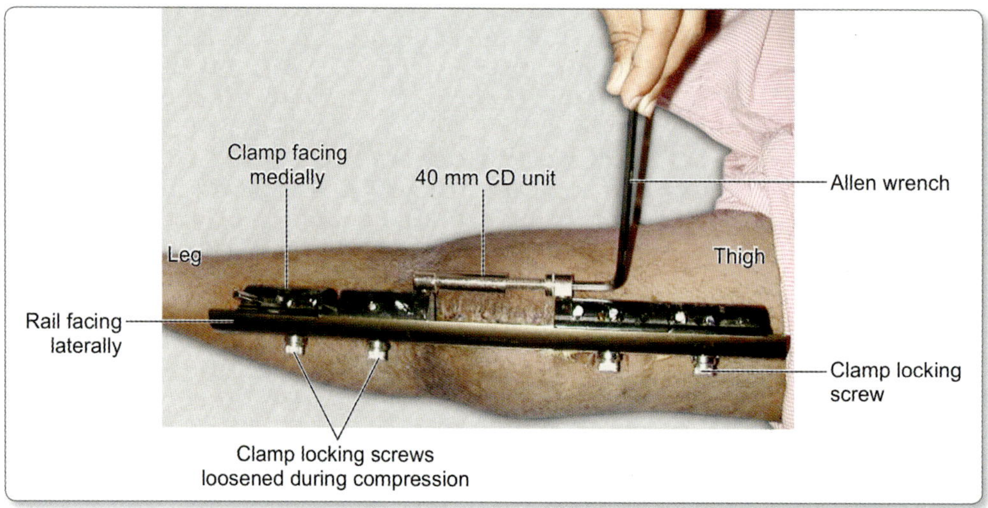

Fig. 5.24 Front view showing compression by Allen wrench applied with CD unit

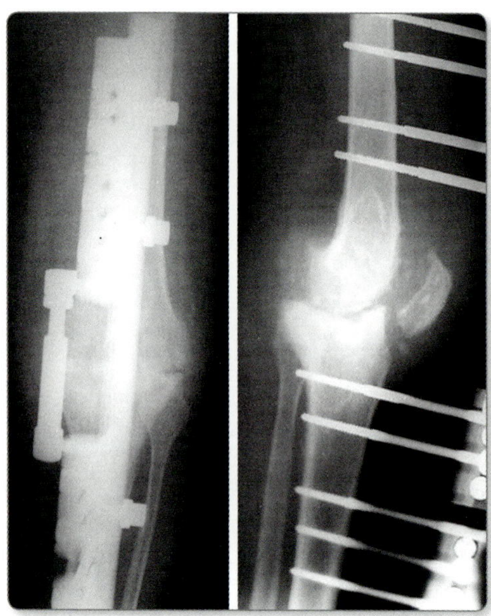

Fig. 5.25 2nd postoperative X-ray AP and lateral views

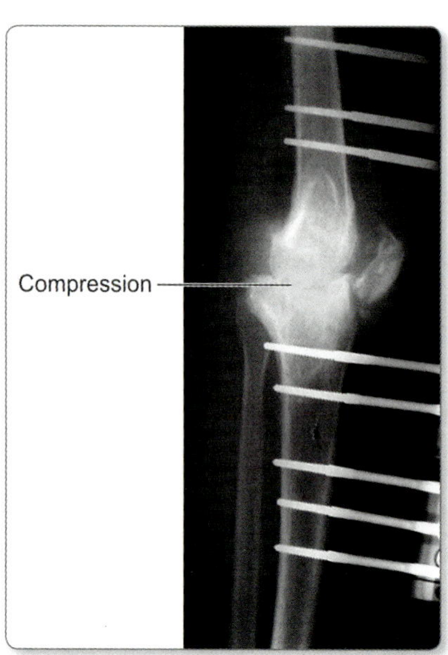

Fig. 26 Lateral view at 3 weeks after compression at arthrodesis site

between the ends of femur and tibia (Arthrodesis) **(Figs 5.26 and 5.27)**. During each compression, both clamp locking screws of 2nd central and distal end clamp are loosened and after compression again tightened. Pin tract dressing is done daily.

Wound Check and Pin Site Care

Forty-eight hours postoperative, the bulk of the dressing is reduced and a small dressing is applied on the operative incision, keeping it separate from the pin sites and thus facilitating daily pin site care. We teach the patient and a relative "our" method of pin site care. The pin site care method that we follow requires the patient to use only preboiled and cooled water or normal saline and sterile gauze pieces. The idea is to keep the pin and skin junction clean and remove any scabs that may form. The process involves first cleaning the pin sites with sterile gauze dipped in boiled and cooled water or normal saline, drying the area with sterile gauze, and then wrapping the pins in sterile gauze soaked in betadine lotion. The first two times (Day 2 and Day 3 postoperative), the pin site cleaning is done by a member of the team (doctor or nurse) and observed by the patient and relative, who is also explained the process.

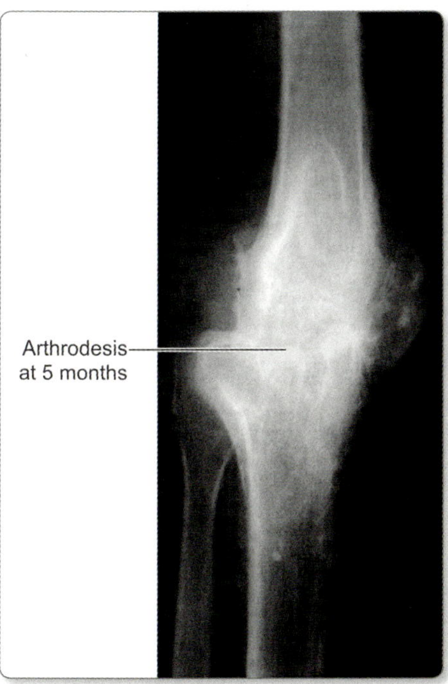

Fig. 5.27 Arthrodesis at 5 months

The next two days the pin site care is done by the patient or relative under supervision of a doctor or nurse who has been previously trained in the method of pin site care. We insist that only the patient or a relative will do the pin-site cleaning. This ensures that pin site care will be done daily, and done in the way that we want it. We make it a point to tell them that even if there is a local doctor/compounder/nurse who is willing to come and do the dressing—we do not allow that. The use of betadine in the gauze pieces is discontinued once the pin sites are relatively dry. The use of any ointment is strictly prohibited, as a combination of ointment and reduction in pin site care leads to the formation of a plug to prevent drainage of fluid from around the pins, which in turn becomes a focal point for the beginning of a pin site infection. Bathing is required. We allow and encourage the patient to take a bath and wash the operated leg along with fixator after about two weeks, as by then suture removal is done, and the pin sites have healed well. Patients are told to bathe the leg, and perform pin site care after that.

At any stage of time, if patient develops pin tract infection, it is controlled by copious irrigation at pin skin junction with betadine solution and gentamicin mixed normal saline and oral antibiotic preferably Amoxicillinclavulanic acid combination or according to swab culture and sensitivity test. Occasionally in few patients, there is skin inflammation due to allergies or irritants (allergic contact dermatitis or irritant contact dermatitis) which are controlled by application of Betnovate (betamethasone) ointment and antihistamine (e.g. cetrizine tablet) but care to be taken not to apply the ointment over the pin tract. In very rare cases, blister formation may occur due to swelling of limb which should be punctured by sterile disposable needle in dependent part and press gently by wet gauze piece to drain the fluid. Postoperative limb elevation avoids blister formation.

Fixator Removal

Check x-ray is taken to confirm the union (see that there is bridging trabeculae at arthrodesis site).

Prior to removal, we like to perform the "stress test" or "gradual disassembly".

1. Make the patient walk, bearing full weight without any support in the clinic. Confirm that there is no pain.
2. Then the fixator is removed and patient is allowed walking full weight bearing again with the half pins still in situ. If there is pain, the fixator just needs to be slipped on again, and maintained for a few days more.
3. Finally, if there was no pain on the previous step, the half pins (schanz screws) are removed. This can be carried out on outpatient basis without any anesthesia. We talk to the patient and make them comfortable, explain to them that it is not going to pain because the pins are threaded and they just need to be unscrewed, that they would be feeling something moving. It is a good idea to remove the pins while explaining them the procedure so that before they know the pins are already out. Thereafter, a compression bandage is applied and the patient is made to rest for 15–20 minutes with the leg elevated to allow coagulation in the pin tracks. This prevents worrisome staining of the bandage after the patient has gone home. The skin at the pin sites generally closes by 2 days, after which the patient can take bath. If they still remain open then a dressing is to be done by the patient just as was being done earlier for the pin site care. However, sometimes, some patient complaints of giddiness just after removal of pins which is relieved after lying down for some period. This is probably due to transient rise in blood pressure due to pain depending upon pain tolerance of the patient. It is a good idea to give intramuscular injection of diclofenac sodium in the gluteal region ½ hour before removal of schanz screws.

Arthrodesis is not easy. It may take a long time even more than 6 months. It may require bone grafting and prolonged antibiotics. Maximum bone contact is extremely important to optimize the outcome of knee arthrodesis. Deficiencies in bone stock and poor bone apposition adversely affect the success of a knee arthrodesis **(Figs 5.28 A and B)**.

Shortening of the limb upto 5 cm is compensated by raising the sole of shoes or sleeper. Lengthening is required if the discrepancy is >5 cm because shoe-lifts become cumbersome with discrepancies of this magnitude.

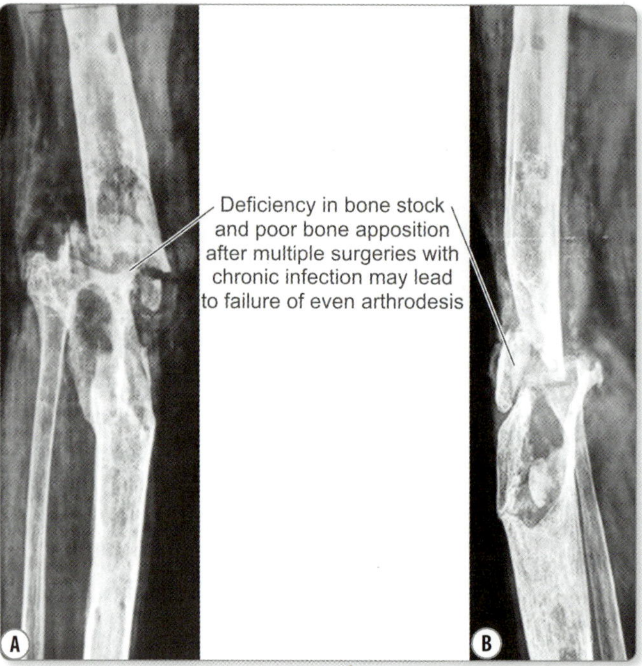

Figs 5.28A and B Failed arthrodesis

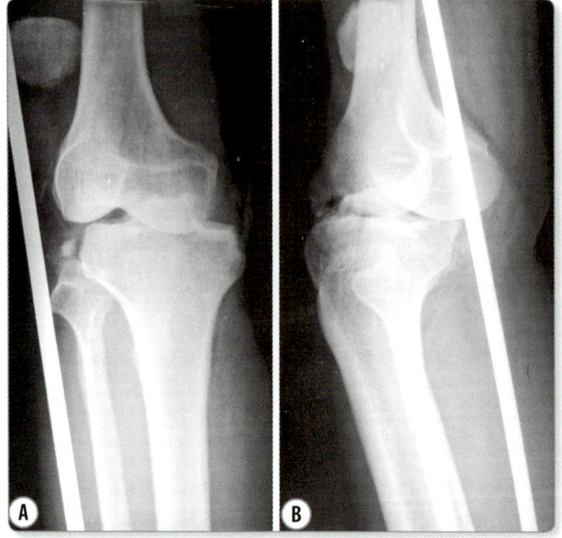

Figs 5.29A and B Internal derangement of knee with dislocation

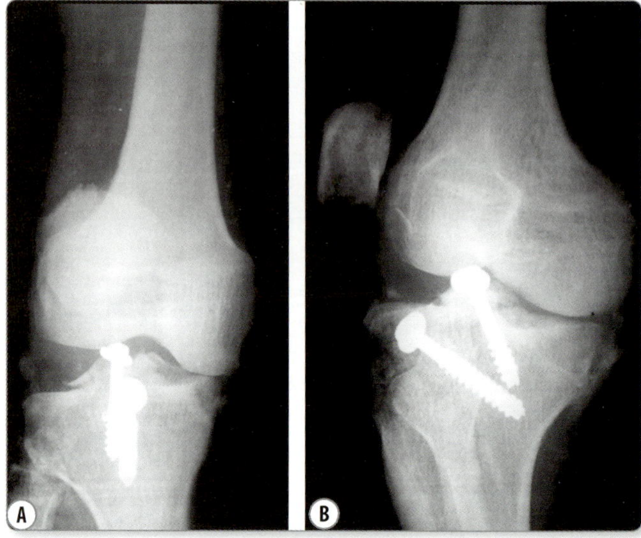

Figs 5.30A and B Reconstruction failed

There is no consensus regarding the optimal alignment of a knee fusion in the sagittal or coronal plane. In order to prevent further limb shortening, the majority of knee arthrodeses are placed in 0° of extension. A 5° to 7° of valgus have been proposed as the ideal normal frontal alignment.

This technique of knee arthrodesis can also be used for post-traumatic internal derangement of knee with dislocation where reconstruction is not possible or failed **(Figs. 5.29 and 5.30)** and painful fibrous healing of infective arthritis of knee with poor skin condition over knee. Tourniquet is applied in the upper third of thigh as high as possible. Knee is exposed by midline skin incision and medial parapatellar approach. Quadriceps snip is usually required for eversion of patella due to a lot of fibrosis. Flex the knee gradually and remove the fibrous tissues, remnants of ACL, PCL and menisci by electrocautery. Resect the upper

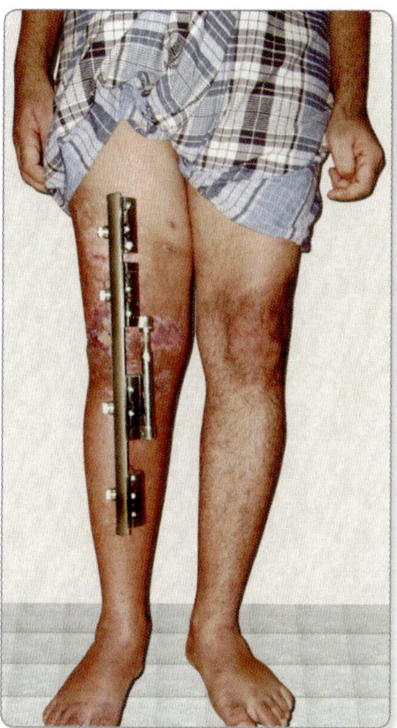

Fig. 5.31 Knee arthrodesis by LRS poor skin condition over knee

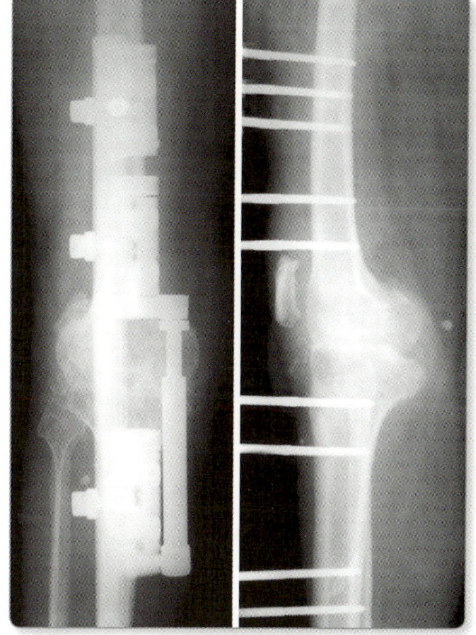

Fig. 5.32 X-ray AP and lateral views

tibia by 0° tibial cutting block with stylus set at 0 mm on less involved condyle (usually on medial condyle) as used for TKR. Resect the distal end of femur 6 to 9 mm by distal femoral cutting block after using the femoral locating device set at 5°–7° valgus as cut for TKR. Denude the cartilage from anterior and posterior part of femoral condyle by nibbler. Patella is resected as in TKR. Resected bone pieces are denuded from cartilage and applied as graft around the approximated bone ends or in bone defects. Approximation of bone ends of femur and tibia with temporary K-wires and technique of application of LRS is same as described above **(Figs 5.31 and 5.32)**.

Extensor Mechanism Patellar Tendon Rupture

Patellar tendon rupture after total knee arthroplasty is a rare, but often catastrophic complication. Many different reconstruction techniques of patellar tendon rupture have been described with variable results. Clinically, there is depression over the patellar tendon **(Fig. 5.33)** and patient is unable to extend the knee actively. X-ray knee shows large gap between lower pole of patella and tibial tubercle due to quadriceps pull of patella **(Fig. 5.34)**.

Repair of Recent Rupture of Patellar Tendon in TKR

A midline skin incision over the previous scar is made on the front of the knee, overlaying the tendon. The site of the tendon rupture is identified **(Fig. 5.35)**. The tendon ends are retracted to allow inspection of the underlying joint. The tendon ends are identified and then repaired together by Ethibond no. 5 **(Fig. 5.36)**. A cylinder cast or knee brace is applied for 6 weeks followed by several weeks of rehabilitation **(Figs 5.37 and 5.38)**.

Repair of Neglected Patellar Tendon Rupture in TKR

Position

Bring the patient down towards the foot end of the operation table. Apply a side support near proximal third of thigh at the level of tourniquet cuff. Apply one foot support at the end of the table in such a way that knee can be flexed at 90. *Dressing* and *draping* are same as used for TKR.

Technique

Expose the patellar tendon rupture through a midline skin incision on previous incision of TKR **(Fig. 5.39)**. Extend the incision below to expose the insertion of semitendinosus tendon. Identify the semitendinosus tendon by palpation. Pass an artery forceps under the tendon near its insertion **(Fig. 5.40)** and pass a small cut piece of ethibond no. 5 to have a better hold **(Fig. 5.41)**.

Separate the tendon from gracilis and adhesions. Keep the insertion point intact. Pass an open tendon stripper and strip the tendon **(Figs 5.41 and 5.42)**.

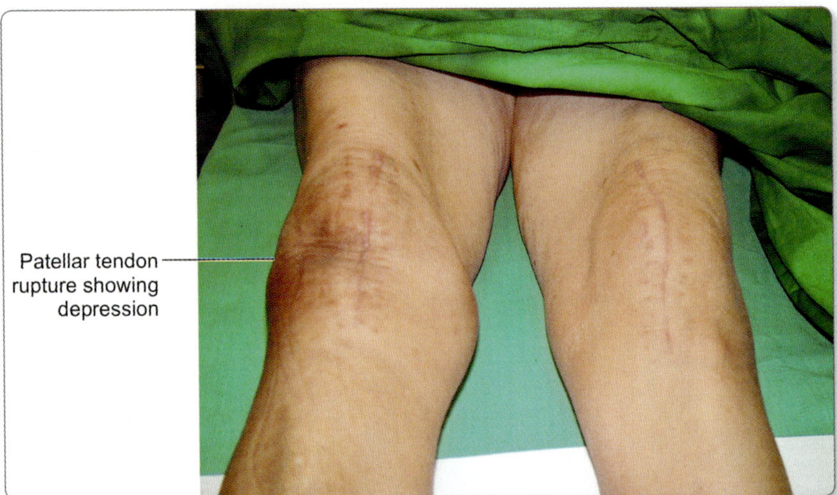

Fig. 5.33 Patellar tendon rupture showing depression

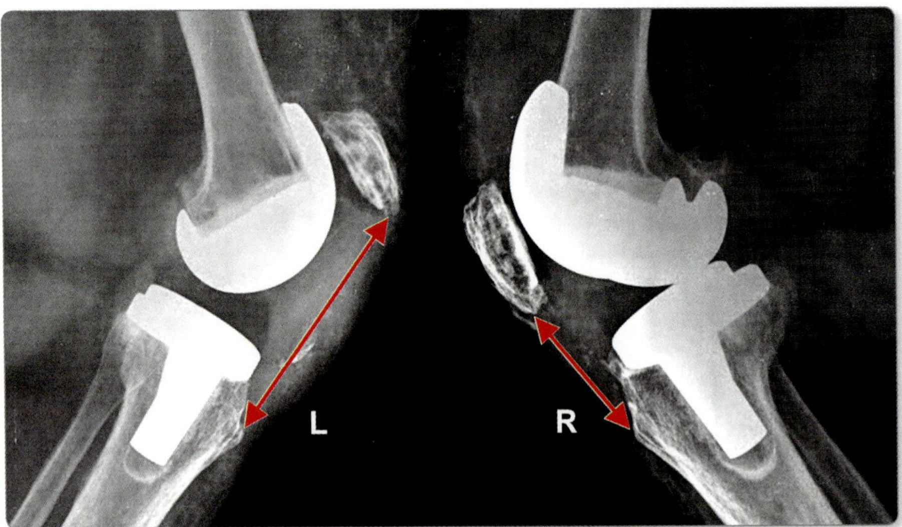

Fig. 5.34 X-ray left knee showing large gap due to tendon rupture as compared to right knee

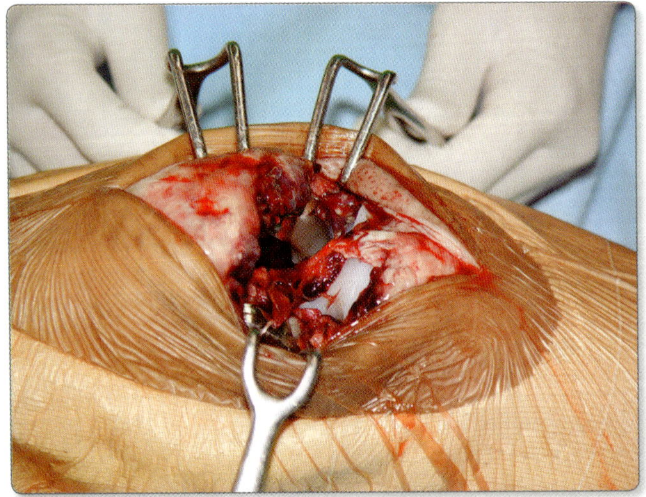

Fig. 5.35 Patellar tendon rupture

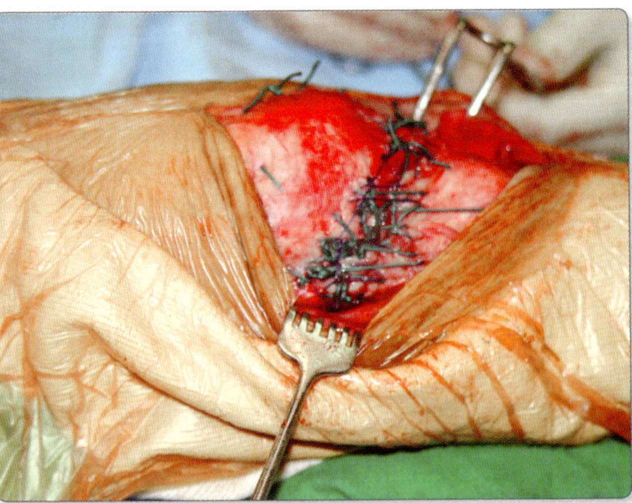

Fig. 5.36 Repaired by ethibond no. 5

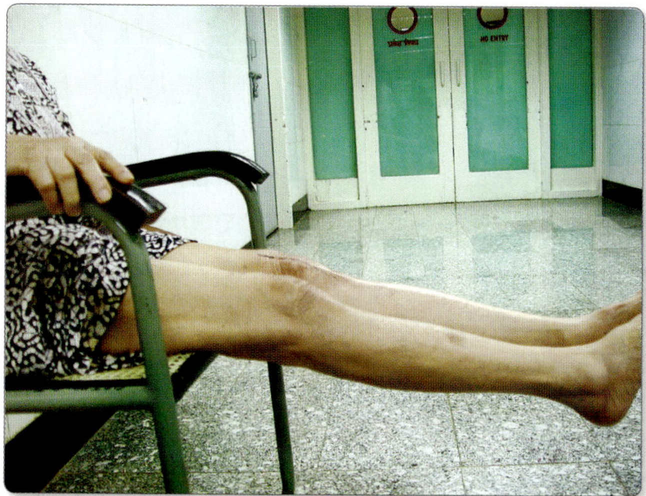

Fig. 5.37 Full extension

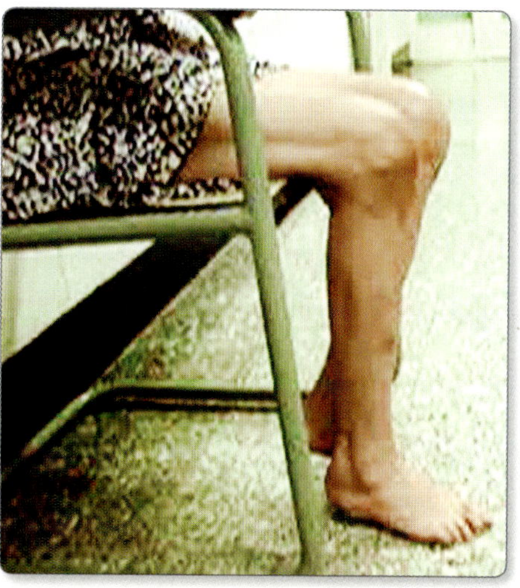

Fig. 5.38 Flexion up to 90°

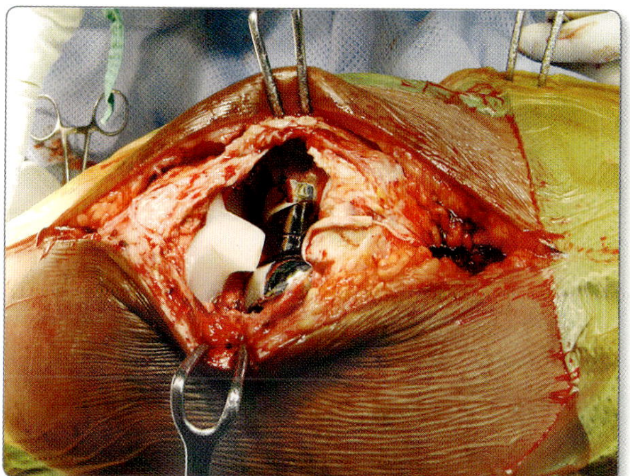

Fig. 5.39 Exposure of knee joint showing patellar tendon rupture

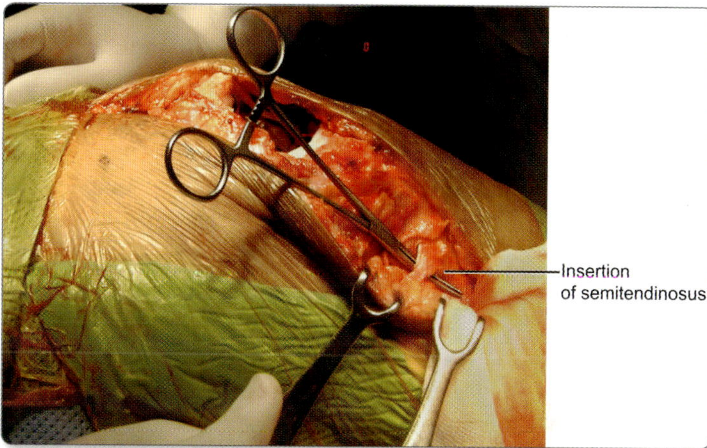

Fig. 5.40 Extension of incision to expose the insertion of semitendinosus

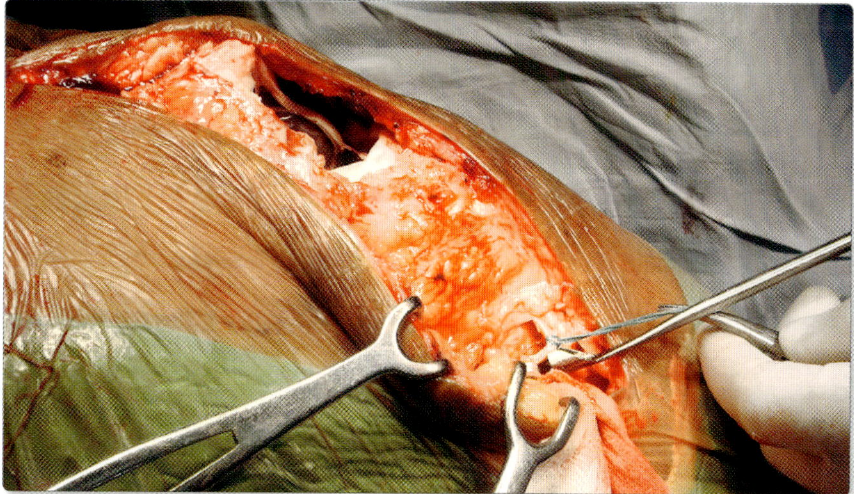

Fig. 5.41 Holding the tendon by ethibond and passing the open tendon stripper

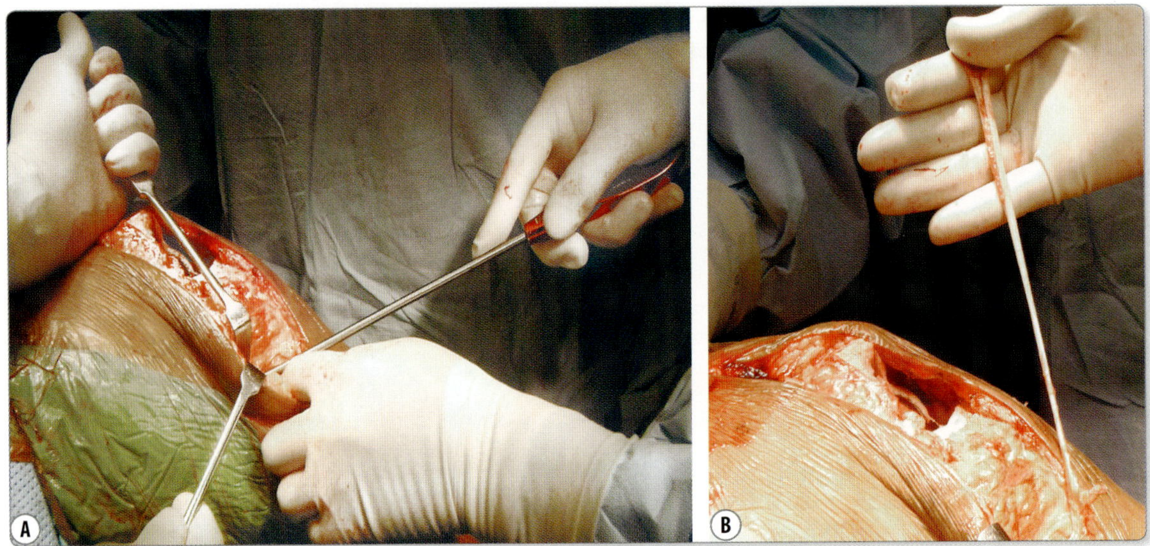

Figs 5.42A and B Stripping the tendon

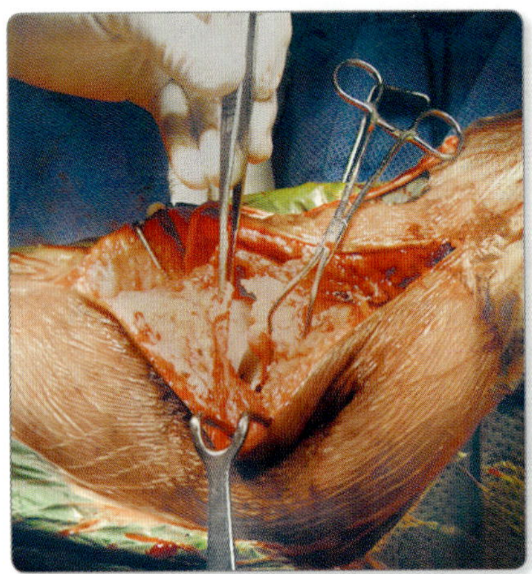

Fig. 5.43 Knee in extension

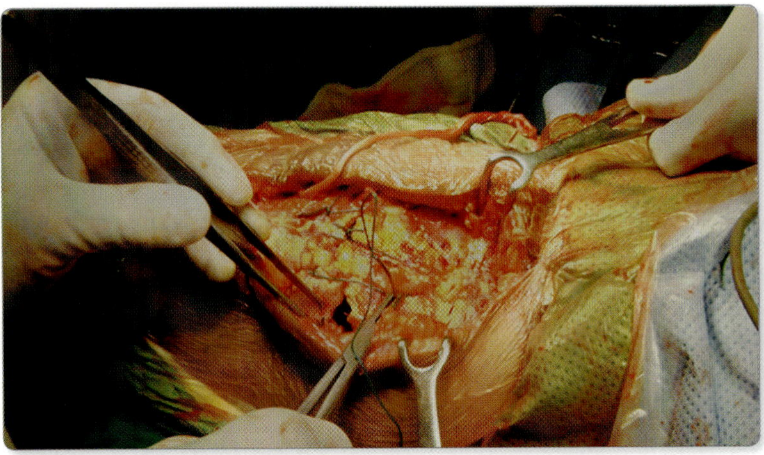

Fig. 5.44 Few stay sutures for maximum approximation of ends

Separate the muscle from the tendon with a periosteum elevator after putting the tendon on the back of kidney tray. Hold the proximal end of the tendon with Allis tissue forceps. Apply a whip stitch to this end of the tendon using ethibond no. 5. Keep the knee in extension by keeping the support (sand bag) underneath the ankle to approximate the rupture ends of extensor mechanism **(Fig. 5.43)**. Apply few stay sutures to bring the ruptured ends in maximum approximation **(Fig. 5.44)**. Few pie-crusting is done in quadriceps tendon to gain some length.

Take a guide wire with eye used during arthroscopic ACL reconstruction. Pass the ethibond through the eye of guide wire. Pass the guide wire along the medial border of patella and bring it out near the superior pole quite close to the bone. Pull the guide wire along with ethibond and subsequently semitendinosus tendon. Pass the guide wire from medial to lateral adjacent to the upper pole of patella through the quadriceps tendon and pull the tendon. Similarly pass the guide wire from superior pole to inferior pole on the lateral border of patella and subsequently the tendon. At every entry and exit point of tendon, fix the tendon by applying sutures of vicryl no.1 **(Fig. 5.45)**.

Make a drill hole by 3.2 mm drill bit from lateral to medial near the inferior part of tibial tubercle taking care to remain away from the stem of tibial tray **(Fig. 5.46)**. Pass the guide wire through this hole and subsequently pull the tendon through this drill hole. Take a deep stitch with another ethibond no. 5 near the insertion. Pull the patella

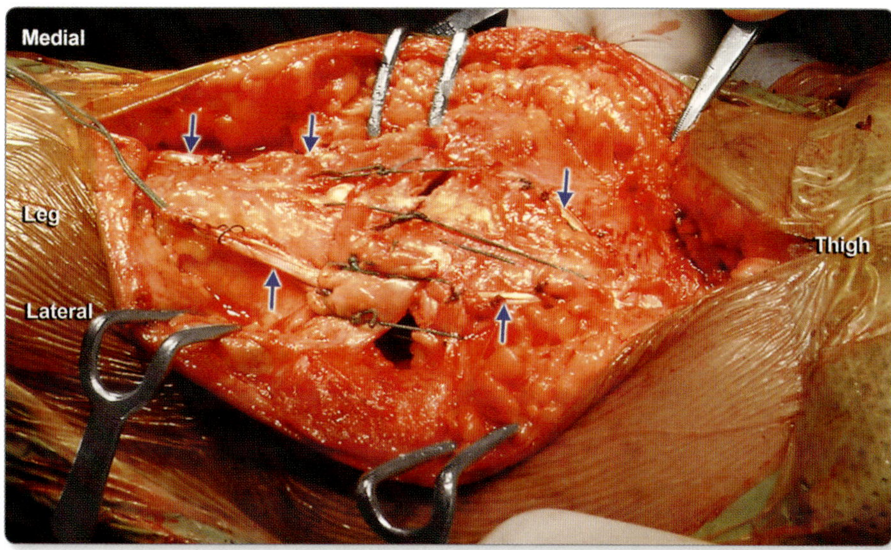

Fig. 5.45 Arrows showing passing of tendon from medial to lateral encircling the patella

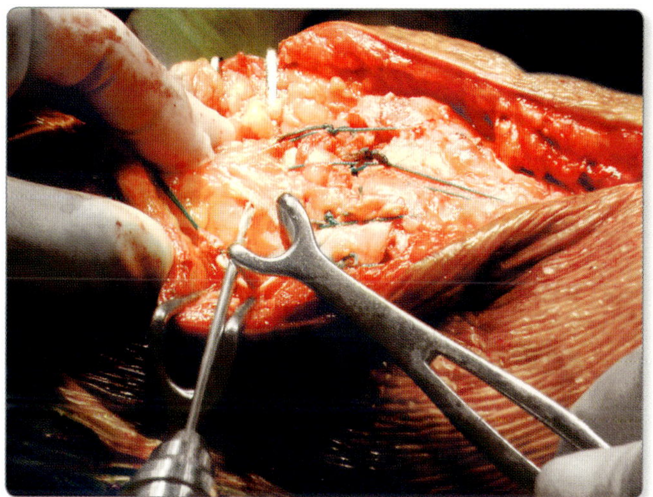

Fig. 5.46 Making a drill hole by 3.2 mm drill bit

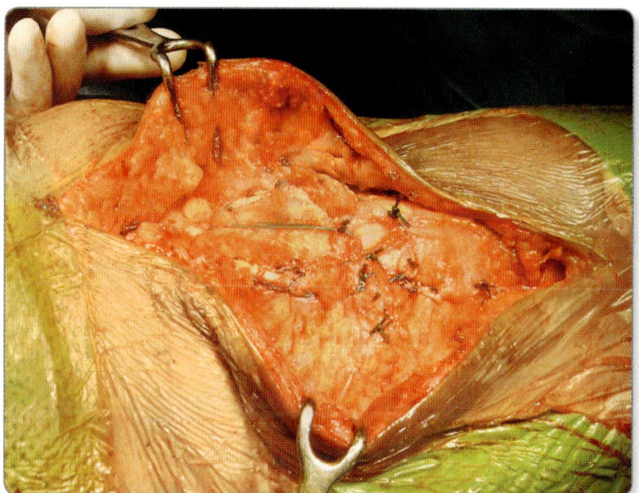

Fig. 5.47 After final repair

down by pulling the tendon through ethibond. Keeping the knee in extension, tie a knot between two ends of ethibond. Secure the tendon near the insertion by multiple stitches with vicryl no. 1. Repair the remnant of patellar tendon by double breasting with ethibind no. 5 **(Fig. 5.47)**. Close the wound in layers under suction drain. Apply the compression bandage.

Apply knee brace or cylinder cast for 6 weeks. Remove the suction drain after 48 hours and skin stitches after 2 weeks. Static quadriceps exercise has to be continued. After 6 weeks, remove the brace or cylinder cast and start gradual knee bending exercise.

Aseptic Loosening (Figs 5.48A and B)

It requires revision total knee replacement. It is sometimes difficult to differentiate aseptic from septic loosening. For aseptic loosening, one stage revision total knee replacement can be planned but for septic loosening two-stage revision TKR is the gold standard. However, one-stage revision TKR for loosening should be planned very cautiously. Recently PET (Positron emission tomography) scan is helpful in differentiating aseptic from septic loosening.

^{18}F-FDG PET (fluorine 18 fluorodeoxyglucose positron emission tomography): It uses fluorine 18 2-fluoro-2-deoxy-

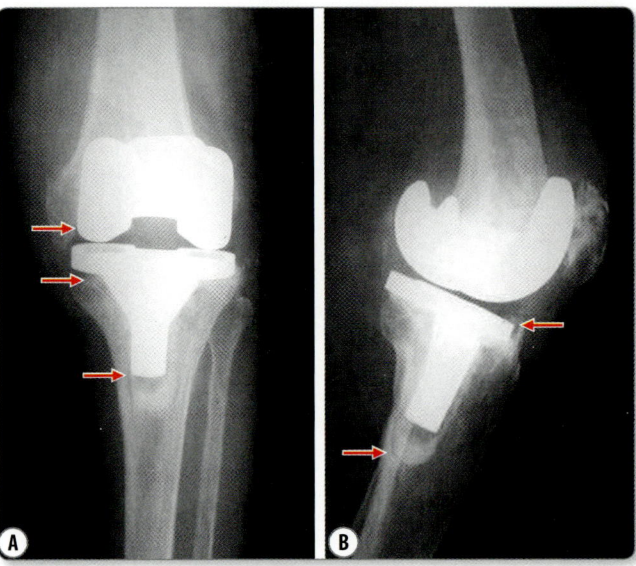

Figs 5.48A and B AP and lateral view X-rays—showing loosening (periprosthetic osteolysis) of the femoral and tibial components 4 years after TKR

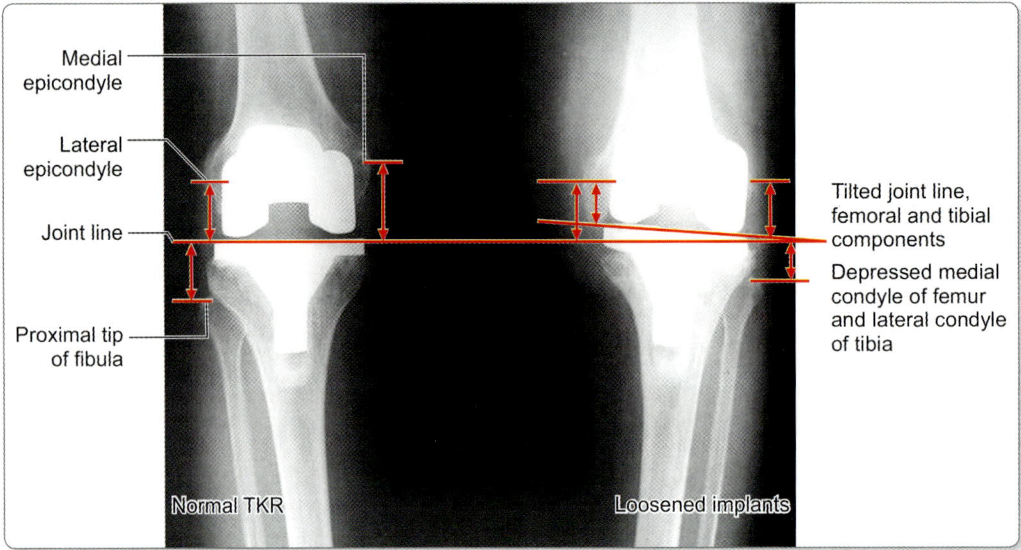

Fig. 5.49 AP view

D-glucose (FDG). Inflammatory cells have a high glucose demand. The detection of periprosthetic inflammation using[18] F-FDG PET has a sensitivity of 100% for septic cases. Because of the high sensitivity, a negative PET eliminates the infection and one stage revision TKR can be planned. In contrast, a positive PET result gives no clear differentiation regarding the cause of inflammation.

Revision TKR

Preoperative Planning for Revision TKR

Take full length standing X-ray of both lower limbs AP view, both knees lateral view and skyline view patella. Review previous X-rays of primary TKR and contralateral knee and compare with the present X-ray to assess the level of joint line, alignment, bone stock and implant fixation **(Figs 5.49 and 5.50)**. The joint line is approximately one fingerbreadth above the proximal tip of the fibula and one fingerbreadth distal to the inferior pole of the patella. It lies approximately 3 cm distal to the medial epicondyle and 2.5 cm distal to the lateral epicondyle.

Technical Difficulties

1. Bone loss
2. Soft-tissue deficiencies
3. Scarring
4. Flexion-extension gap imbalance
5. Changes in anatomic joint line

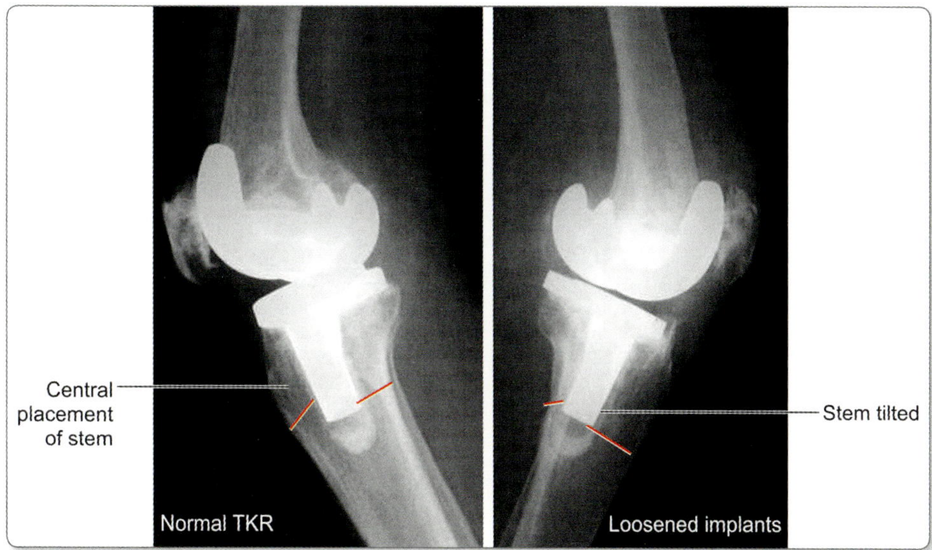

Fig. 5.50 Lateral view

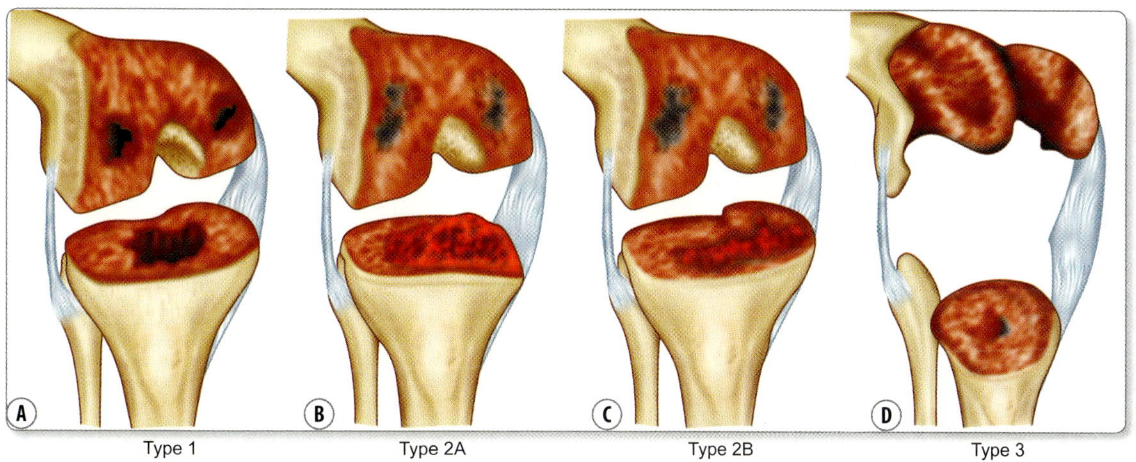

Figs 5.51A to D Classification of bone loss

Stress views are helpful in evaluating ligamentous instability and 3D CT is of value in cases of major bone loss. Failure of a total knee replacement is often associated with bone loss from either the proximal aspect of the tibia or the distal aspect of the femur. Classification of bone loss will help to anticipate the requirement of implants and bone grafts during revision surgery **(Figs 5.51A to D)**. Anderson Orthopedic Research Institute (AORI) classifies the femur (F) and tibia (T) as follows:

1. Type 1: **Intact** metaphyseal bone with minor defects which will not compromise the stability of a revision component.
2. Type 2: **Damaged** metaphyseal bone. Loss of cancellous bone in the metaphyseal segment which will need to be filled with cement, augments, sleeves or bone graft to restore the joint line. Defect can occur in one femoral condyle or tibial plateau (2A) or in both condyles or plateaus (2B).
3. Type 3: **Deficient** metaphyseal bone. Bone loss which comprises a major portion of either condyle or plateau. These defects are occasionally associated with detachment of the collateral or patellar ligaments and usually require structural bone graft, long-stemmed hinged implant (e.g. S-ROM Noiles rotating hinge knee system), metaphyseal sleeve or custom component.

The difference in primary and revision TKR is that in primary TKR, the laxity of knee is balanced by using a thicker plastic insert while in revision TKR, it is balanced by using larger femoral component with distal and posterior metal augmentation to avoid the joint line elevation.

Goals

1. Avoid joint line elevation.
2. Equalize flexion-extension gap.
3. Reconstruct bone defects.
4. Restore knee stability.
5. Maintain limb alignment.
6. Rigid fixation.

For achieving the above goals, there are various types of wedges and step augmentations, metaphyseal sleeves, and extension rods. Limb alignment is maintained by using femoral and tibial extension rods by using the medullary canal of femur and tibia as reference point.

Flexion and extension gap balance and joint line determination

	Flexion gap equals extension gap	Flexion gap > Extension gap	Extension gap > Flexion gap
Joint line—Normal	Adjust tibial insert thickness to achieve stability	Consider distal resection (small amount only); Beware of raising the joint line	Downsize femoral component or use –2 stem position
Joint line—elevated	Equal distal and posterior augmentation	Use larger femur, augment posterior condyles and consider a +2 stem position	Augment distal femur

Once the flexion-extension gaps are balanced and joint line is restored, the stability is achieved by adjusting the tibial insert thickness.

Techniques of Revision TKR

1. Standard condylar revision knee system—in cases of type 1 and 2A bone loss.
2. TC3 RP (rotating platform) and MBT (mobile bearing tibial) revision tray system (*TC3 RP system and metaphyseal sleeve fixation)*—in cases of Type 2A and 2B bone loss.
3. S-ROM Noiles rotating hinge knee system—in cases of Type 3 bone loss.

Standard Condylar Revision Knee System

Procedure

Preoperative advice, anesthesia, bladder catheterization, tourniquet application, positioning, dressing and draping are similar to primary TKR.

Midline skin incision is given over the previous scar with proximal extension for mobilization of extensor mechanism. Do not undermine the skin. Knee is opened by medial parapatellar incision. Make a periosteal sleeve at anteromedial, medial and posteromedial part of upper tibia. Eversion of patella is difficult due to lot of fibrosis. Remove the infrapatellar and suprapatellar fibrous tissue. Apply a hohmann around lateral femoral condyle to displace patella laterally without making any effort to evert it. Release the fibrous adhesions from the lateral gutter and margin of lateral tibial plateau by electrocautery. Put a pin over the tibial tubercle to avoid avulsion of patellar tendon. Evert the patella with knee in extension. Holding the patella in eversion, gradually flex the knee fully keeping the constant watch over the insertion of patellar tendon to avoid avulsion. If unable to evert the patella, then do lateral retinacular release. Even if there is difficulty in patellar eversion, a quadriceps snip, a proximal inverted quadriceps incision or a tibial tubercle osteotomy is done. For doing tibial tubercle osteotomy, extend the incision 10 cm distal to tibial tubercle and make a flap of proximal tibia anteriorly 1 cm thick and 8 cm long cutting by oscillating saw from medial aspect. It is hinged to the lateral periosteum. Keeping the patella in everted position, gradually flex the knee till the leg is perpendicular to the table. Remove the plastic insert by plastic insert remover. If the components are loose, remove the femoral, tibial and patellar components. Gigli saw is used for separation of the components from bone to avoid bone loss and iatrogenic fracture of condyles. Oscillating saw with a thin and flexible blade, osteotome, punch and hammer are used for gradual removal of tibial tray, femoral and patellar components. The osteotome is directed at the prosthesis-cement interface. After disruption of the fixation surfaces, the femoral component is removed with extraction device that uses a slap hammer which delivers longitudinal force to the component. Gently remove the bone cements. Assess the size of tibial tray and same size of femoral component is initially chosen.

Extend the knee. Evaluate the level of joint line. Usually the joint line is elevated. The normal joint line is approximately one fingerbreadth above the proximal tip of the fibula and one fingerbreadth distal to the inferior pole of the patella. It lies approximately 3 cm distal to the medial epicondyle and 2.5 cm distal to the lateral epicondyle. Remnant meniscus also determines the level of joint line. Assess the flexion-extension gap by series of spacer blocks which will indicate the requirement of prosthetic augmentation as per guideline given in the chart above to equalize the flexion-extension gap and to restore the joint line.

Tibial Cut

Flex the knee fully. Put a small curved Hohmann on the lateral aspect of tibial condyle to retract the everted patella. Put a small Hohmann on the medial aspect of tibial condyle also to retract the medial collateral ligament and soft tissues on the medial side. The canal is initially opened by 8 mm drill upto 2–4 cm. A small diameter reamer (10 mm) is introduced up to the predetermined depth and then sequentially opened with progressively larger reamers till snugly fitting (Sizes of reamers are 10 mm, 11 mm, 12 mm, 13 mm, 14 mm, 15 mm, 16 mm, 17 mm and 18 mm). Avoid over reaming in cases of osteoporosis. Reamers for tibial and femoral rods are same with different marking of tibial rod length and femoral rod length. (Tibial IM rods are available in 3 lengths—75 mm, 115 mm, 150 mm and diameter 10 mm, 12 mm, 14 mm, 16 mm). The intramedullary rod has three length markings for tibia, A-75 mm, C-115 mm and E-150 mm. Select the sleeve of predetermined length and corresponding to the size of the final reamer. The IM rod is inserted through the selected sleeve and advanced to the distal end. The T-handle is applied to the rod. The sleeve is rotated 180^0 clockwise on the rod and retracted towards the handle until locked in position. The rod and sleeve assembly is advanced into the medullary canal till the predetermined depth as indicated on the rod is aligned with the proximal surface of the tibia. After putting the sleeve, the IM rod is retracted about 15 mm and rotated 180° clockwise by the handle to disengage from the sleeve and advance the rod beyond the sleeve until its tip is engaged at the diaphyseal isthmus to increase the stability. Leave about 12 cm of rod extending out of the proximal tibia to accommodate the IM tibial alignment device. The T-handle is removed and the rod remains in place. Attach the 3° posterior sloped tibial cutting block with the IM tibial alignment device and apply over the IM rod and allow to descend to the proximal tibial surface keeping the center of the tibial cutting block on the medial third of the tibial tubercle. The assembly is locked in position with the lateral setscrew. The cutting block is advanced to the anterior tibial cortex and locked into position by tightening the knurled knob on the outrigger. Take the tibial stylus with slotted mark on the outrigger and insert the footplate of tibial stylus into the slot of tibial cutting block with height set at 2 mm on less deficient condyle while keeping the tip of outrigger at the center of tibial plateau for minimal resection. Fix the tibial cutting block with two pins introduced through the central holes marked with square. The IM alignment device is unlocked from the cutting block and IM rod with sleeve is removed from the tibia. Check the amount of cut with the help of visualization guide. Put the oscillating saw (1.25 mm thick saw blade No. 519.115) in the slot of tibial cutting block and resect the tibia. Lift the resected part of tibia with osteotome and remove it from soft tissue on posterior aspect with help of electrocautery keeping it adjacent to the resected bone. Apply the decided size of trial tibial tray with extension rod on the prepared surface of tibia and gently hammer to seat in position.

If there is bone defect in the tibia and require tibial augmentation, the bone defect preparation is delayed until after initial trial reduction is performed and exact rotational position of the tibial component is confirmed.

If full wedge resection is required, then assemble appropriate full wedge cutting guide to the outrigger of the IM tibial alignment device in place of tibial cutting block and adjusted to the level which cut minimum bone. Confirm the rotational alignment and advance to the anterior cortex of upper tibia and fix with pins through square holes. Alignment device, IM rod and sleeve are removed. Cut the tibia with oscillating saw keeping it flushed to the cutting surface.

Femoral Preparation

Keep the knee flexed fully. The femoral canal is initially opened by 8 mm drill upto 3–5 cm. A small diameter reamer (10 mm) is introduced up to the predetermined depth and then sequentially opened with progressively larger reamers until firm endosteal engagement is established (Sizes of reamers are 10 mm, 11 mm, 12 mm, 13 mm, 14 mm, 15 mm, 16 mm, 17 mm, 18 mm). Femoral IM rods are available in 2 lengths—125 mm, 175 mm and diameter 10 mm,12 mm, 14 mm, 16 mm, 18 mm with 5° and 7° valgus angles, bolts for fixing IM rod with femoral component—0 mm and 2 mm offset).

The intramedullary rod has three length markings for femur, B-125 mm stabilized fluted femoral stem, B-125 mm TC3 fluted stem, E-175 mm stabilized fluted stem and F-175 mm TC3 fluted stem. Select the sleeve of predetermined length and corresponding to the size of the final reamer. The IM rod is inserted through the selected sleeve and advanced to the distal end. The T-handle is applied to the rod. The sleeve is rotated 180° clockwise on the rod and retracted towards the handle until locked in position. The rod and sleeve assembly is advanced into the medullary canal till the predetermined depth as indicated on the rod is aligned with the distal surface of the femur. After putting the sleeve, the IM rod is retracted about 15 mm and rotated 180° clockwise by the handle to disengage from the sleeve and advance the rod beyond the sleeve until its tip is engaged at the diaphyseal isthmus to increase the stability. Leave about 12 cm of rod extending out of the distal femur to accommodate the femoral locating device. Attach the femoral locating device fixed at 5° or 7° valgus on operating side (R or L) over the IM rod advance to contact the distal femur. The calibrated outrigger is centered at the femoral trochlea and raised fully in relation to the prepared anterior surface. The distal femoral cutting block is assembled onto the calibrated outrigger by depressing the button located on the right proximal end. Adjust the distal femoral cutting block at 0 mm marked on the calibrated outrigger. The cutting block has slots to allow for a 0 mm, 4 mm, or 8 mm resection level. The outrigger and distal femoral cutting block is lowered onto the anterior cortex by depressing the button on left hand side of the locating device. Fix the distal femoral cutting block with two pins in the square marked holes. If bone is hard, make 2.5 mm drill before passing the pins. The distal femoral cutting block and outrigger are removed from the locating device. The locating device is removed from the IM rod. The distal femoral cutting block is removed from the outrigger and placed back over the Steinmann pins. The rod and sleeve remain in place. Check the amount of cut with the help of visualization guide. The assistant will retract the medial and lateral collateral ligaments and press the distal femoral cutting block with Kocher. Make the distal cut by oscillating saw (1.25 mm thick saw blade, No. 519.115) passed through the 0 mm marked slot in distal femoral cutting block. Little or no bone is resected from the distal femur. Remove the distal femoral cutting block. Take the revision A/P cutting block and assemble the appropriate 5° or 7°, 0 mm or +/– 2 mm offset bushing which corrects for the normal stem position at the selected femoral valgus angle and interior bone loss. Where indicated, the appropriate distal spacer (4, 8, 12, or 16 mm) is assembled to the proximal side of the cutting block to compensate for the condylar discrepancy as determined during spacer block assessment. The block is assembled onto the IM rod through the appropriate right/left opening and seated flush to the prepared distal surface. Apply the spacer block between the upper surface of trial tibial tray and posterior surface of the revision A/P cutting block in 90° flexion of knee and rotate the cutting block in such a way that there will be rectangular flexion gap and thus keeping the equal tension on medial and lateral ligaments. The rotational positioning of revision A/P cutting block is further confirmed by checking that the cutting block is parallel with the transepicondylar axis. Fix the cutting block with two pins. Set the stylus at 0 mm height, apply the foot-plate of the stylus in the anterior slot of the cutting block. The slotted marked arm of stylus will touch the anterior cortex. If there is obstruction then there are two options depending on the flexion gap. If the flexion gap is more than extension gap then use larger size femoral component and augment posterior condyle. If the flexion gap is less than extension gap then replace the 0 mm bushing in AP cutting block with +2/–2 mm bushing in the -2 mm position which translates the femoral component 2 mm anteriorly. If there is no obstruction to the arm of stylus then 0 mm bushing in AP cutting block is replaced with +2/–2 mm bushing in +2 position which translates the femoral component 2 mm posteriorly and hence, decreases the flexion gap by 2 mm. Remove the stylus. Where unilateral distal augmentation is required, keep the appropriate spacer between the block and the deficient condyle. Where bilateral distal augmentation is required, keep the larger spacer on more deficient condyle and apply two extra pins through the anterior holes for firm fixation of the cutting block. Check the amount of anterior and posterior cut by visualization guide. Do the anterior cut by oscillating saw (1.25 mm thick saw blade, No. 519.115) through the anterior slot and posterior cut through the posterior slot designated 0 mm. If there is posterior condylar deficiency, do posterior cut through the posterior slot designated 4 or 8 mm depending upon the amount of posterior augmentation.

Apply appropriate size trial spacer over the appropriate size notch cutting guide. Select the appropriate bushing right/left and 0 mm, +2 mm or -2 mm according to bushing used for A/P cutting block. Lock the bushing over the notch cutting guide by rotating the tabs anteriorly to the stop. The notch cutting guide is applied over the IM rod and advanced to the prepared distal surface. Fix it with 4 pins after making 2.5 mm drill holes. Sequence of putting pins is 1st pin in superolateral, 2nd pin in inferomedial, 3rd pin in superomedial and 4th pin in inferolateral, i.e. contralateral) to avoid rotation or tilt of femoral notch cutting guide. The notch and chamfer cuts are done with oscillating saw. Remove the bushing. Assemble the T-handle over the IM rod and remove the IM rod with sleeve. If TC3 femoral component has to be applied, do notch cut through the slot designated TC3 on anterior surface of the guide. Remove the pins and notch cutting guide.

Assemble the appropriate size trial femoral component with appropriate box. For making the femoral component box assembly, place the two outrigger tabs of the box trial into the recesses of the posterior condyles, insert the anterior tabs into the recesses of the anterior flange and turn the angled screw, located in the side of box until tight. Select the appropriate size (both length and diameter) extension rod, appropriate bolt (0, +2/–2 mm) and appropriate trial femoral stem collar assembly, 5° or 7°, corresponding to the bushing used on the A/P cutting block and the notch/ chamfer guide **(Figs 5.52 and 5.53)**. The direction of arrow over the bolt indicates the direction of stem which will be placed **(Figs 5.54 and 5.55)**. When the arrow is pointing to the anterior part of the femoral component the stem is shifted 2 mm anterior to the 0 mm position and thereby shifting the femoral component 2 mm posteriorly (+2 mm position) **(Figs 5.56 to 5.58)**. When the arrow is pointing to the posterior part of the femoral component the stem is shifted 2 mm posterior to the 0 mm position and thereby shifting the femoral component 2 mm anteriorly (–2 mm position) **(Fig. 5.59)**. The stem collar, 5° or 7° has left orientation and right orientation mark (5°L and 5°R, 7° L and 7°R) **(Figs 5.60 and 5.61)**. This mark has to be tallied with the marking facing the posterior trial femoral component.

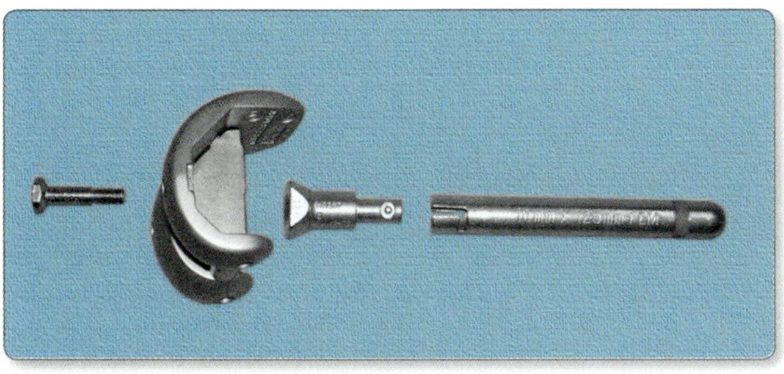
Fig. 5.52 Trial bolt, TC3 femoral component, femoral stem trial adapter and extension rod

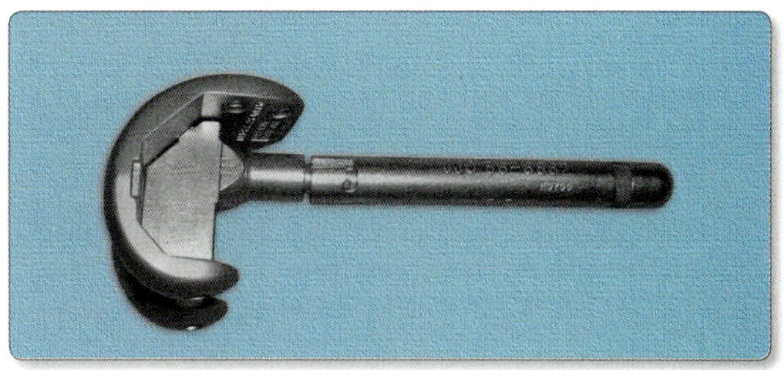
Fig. 5.53 After assembling the trial femoral component, femoral stem trial adapter with bolt and extension rod

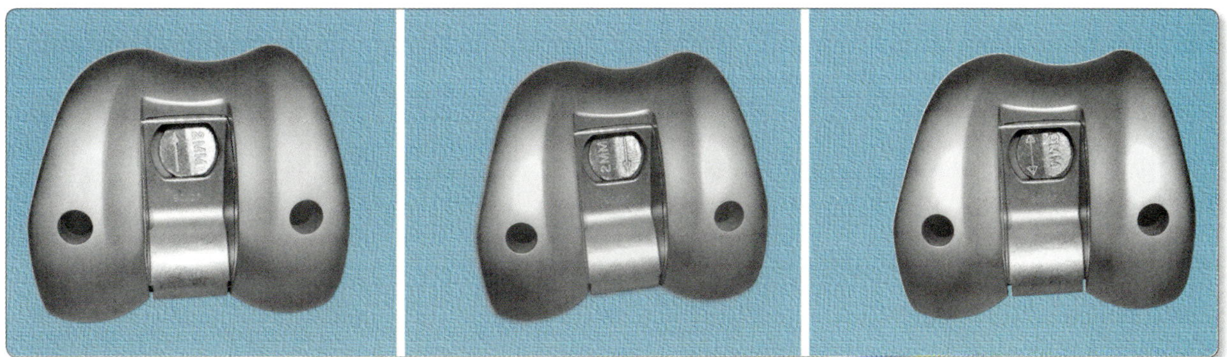
Fig. 5.54 Arrow indicates magnitude and direction of offset

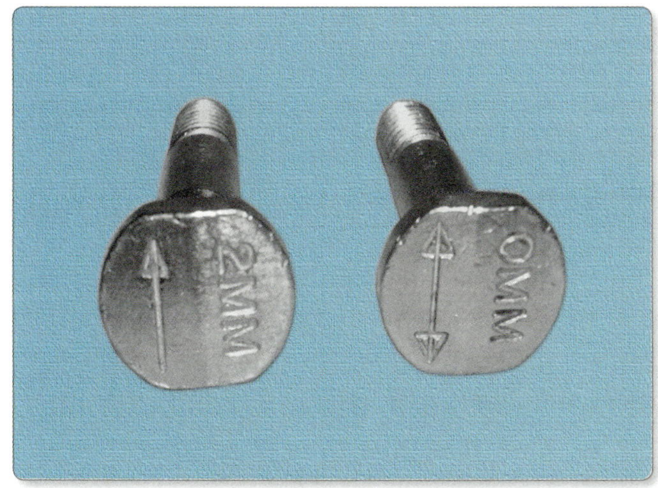

Fig. 5.55 Offset (± 2 mm offset) bolt

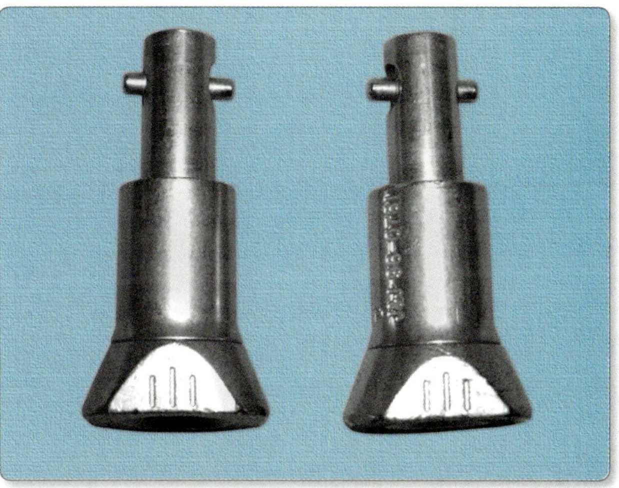
Fig. 5.56 Marks for verifying offset position

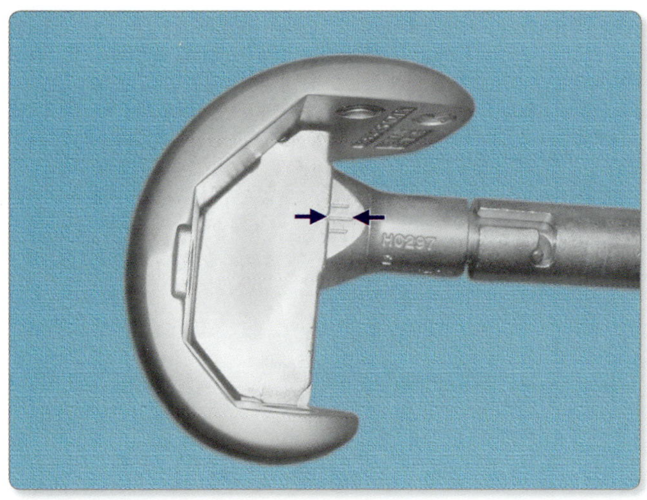

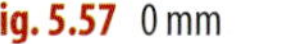

Fig. 5.57 0 mm

Fig. 5.58 +2 mm

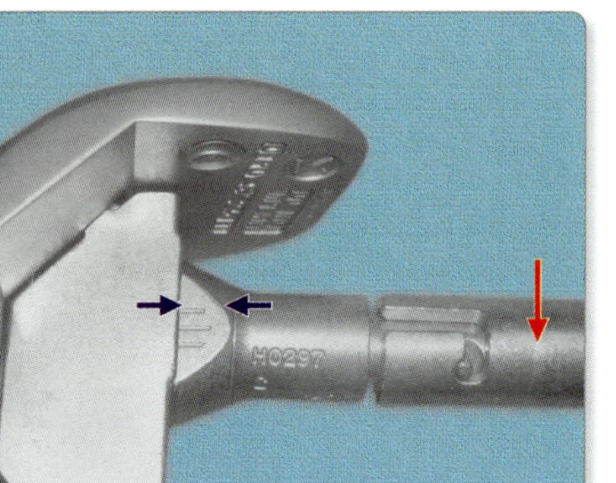

Fig. 5.59 –2 mm

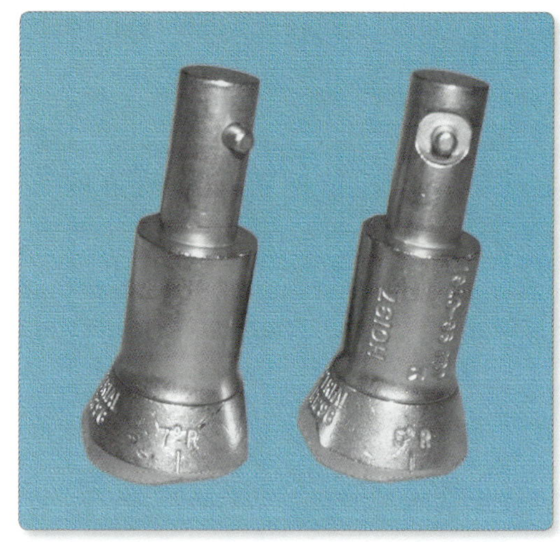

Fig. 5.60 Femoral stem trial adapter assembly (Right orientation marks)

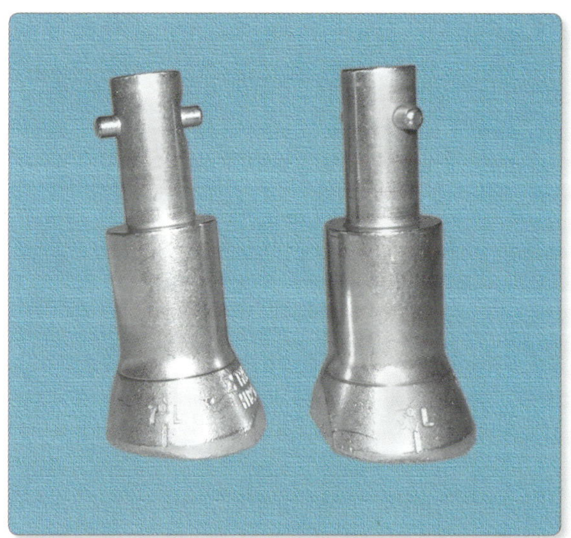

Fig. 5.61 Femoral stem trial adapter assembly (Left orientation marks)

The bolt is tightened with the trial femoral stem assembly by femoral trial assembly wrench.

Finally the proper assembly is checked by the direction of arrow of the bolt, alignment of the lateral side of the collar with the box trial and viewing the angle and right/left orientation tallies with the posterior trial femoral component **(Fig. 5.62)**. Apply the selected trial extension rod over the trial femoral component. Apply the appropriate size and thickness distal and posterior trial augmentation over the trial femoral component. The trial assembly is gently impacted over the femur. Apply the 10 mm appropriate size trial tibial insert over the trial tibial tray and joint is reduced and extended. The trial tibial tray will take the position according to kinematics of the knee which can further be adjusted by applying the tibial alignment handle with the tray and rotated into congruency with the femoral trial. Check the mediolateral stability both in extension, mid-flexion and flexion at 90° and correct the ligament balance accordingly. If lax, use thicker plastic insert or if tight then release the ligament. Check the flexion and extension gap and the restoration of anatomic joint line. Check the alignment with alignment rod passing through the hole in the tibial tray alignment handle attached with the tibial tray. This will pass through the centers of hip, knee and ankle. Usually the femoral component and tibial tray are of same size but sometimes one size down or up may be selected as per requirement. Remove the alignment rod. Mark by electrocautery over the anterior aspect of upper tibia in center and on medial according to the marks on the center of tibial tray alignment handle and trial tibial tray, respectively. Remove the tibial alignment handle.

Resurfacing of Patella

Remove the cement with thin osteotome and thin oscillating saw blade. Apply the patellar template which covers the resurfaced patella along the horizontal axis. Hammer the patellar template, hold it firmly and drill the holes for pegs of patellar implant. Apply the patella trial and check the patellar tracking. The patella trial should stay without holding it.

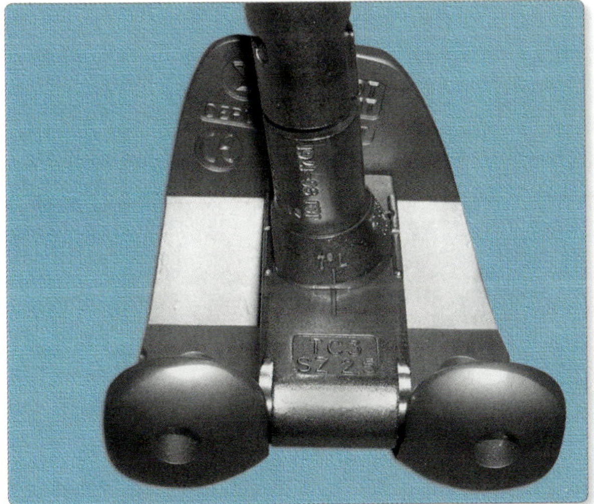

Fig. 5.62 Orientation system to verify angulation and left/right orientation

Tibial Preparation

Flex the knee fully. Remove the tibial insert with tibial insert remover. Apply the big Hohmann posterior to the upper tibia to dislocate the tibia anteriorly and two small Hohmann one on the medial and other on the lateral aspect. Hemiwedge or step resection is done depending upon the defect in upper tibia. After confirming the rotational alignment of the tibial tray stem trial with checking the electrocautery marks, fix the tibial tray by two short fixation pins. Appropriate hemiwedge (10° or 20°) or step (10 mm or 15 mm) cutting guide with appropriate cutting surface positioned at the deficient condyle is attached with wedge cutting attachment device and applied with trial tibial tray. The hemiwedge or step cutting guide is slided towards the anterior aspect of upper tibia and fixed with two pins passed through the holes marked with square. After fixing the cutting guide, it is unlocked and the assembly slides out of the cutting guide and the handle is disconnected from the trial tibial tray. Short fixation pins are removed. The trial tibial tray with extension rod is removed. Check the amount of cut with the visualization guide. Cut the hemiwedge or step with oscillating saw but the cut does not extend beyond the central riser. The cutting guide and pins are removed. The selected wedge or step is attached with the trial tibial tray and with extension applied over the tibia. Make the cut smooth with bone file where indicated to ensure maximal contact. Fix the trial tibial tray with two short fixation pins. Widen the bone area of slot of trial tibial tray by oscillating saw and osteotome to avoid shattering of upper tibia. The appropriate size revision tibial keel punch is positioned at the tray and impacted with hammer until the shoulder of the punch is in contact with the trial tibial tray. The keel punch is subsequently removed with slap hammer moving up. Apply the antifin over the trial tibial tray. Remove the short fixation pins. Apply the appropriate size and thickness of trial insert. Remove the small and big Hohmann. Reduce the knee joint and extend it.

Keep the vertical sand bag under the heel. Check the overall alignment, stability, movement and patellar tracking. If there is any instability, exchange the tibial insert trial with the next greater thickness and repeat reduction. Select the insert that gives the greatest stability in flexion and extension and allowing full extension. Flex the knee. Remove the insert with insert remover. Apply the big hohmann posteriorly to the upper tibia to dislocate anteriorly. Apply small hohmanns on medial and lateral aspect of upper tibia. Remove the trial tibial tray assembly.

Remove the hohmanns and trial femoral component box assembly. Make some drill holes by 2.5 mm drill bit in the hard area of the bone for better penetration of the cement. Thoroughly wash with pulse lavage (Normal saline mixed with Gentamicin).

If the tourniquet time exceeds 2 hours, then deflate the tourniquet for 15 minutes to take place the complete blood perfusion and re-inflate the tourniquet.

Assembling the Prosthesis

For preparing the tibial component assembly, hold the appropriate tibial tray with tibial holding clamp. Remove the plastic plug from the lower end of the tibial tray. Extension rod is held with press-fit rod wrench and completely tightened with the tibial tray. Remove the tibial holding clamp and press-fit rod wrench. After locking the stem in position, assemble the wedge or step augmentation. Remove the plastic plug from the modular plus tibial tray by plug puller. The selected wedge or step is assembled to the tibial tray and fixed by the screws with modular plus torque driver attached with torque driver handle extension till the click sound is heard indicating permanent interlock **(Figs 5.63A and B)**. For preparing the femoral component assembly, hold the box of appropriate femoral component with femoral holding clamp. Hold the appropriate extension rod with press-fit rod wrench and apply over the femoral component and fixed with bolt keeping the arrow on the bolt pointing to the required position as decided. Check that the lateral side of the collar and the femoral box are aligned and angle and orientation are viewed from the posterior end of the femoral component. After assembling the rod, install the posterior and distal augmentation and fix the augmentation by wobble hex bit with torque driver. The torque driver is turned until an audible click is heard, ensuring a full and permanent interlock **(Figs 5.64A and B)**.

Cementing, final insert selection and application, closure of the wound and post-operative advice are similar to primary TKR. Bone cement is applied carefully so that it should not enter in the medullary canal.

If tibial tubercle osteotomy has been done, then reattach the tibial tubercle with 2 or 3 wires. Drill holes are made in

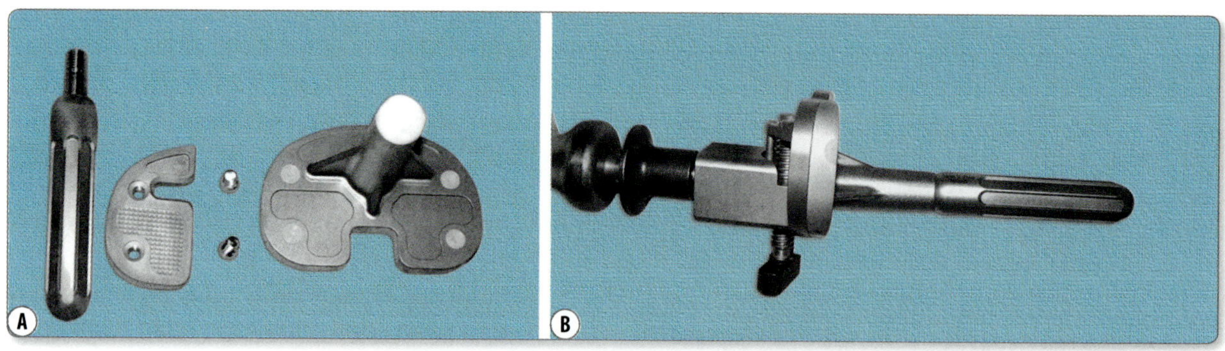

Figs 5.63A and B Extension rod, wedge, screws, modular plus tibial tray before and after assembly

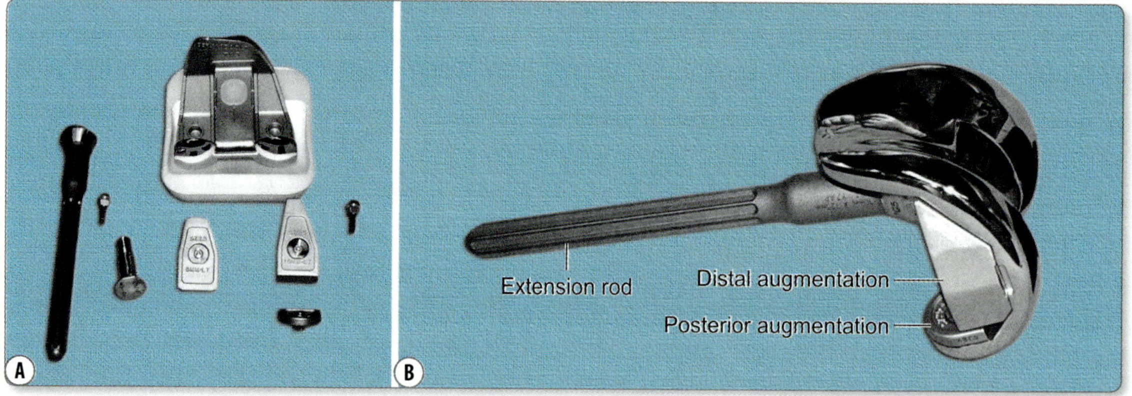

Figs 5.64A and B TC3 femoral component, extension rod, femoral stem bolt, distal and posterior femoral augmentations before and after assembly and wobble hex bit

medial tibia little distally and corresponding drill holes are made in lateral aspect of tibial tubercle fragment. After passing the wires, tibial tubercle is rotated back into its bed and the wires are tightened keeping the knots on medial side. As the drill holes in medial tibia is slightly distally, the wire passed is at 45° angle to long axis of tibia and this gives tension effect to wires and enhances stability of fixation. Postoperative knee mobilization is slow to protect the tibial tubercle osteotomy. Only active and assisted flexion and passive extension is allowed in the beginning. Active extension and straight leg raise are not allowed for 6 weeks.

Implants Required during Revision TKR

1. Stabilized femoral components—1.5, 2, 2.5, 3, 4, 5—right and left.
2. TC3 femoral components (2 mm more depth of box than the box of stabilized femoral component)—2, 2.5, 3, 4—right and left.
3. Modular plus tibial tray component—2, 2.5, 3, 4.
4. Tibial insert:
   i. Posterior stabilized—8, 10, 12.5, 15, 17.5 and 20 mm.
   ii. Stabilized plus—10, 12.5, 15, 17.5, 20 and 22.5 mm.
   iii. TC3—10, 12.5, 15, 17.5, 20 and 22.5 mm.
5. Femoral augmentation component:
   i. Posterior augmentation:
      - 4 mm and 8 mm for sizes 2, 2.5, 3, 4, 5.
      - 4 mm only for size 1.5.
   ii. Distal augmentation for right and left:
      - 4 mm, 8 mm, 12 mm,16 mm for sizes 2, 2.5, 3, 4, 5.
      - 4 mm, 8 mm, 12 mm for size 1.5.

   Note:
   i. For size 1.5 femoral component, if distal augment has to be used with posterior augment, then install the posterior augment first.
   ii. If 4 mm or 8 mm distal augment has to be used with posterior augment, then install the distal augment first. The 4 mm and 8 mm distal augmentations are fully interchangeable.
   iii. If 12 mm or 16 mm distal augmentation has to be used with posterior augment, then install the posterior augment first.
   iv. With 12 mm and 16 mm distal augment, femoral stem is indicated.
   v. 16 mm distal augmentation is used with TC3 femoral component only.
   vi. If 12 mm or 16 mm distal augmentation has to be used with size 2, 2.5, 3 femoral components, then use 4 mm posterior augment.
   vii. If 12 mm or 16 mm distal augmentation has to be used with size 4, 5 femoral components, then use either 4 mm or 8 mm posterior augment.
6. Tibial wedges—Modular plus tibial wedges
   i. Half wedges and steps:
      Size 2-10° Hemi × 8 mm height (Ht)
      20° Hemi × 13 mm Ht
      10 mm step, 15 mm step
      Size 2.5-10° Hemi × 8 mm Ht
      20° Hemi × 13.5 mm Ht
      10 mm step, 15 mm step
      Size 3-10° Hemi × 8.5 mm Ht
      20° Hemi × 14.5 mm Ht
      10 mm step, 15 mm step
      Size 4-10° mm Hemi × 9 mm Ht
      20° Hemi × 15 mm Ht
      10 mm step, 15 mm step
   ii. Full wedges:
      Size 2-10° Full × 15 mm Ht
      15° Full × 20 mm Ht
      Size 2.5-10° Full × 15.5 mm Ht
      15° Full × 21 mm Ht
      Size 3-10° Full × 16 mm Ht
      15° Full × 21.5 mm Ht
      Size 4-10° Full × 17 mm Ht
      15° Full × 23 mm Ht.
7. Extension rods:
   i. Tibial IM rods (Fluted tibial stem) are available in 3 lengths—75 mm, 115 mm, 150 mm and diameter 10 mm, 12 mm, 14 mm and 16 mm.
   ii. Femoral IM rods (Fluted femoral stem) in 2 lengths—125 mm, 175 mm and diameter 10 mm,12 mm, 14 mm, 16 mm, 18 mm with 5° and 7° valgus angles.
   iii. Bolts for fixing IM rod with femoral component—0 mm and 2 mm offset.
8. Oval dome patella:
   Size—32 mm (8 mm thick), 35 mm (8.5 mm thick), 38 mm (9 mm Thick) and 41 mm (11.5 mm thick)
   CMW1 Gentamicin—40 g and 20 g.

Instruments Required for Revision TKR (Figs 5.65 and 5.66)

Tibial peg trial
Torque driver handle extension
Modular plus torque driver
Wedge cutting tibial attachment device
IM tibial alignment device
Plug puller
Anti-fin
Full wedge trials 100 and 200
Tibial holding clamp
Step trial 10 and 15 mm
Full wedge cutting blocks
Step wedge cutting block
Tibial fluted Rod trial
Hemiwedge trials 10° and 20°
Modular plus wedge trial screw driver
Hemiwedge cutting block

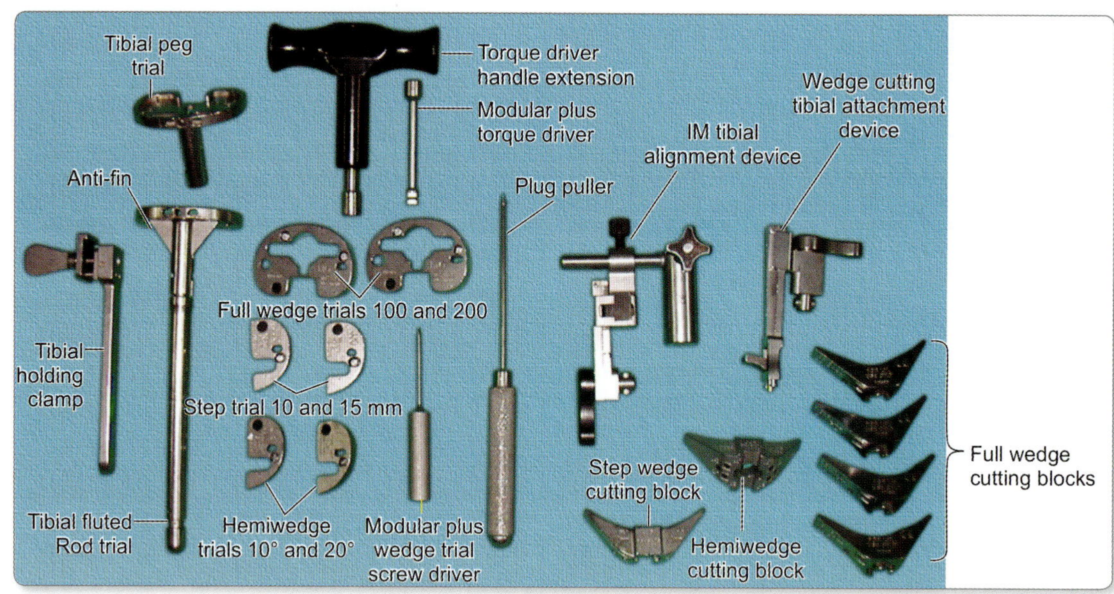

Fig. 5.65 Instruments required for application of extension rod, wedges and steps with tibial tray
Abbreviation: IM, intramedullary

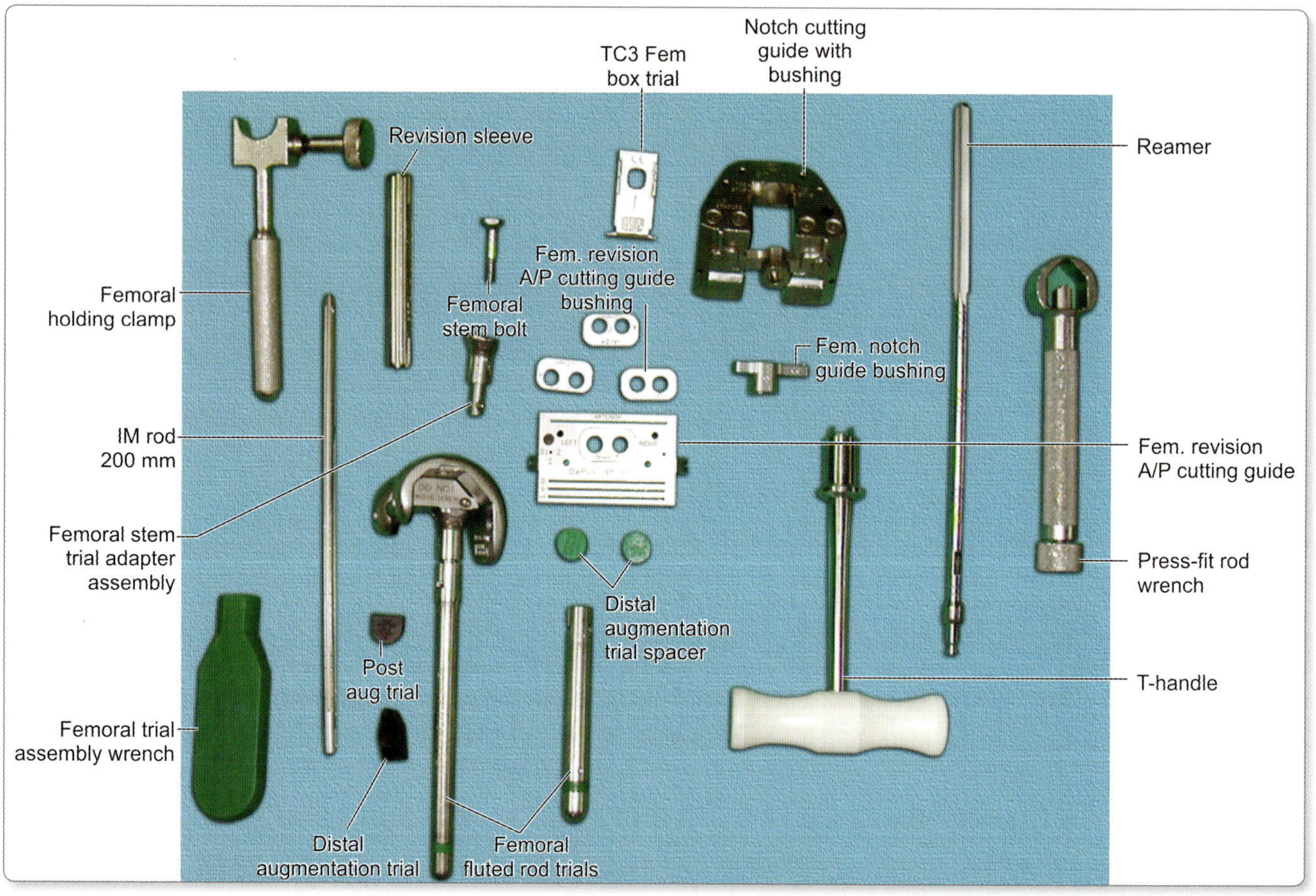

TC3 Fem box trial
Notch cutting guide with bushing
Revision sleeve
Reamer
Fem. revision A/P cutting guide bushing
Femoral holding clamp
Femoral stem bolt
Fem. notch guide bushing
IM rod 200 mm
Fem. revision A/P cutting guide
Femoral stem trial adapter assembly
Press-fit rod wrench
Distal augmentation trial spacer
Post aug trial
T-handle
Femoral trial assembly wrench
Distal augmentation trial
Femoral fluted rod trials

Fig. 5.66 Instruments required for application of extension rod with femoral component and femoral augmentation
Abbreviations: Fem, femoral; A/P, anteroposterior; Aug, augmentation

Two-stage Revision TKR for Late Infections (Figs 5.67 to 5.74)

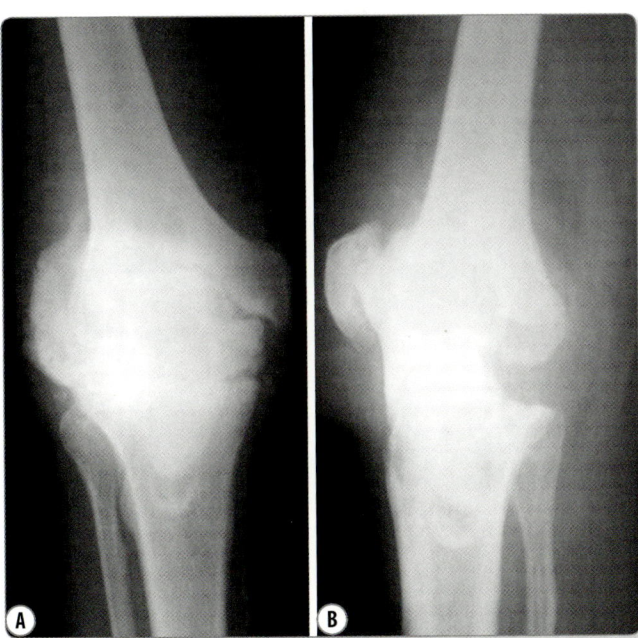

Figs 5.67 Stage 1—Application of antibiotic (gentamicin and vancomycin) impregnated static cement spacer

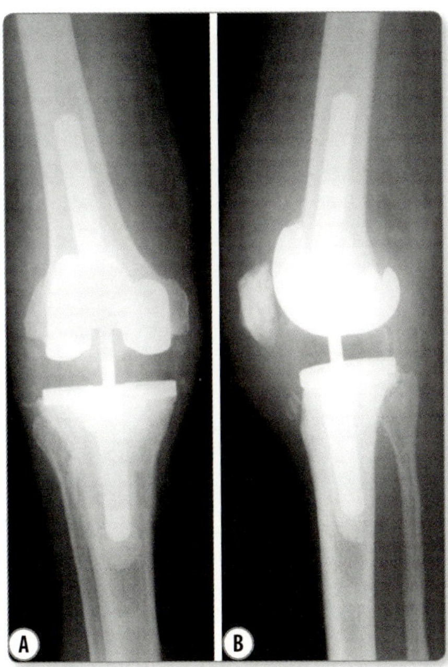

Figs 5.68A and B Stage 2—Revision TKR by standard condylar revision knee system for type 1 defect

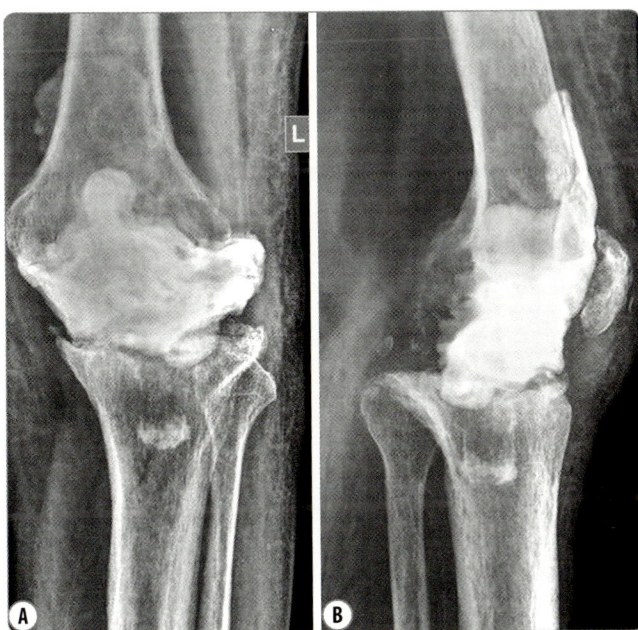

Figs 5.69A and B Stage 1 revision TKR

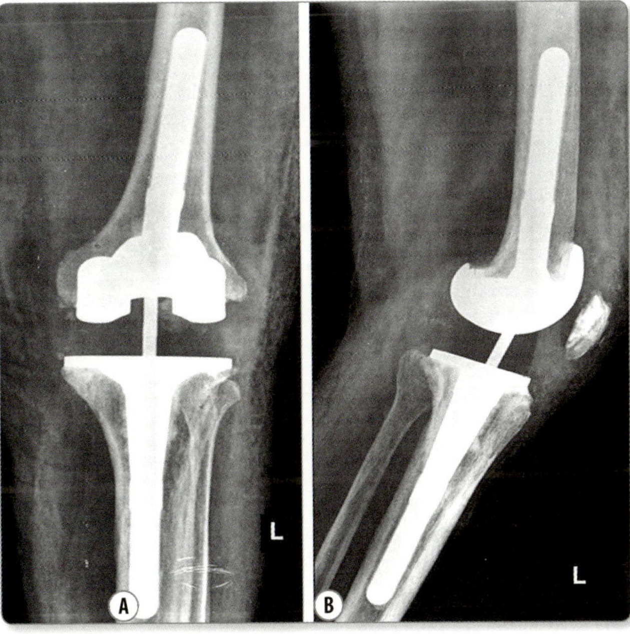

Figs 5.70A and B Stage 2 revision TKR by standard condylar revision knee system for type 2A defect after control of infection

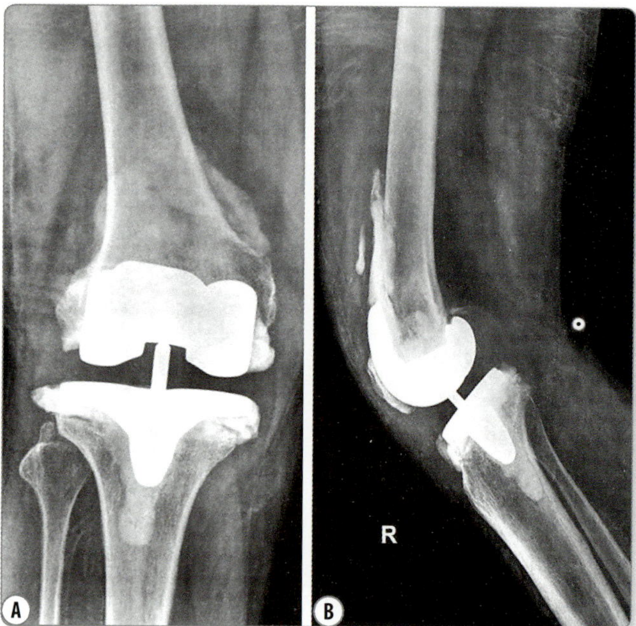

Figs 5.71 A and B Stage 1 with dynamic articulating spacer

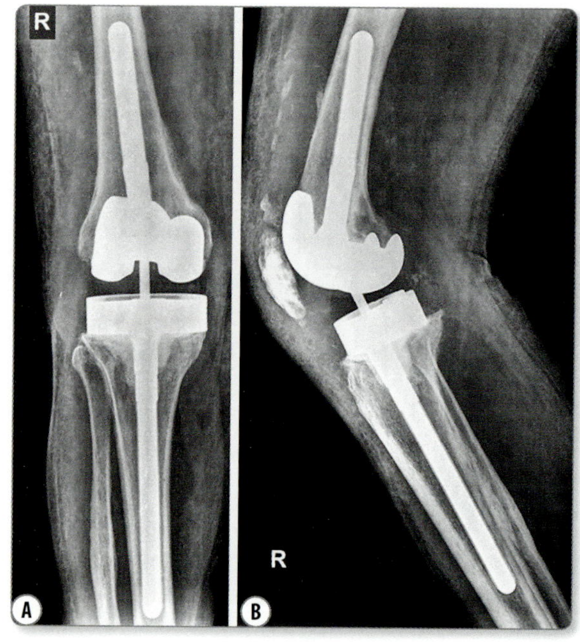

Figs 5.72 A and B Stage 2 revision TKR by standard condylar revision knee system

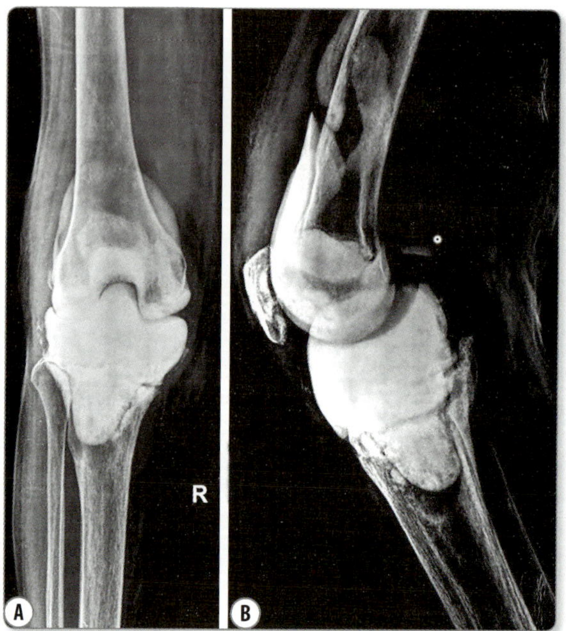

Figs 5.73A and B Stage 1 TKR with dynamic cement spacer

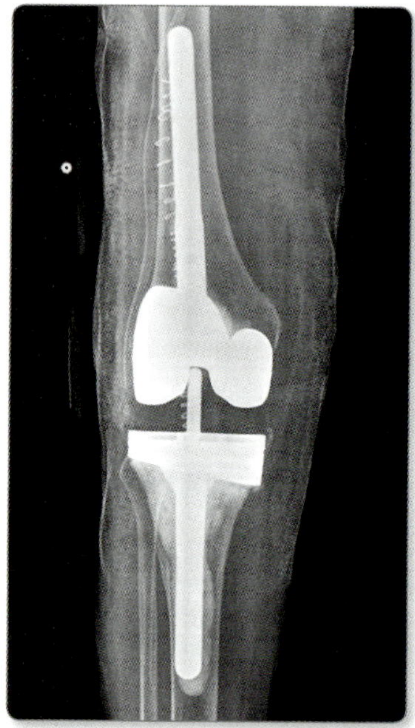

Fig. 5.74 Stage 2 revision TKR by standard condylar revision knee system with full wedge

TC3 RP and MBT Revision Tray System (TC3 RP System and Metaphyseal Sleeve Fixation)

Fixation modalities currently available for revision TKR implants include those for the distal femoral and proximal tibial bone surface, as well as the bones' diaphysis and metaphysis.

This system offers rotating platform to minimize post wear and reduce loosening forces and use of metaphyseal sleeves on femoral and tibial side provide implant stability. The design of the rotating-platform mobile-bearing knee translates complex input motion into more unidirectional motion, resulting in a reduced wear rate due to decreased shear in the polyethylene. In published studies, a mobile bearing construct has been shown to decrease loosening forces by 68–73% and reduction in wear by 94%. Acting as a universal tray, it is compatible for all rotating platform inserts from primary, constrained and hinged inserts. This MBT revision tray accepts fluted and cemented stems, step wedges and metaphyseal sleeves and its universal cone allow upsizing and downsizing between insert and tray.

MBT revision tray can be used in all defects. It can be used with:

1. Metaphyseal sleeve alongwith fluted tibial rod.
2. Step wedge alongwith fluted tibial rod or cemented stem.
3. Cemented stem.

The metaphyseal sleeves compressively load the bone to form a strong foundation, avoiding excessive bone resection and aid in preserving true joint line restoration. Metaphyseal sleeves are modular and provide optimal fit and fill of cavitary bone defects with excellent stability and equal stress distribution. All improved metaphyseal fixation methods aim to create a better cemented or uncemented interface with bone. The sleeves are textured with beads (porous coated) allowing for possibility of bone ingrowth. The sizes of tibial sleeves are 29, 37, 45, 53 and 61 mm (M/L) with 20° internal or external rotation. The sizes of femoral sleeves are 37, 45, 53 and 61 mm (M/L).

Tibial step wedges are universal for use on medial, lateral or both sides and may be downsized to prevent overhang. These are available in 5, 10 and 15 mm thickness in all sizes.

Tibial stems—cemented tibial stems are 30 and 60 mm lengths of diameter 13 mm and fluted tibial rods are 75, 115 and 150 mm lengths of diameters 10 through 24 mm in 2 mm increments.

The MBT revision tray will accept either a tibial metaphyseal sleeve or tibial step wedge if using sleeve sizes 37, 45, 53 and 61 mm, but not both. Sleeves and wedges can only be used together if using a 29 mm sleeve. It is imperative to assemble the sleeve or step wedge prior to stem attachment.

Procedure

Exposure of knee, removal of spacer, assessment of level of joint line, joint space and bone loss, opening and reaming the medullary canal is similar as described for standard condylar revision knee system. The steps differ in preparation of the metaphyseal bone by tapered reamer and broach.

Tibial Preparation for Metaphyseal Sleeve

Attach the T-handle on the top of tapered reamer and the appropriately sized stem trial to the end of the reamer. Use tapered reamer to the planned proximal tibial resection level. Decide the use of metaphyseal sleeve or step wedge peroperatively depending upon the loss of metaphyseal bone. Do not reverse ream while removing the reamer to avoid stem trial disengagement. Attach the MBT revision roach handle to the smallest broach and then attach the appropriately sized stem trial. As the broaches are asymmetrical, position the "ANT" written surface of broach anteriorly and insert into and then out of the tibia until the top surface of the broach is at the desired proximal tibial resection level. Check for the rotational stability. If the broach is unstable or the defect is unfilled, repeat with consecutively larger broaches until the desired fit is achieved **(Fig. 5.75)**. Leave the last broach in place and remove the broach handle. Resect the proximal tibia parallel to the top of broach which has 2° inbuilt posterior slope. Slide the tibial view plate (which is transparent and visualize the tibial coverage) which best covers the proximal tibia over the broach post. Note the view plate size, as it will dictate the size of tibial base plate.

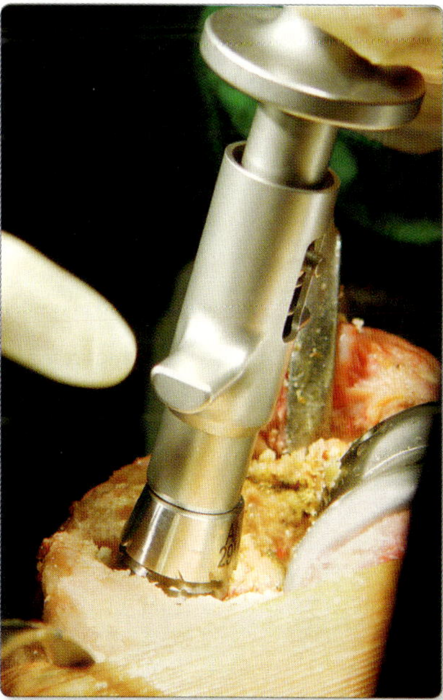

Fig. 5.75 Broaching of tibia for metaphyseal sleeve

Joint Space Assessment

The joint space is evaluated with spacer blocks to determine the flexion-extension gaps. Balance the flexion and extension gaps and restore the joint line as per chart.

Femoral Preparation for Metaphyseal Sleeve

1. Reaming of medullary canal
2. Reaming of metaphysis
3. Broaching of metaphysis
4. Femoral cuts - distal, anterior, chamfer and box cuts
5. Femoral trial

Femoral preparation involves reaming the canal and metaphysis to size **(Fig. 5.76)**, broaching with sized medullary pilots to metaphyseal fill **(Fig. 5.77)** and bone cuts made off the stem-sleeve aligned guides. Attach the pilot shaft with femoral sleeve trial and assemble with TC3 femoral component trial by femoral sleeve adapter trial and femoral bolt trial. Use wedge trial spacer whenever required. Remove the broach and apply the femoral component, sleeve and pilot shaft trial assembly over the prepared femur for trial reduction. The trial assembly is gently impacted over the femur.

Attach the alignment handle with appropriate size MBT tibial trial and apply over the broach. Put appropriate size and thickness of trial insert. Reduce the joint and place the knee in full extension and determine appropriate rotation of the tibial tray. The trial tibial tray will take the position according to kinematics of the knee which can further be adjusted by applying the tibial alignment handle with the tray and rotated into congruency with the femoral trial. Mark the appropriate rotation with electrocautery on the anterior tibial cortex at the center and sides of the alignment handle.

Resurfacing of patella is done as described for standard condylar revision knee system.

Flex the knee. Remove the insert and trial tibial tray alongwith alignment handle. Apply the hohmann posteriorly to dislocate the tibia anteriorly. Remove the broach alongwith pilot shaft. Assemble the tray trial with stem, sleeve trial and tibial rod trial. Position the assembly into the prepared tibial canal. Sleeve trial allows 20° of rotation. Assess the proximal tibial coverage and rotation of tibial component. Impact the appropriate keel punch. Disconnect the universal handle, leaving the keel punch in place for trial reduction.

Remove the trial component from tibia and femur. Make multiple drill holes in the hard area of bone. Thoroughly cleanse the site with gentamicin mixed nomal saline by pulse lavage.

Assembling the Prosthesis

Place the MBT revision tray on a firm, stable, padded surface. Set the tibial sleeve in an orientation that matches the prepared canal. Matching the orientation of the tray/sleeve trial is helpful in determining appropriate rotation of the final tibial tray/sleeve implant. The sleeve can rotate 20° internally or externally. Using the sleeve impactor and a mallet, impact the sleeve onto the MBT revision tray. Deliver several strikes to engage the two components.

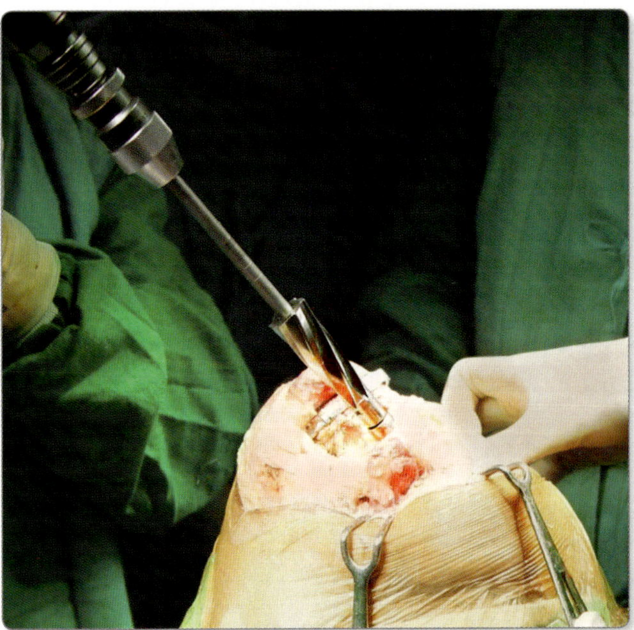

Fig. 5.76 Femoral reaming for metaphyseal sleeve

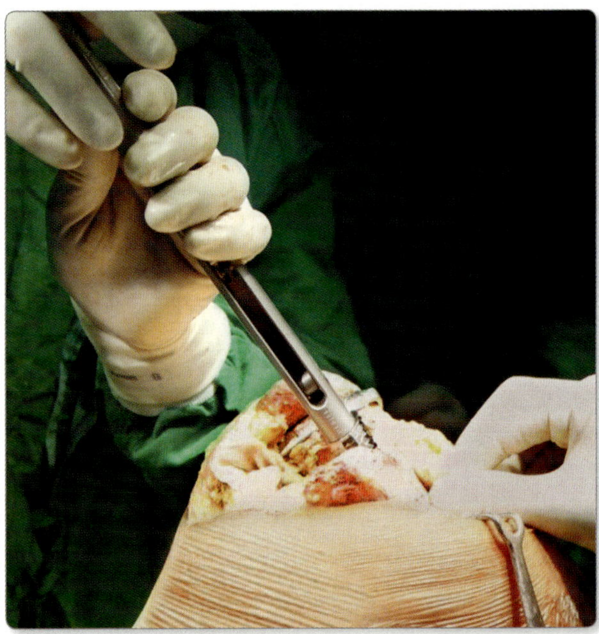

Fig. 5.77 Femoral broaching for metaphyseal sleeve

Hold the stem of MBT revision tray by revision femoral/tibial/sleeve clamp and attach the stem extension by pressfit rod wrench to ensure full engagement. Hold the Femoral sleeve by Revision femoral/tibial/sleeve clamp and attach the fluted tibial rod by press-fit rod wrench to ensure full engagement. Sleeve with extension rod is attached with femoral component by femoral adapter and bolt. After assembling the rod, install the appropriate augmentations and fix the augmentation by wobble hex bit with torque driver. The torque driver is turned until an audible click is heard, ensuring a full and permanent interlock.

Cementing

Apply the bone cement to the underside of the patellar implant, femoral component and tibial tray. Apply the bone cement on the resected surface of patella and apply the patellar implant with patellar clamp. Apply the bone cement on the surface of femur. Put the femoral component assembling on prepared femur and pressurize it first by thumb and palm and then by femoral impactor and gentle blow of hammer. Remove the extruded cement. Apply a Hohmann on the posterior aspect of upper tibia to dislocate it anteriorly. Apply bone cement to the proximal tibial surface and put the tibial tray assembly in proper orientation on the prepared tibia by manual pressure. Put a swab over the tibial tray in order to protect the bearing surface. Place the MBT tray impactor and deliver several gentle blows. Remove the extruded cement by curette. Bone cement is applied carefully so that it should not enter in the medullary canal. Apply the revision trial post into the cone of the MBT revision tray. Seat the appropriate trial insert in the trial post/tray and reduce the knee and extend it. Keep the sand bag under the heel and maintain even pressure across bone/tibial implant interface. Avoid hyperextension which may cause posterior lift-off. Assistant will keep the ankle dorsiflexed. Maintain the position till cement sets. Femoral and tibial components are pressurized against each other. Release the tourniquet. Achieve the hemostasis specially coagulate the lateral inferior genicular artery by electrocautery. Check the stability, movement and patellar tracking and decide the thickness of insert.

Application of Tibial Insert

Flex the knee. Remove the tibial insert trial and MBT revision trial post. Apply Hohmann on the posterior aspect of upper tibia and small Hohmann on the lateral and medial aspect of upper tibia. Remove the extruded cement with small osteotome and mallet or nibbler. Cleanse with gentamicin mixed normal saline by pulse lavage. Apply the appropriate size (according to size of femoral component) and thickness of RP revision tibial insert. Remove the Homann and reduce the knee as described. Check the stability, movement and patellar tracking. Close the wound under two suction drains as described for fixed bearing TKR.

Tibial Preparation for Step Wedge

Attach the 2 degree tibial cutting block to the IM tibial referencing device. Attach the IM tibial referencing device to the shaft of tapered reamer and allow it to descend to the proximal tibial surface. Resect the most prominent condyle (not more than 1–2 mm) and plan to manage residual defect of other condyle by step wedge. Assess whether one condyle requires wedge augmentation or both to restore the joint line. If step wedge is required on one side, then step wedge preparation is done after checking the rotational position of both femoral and tibial components after trial reduction. Fix the tibial tray stem trial with two fixation pins according to the rotational alignment. Attach the wedge cut attachment with the step wedge cutting block to the trial tray. Slide the step wedge cutting block to the anterior proximal tibia and fix by two Steinmann pin through square marked holes. Unlock the step wedge cutting block and remove the wedge cut attachment with trial tray. Resect the tibia with oscillating saw taking care not to extend beyond the central riser. Remove the step wedge cutting block and pins. Assemble the trial wedge to the appropriate tibial tray trial and apply into the prepared tibia. Fine adjustment can be done by bone file to ensure maximum contact. Do broaching by MBT revision tibial keel punch. Leave the punch in place and do final trial reduction.

Tibial Preparation for Cemented Tibial Stem

30 or 60 mm length cemented stem of diameter 13 mm only is used with MBT revision tray to avoid a step off at the stem/tray junction. Fix the MBT tibial trial with two fixation pins after determining the appropriate rotation of tibial tray following reduction of knee and full extension. Apply the MBT revision drill bushing over the MBT tibial trial. Apply the cemented drill bushing into the MBT revision drill bushing. Pass the cemented reamer to the appropriate length (30 mm or 60 mm). Remove the reamer and cemented drill bushing but leave the MBT revision drill bushing in place. Attach the selected size cemented stem trial with cemented tapered reamer. Assemble the revision reamer adapter over the cemented tapered reamer. Ream until the revision reamer adapter is flushed with the MBT revision drill bushing. Remove the tapered reamer but taking care not to reverse the ream to avoid stem trial disengagement. Remove the MBT revision drill bushing and tibial trial. Assemble the appropriate sized cemented stem with MBT revision tray trial and apply over the prepared tibia. Fix by two fixation pins. Assemble the universal handle

to the cemented keel punch and insert it into MBT revision tray trial. Disconnect the universal handle, leaving the MBT keel punch in place. Remove the two fixation pins. Apply the appropriate size and thickness of rotating platform trial tibial insert according to size of femoral trial. Apply the trial patellar implant. Reduce the knee and extend it fully.

Assembling the Prosthesis

Assemble the appropriate sized femoral component with wedge and stem and MBT revision tibial tray with appropriate size wedge and cemented stem. For assembling the wedge and stem, attach wedge prior to stem attachment. Assemble the selected wedge to the MBT revision tray and fix with appropriate screw. Tighten the screw with T-handle torque driver until audible click is heard to ensure full and permanent interlock. Hold the stem of MBT revision tray by Revision femoral/tibial/sleeve clamp and attach the stem extension by press-fit rod wrench to ensure full engagement.

Cementing

Dislocate the knee and remove the all trial components. Cleanse the prepared femur, tibia and patella by gentamicin mixed normal saline by pulse lavage. Apply the CMW1 gentamicin bone cement over the prepared surfaces of patella and femur and tibia and under surface of prosthesis and stem. Cementing, insert application, reduction of knee and closure are same as described.

Two-stage Revision TKR with Metaphyseal Sleeve for Late Infections in Type 2B Defect (Figs 5.78 to 5.85)

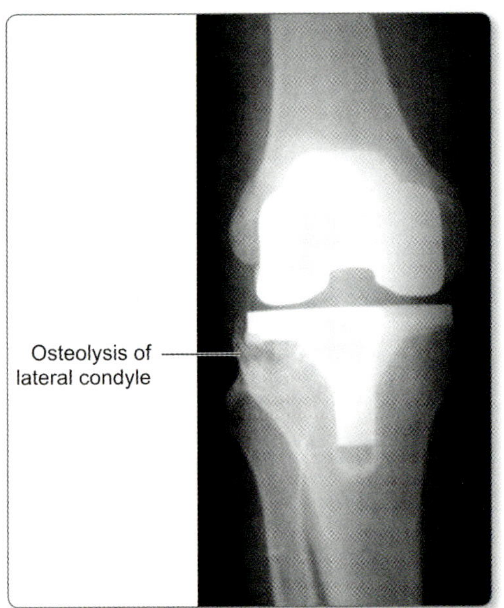

Fig. 5.78 Infection with periprosthetic osteolysis of lateral condyle

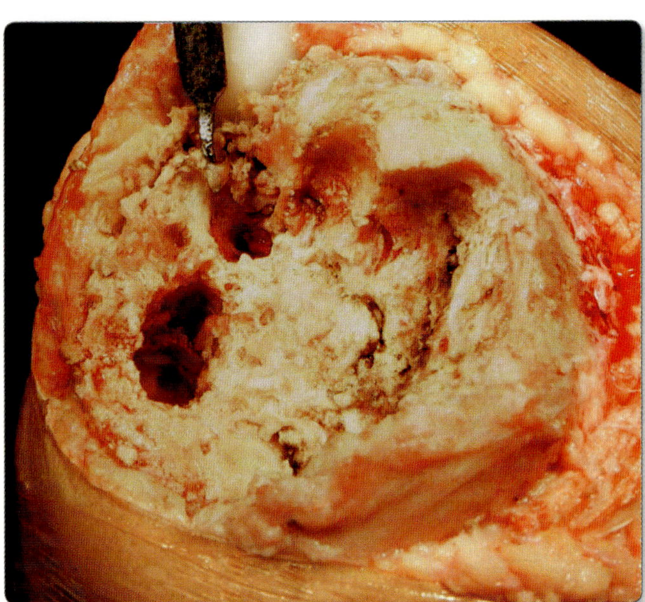

Fig. 5.79 Type 2B defects

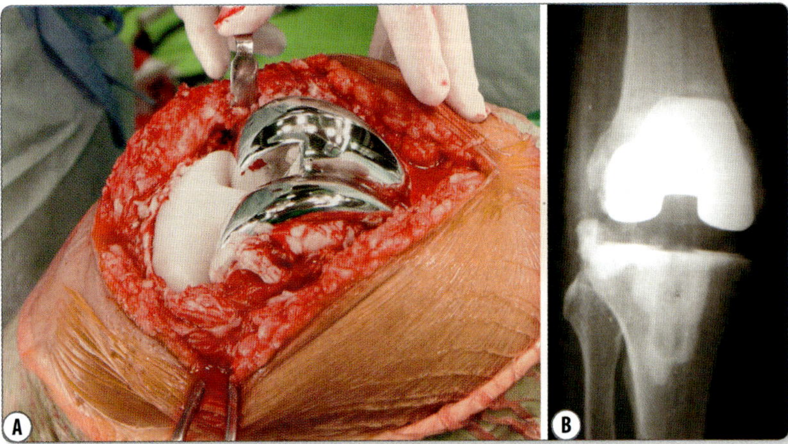

Figs 5.80A and B Stage I—Application of dynamic articulating spacer (same femoral component after autoclaving and new plastic insert) with antibiotic (gentamicin and vancomycin) impregnated bone cement

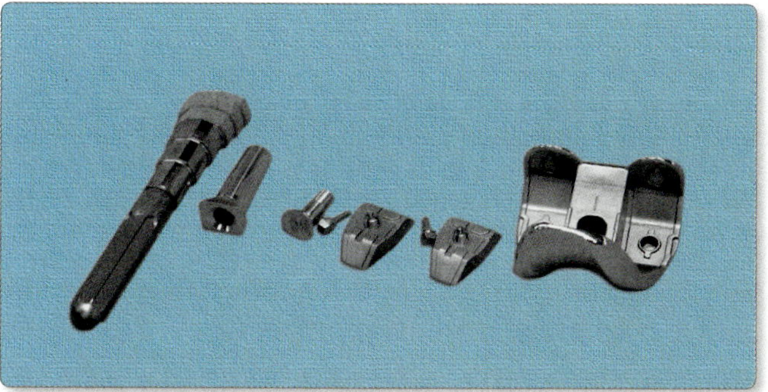

Fig. 5.81 Femoral metaphyseal sleeve with fluted rod, adapter, bolt, step wedges, wobble hex bit and TC3 femoral component

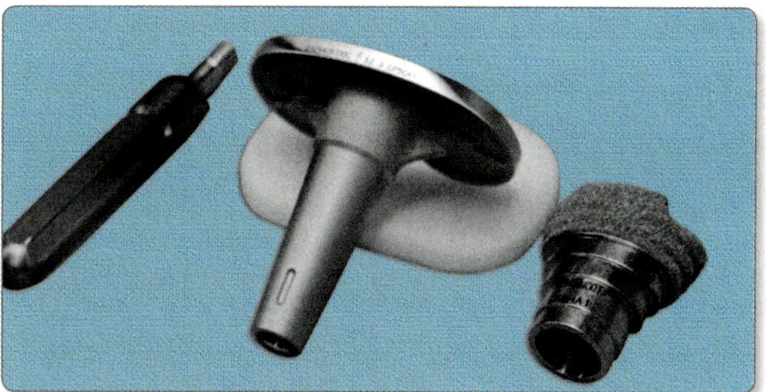

Fig. 5.82 Fluted rod, MBT revision tray and tibial metaphyseal sleeve

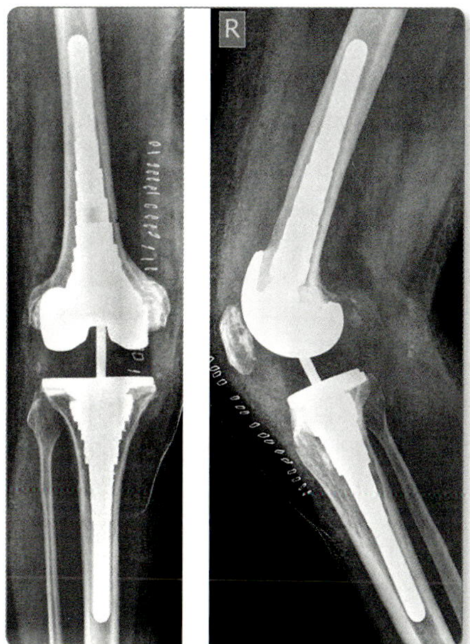

Fig. 5.83 Stage II—Revision TKR with TC3 femoral component and MBT revision tray, metaphyseal sleeves, fluted femoral and tibial rods and rotating platform insert

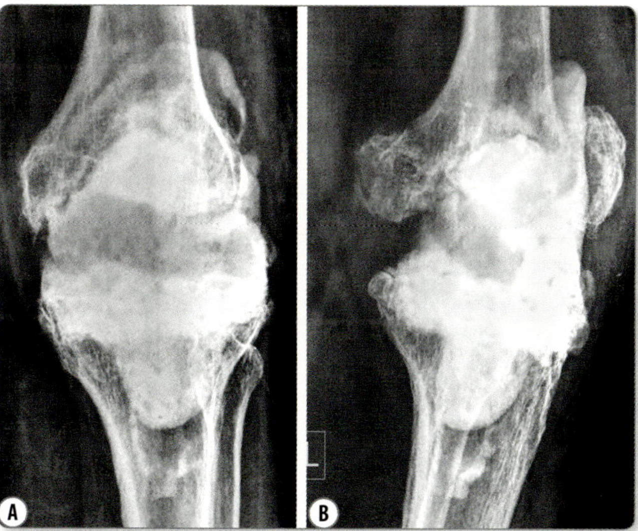

Figs 5.84A and B Stage 1 revision TKR with static cement spacer for infected TKR

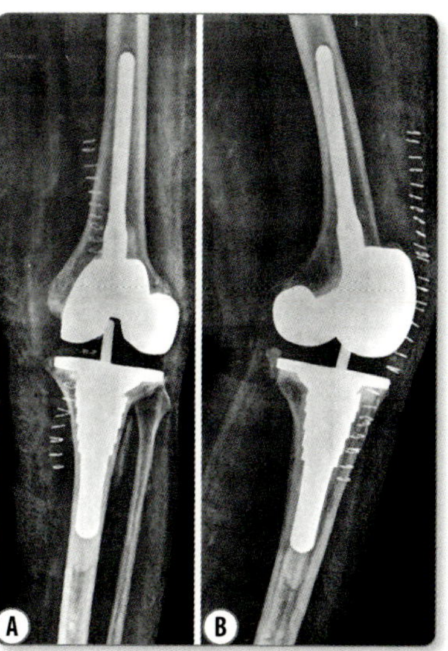

Figs 5.85A and B Stage 2 revision TKR with MBT revision tray, metaphyseal sleeve in tibia, standard femoral condyle with fluted femoral rod and rotating platform insert

Instruments Required for TC3 RP and MBT Revision Tray System (Figs 5.86 and 5.87)

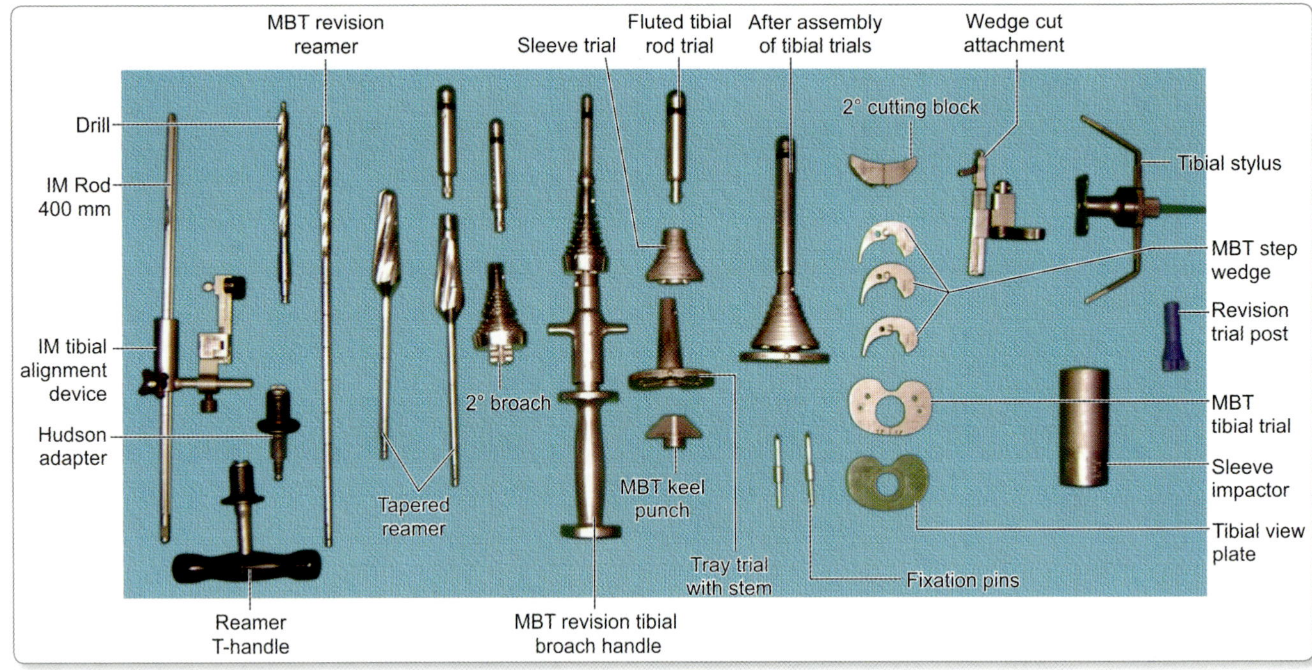

Fig. 5.86 Instruments required for application of metaphyseal sleeve with MBT revision tray and step wedge trials

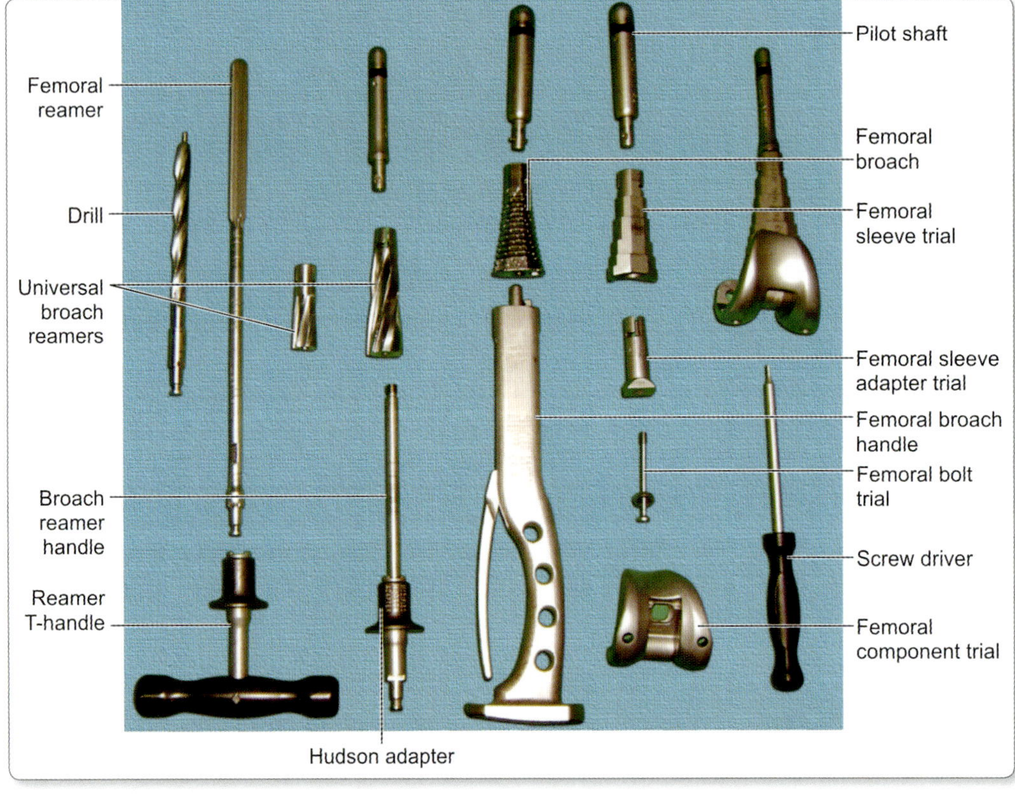

Fig. 5.87 Instruments required for application of metaphyseal sleeve and rod with femoral component

S-ROM Noiles Rotating Hinge Knee System

This is third generation modular rotating hinge knee system. This system has following features:

1. The femoral component and the tibial tray (modular tibial base) are made up of cobalt-chromium (CoCr) alloy. The articulating surfaces on the top of tibial tray and inside of the stem receptor area are highly polished to provide a broad mobile surface for the ultrahigh molecular weight polyethylene tibial bearing component.
2. 7° physiologic valgus, fixed in the femoral component.
3. Deepened femoral trochlear groove enhances physiologic patellar tracking.
4. Modular metaphyseal filling and loading sleeves which provide metaphyseal fit and fill, facilitating load sharing and load transfer in cases of metaphyseal deficiencies and poor bone quality. The metaphyseal sleeves are stepped for progressive loading and textured with beads (porous coated) having interbead pour diameters of approximately 200 micron allowing for the possibility of bone ingrowth (osseointegration). Sizes of femoral metaphyseal sleeves are 20 mm, 31mm, 34 mm, 40 mm and 46 mm.
5. Modular femoral and tibial stems which are splined to enhance rotational stability and slotted to more closely match bone stiffness and eliminate end-stem pain. The stems are 100 or 150 mm to bypass defects and stable fixation into intact medullary bone.
6. Broad, congruent contact areas between femoral and tibial components to best distribute surface and subsurface stresses in the polyethylene.
7. Rotating hinge with an axle-yolk assembly that accommodates axial rotation reducing stresses at the bone-cement-implant interface.
8. Distal femoral augments are available in 5 to 10 mm sizes to help better store the joint line.
9. Enhanced tibial base plates can add 14–24 mm to the base plates.
10. Polyethylene bearing thickness is available up to 31 mm.
11. Selection of sizes to match condylar, metaphyseal and diaphyseal anatomy and provide fit and fill of hard tissue.

Indications

1. Revision TKR in:
   i. Type 3 bone loss.
   ii. Medial or lateral collateral ligament loss.
   iii. Severe flexion gap imbalance.
   iv. Joint jack phenomenon.
2. Primary TKR in patients with:
   i. Neuromuscular deficits such as polio, flail knee which require hyperextension stop.
   ii. Extension arthrodesis.
   iii. Severe traumatic arthrosis.
   iv. Extension arthrofibrosis.

Technique

1. Skin incision and exposure of knee.
2. Tibial preparation.
3. Femoral preparation.
4. Trial reduction.
5. Component assembly.
6. Cementing.
7. Bearing and hinge pin insertion.

Incision and Exposure of Knee

Open the joint by previous skin incision and medial parapatellar approach. Remove prosthesis and do debridement as described. Assess the bone loss and soft tissue support.

Tibial Preparation

1. Reaming.
2. Broaching.
3. Tibial cut.
4. Tibial trial.

Ream the proximal tibia to the correct size using sequential straight reamers by cortical diaphyseal fill. For larger tibial defects, the 150 mm may be more appropriate than the standard 100 mm stem. Intramedullary pilots are placed on the tibial broaches and used progressively until rotational stability is achieved. Do the proximal tibial resection using the top of the tibial broach as a guide. Do tibial trial over tibial broach by using tibial view plate and tibial plateau trial. The tibial plateau size must match femoral component size.

Femoral Preparation

1. Reaming of medullary canal.
2. Reaming of metaphysis.
3. Broaching of metaphysis.
4. Femoral cuts with stem-sleeve aligned guides.
5. Femoral trial.

Femoral preparation involves reaming the canal and metaphysis to size, broaching with sized medullary pilots to metaphyseal fill and bone cuts made off the stemsleeve aligned guides. Ream the femur to cortical fill. The appropriate depth for 20, 31 and 34 mm sleeves and 40 and 46 mm sleeves with 100 mm stem extensions are indicated by grooves on the reamer. Use 150 mm stem for large femoral defect. Use the flexible reamer for 150 mm stem and ream 1-1.5 mm over the straight ream size to accommodate the bowing in the stem. Use reaming depth for 150 mm extensions—245 mm for 20 mm femoral sleeve, 245 mm for 31 mm, 250 mm for 34 mm, 260 mm for 40 mm and 265 mm for 46 mm femoral sleeves. Attach the sized pilot shaft to metaphyseal broach and do broaching till rotational stability is achieved. Apply the stem sleeve-aligned intramedullary guide and make the bone cuts. Apply the appropriate distal femoral step wedges to adjust the joint line and to improve kinematics. Assemble the trial components and appropriate trial insert and reduce the joint and extend it. Remove the trial components. Cleanse the prepared femoral, tibial and patellar surfaces. Assembling the components and cementing Assemble the final component according to matched trial components and do cementing as described. Place the condyles of the femoral component into the corresponding recesses in the tibial plateau. Squeeze the clothespin end of the hinge pin and insert through the hole on the medial side of the femoral component. Close the wound in layers.

Total Knee Replacement by Navigation System

6

CHAPTER

CHAPTER OUTLINE

- Steps
- Additional Instruments Required during TKR by Naviagation System

Introduction

The nagivation system works by implanted sensors in the femur (Y-femoral array) and tibia (T-tibial array) **(Fig. 6.1)**. These sensors allow the computer to track the position of the knee with infrared technology **(Fig. 6.2)**. A probe with another infrared sensor (pointer) marks out the bony anatomy. This technique requires registering of center of hip, bony landmarks of tibia, fibula (lateral malleolus), femur and surfaces of upper end of tibia and lower end of femur by distant camera with the help of Y-femoral array and T-tibial array fixed on anteromedial surfaces of femur and tibia on Schanz screws respectively and by pointer. By all these registration data, the computer prepares the 3—dimensional bone models. Surgeon determines the amount of tibial cut and femoral cuts by help of cutting block adapter applied on tibial cutting block and femoral cutting blocks (Distal and AP and chamfer cutting block) respectively. Verify the data for accuracy after each cut and adjust accordingly.

Positioning, draping, exposure of knee, bony resection, implants trial, tibial preparation and cementing are similar to conventional technique. Only the technique of assessment of bony resection, ligament balancing and patellar tracking differ from conventional technique which is assessed directly under vision by navigation system. However, eye balling is very important while doing TKR by navigation system because the navigation system works on feeding of data and wrong data feeding may land up into wrong resection.

First check the camera setup for position of femoral and tibial arrays in full flexion and extension of knee.

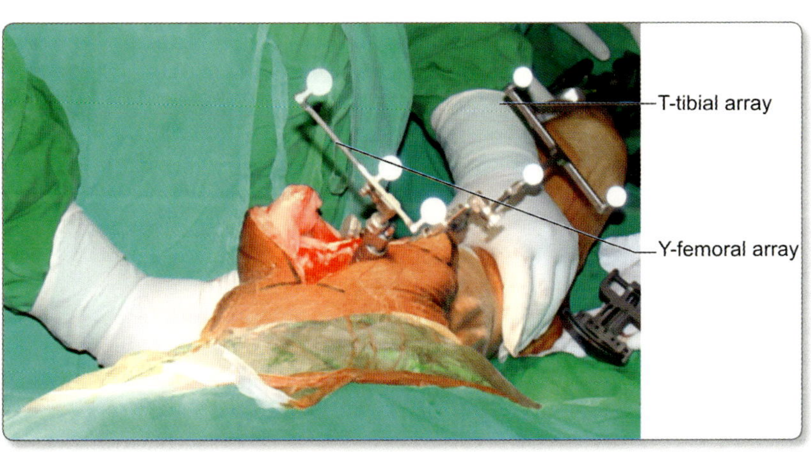

Fig. 6.1 Position of tibial and femoral arrays

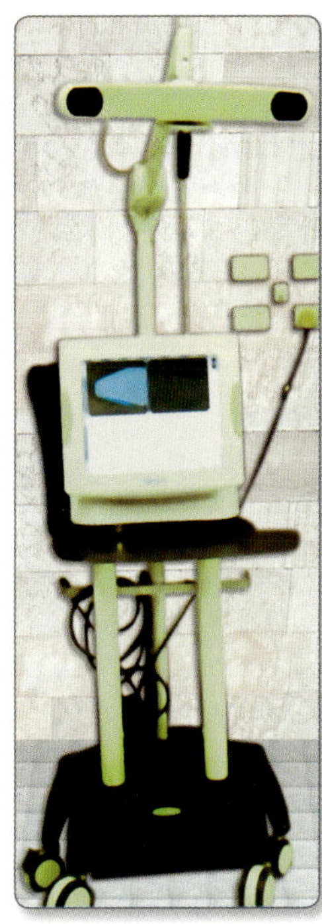

Fig. 6.2 Distant camera with computer (Navigation system)

Steps

Following steps are involved which are shown on monitor:

- Femoral registration
- Tibial registration.

1. *Femoral head center*: Pivot the head in the acetabulum **(Fig. 6.3)**. For this, the assistant will fix the pelvis and surgeon will hold the leg and knee and rotate the femur till the computer registers the femoral head center within 3 mm of accuracy.
2. *Initial leg alignment*: Note the initial leg alignment in full extension and flexion **(Fig. 6.4)** and store the data for comparison with final leg alignment.
3. *Mechanical axis point of femur*: Pivot the pointer on the distal femoral mechanical axis point.
4. *Malleoli registration*:
   i. Medial malleolar point: Pivot the pointer on the medial malleolar point.
   ii. Lateral malleolar point: Pivot the pointer on the lateral malleolar point.
5. *Tibial landmark registration*:
   i. Mechanical axis point.
   ii. Medial tibial contour point.
   iii. Lateral tibial contour point.
   iv. Anterior tibial contour point.
   v. Tibial AP direction.
6. Tibial surface registration:
   i. Medial tibial plateau: Pivot the pointer at the lowest point on the medial plateau and glide the tip along the surface till it is registered **(Fig. 6.5)**.
   ii. Lateral tibial plateau: Pivot the pointer at the lowest point on the lateral plateau and glide the tip along the surface till it is registered **(Fig. 6.6)**.

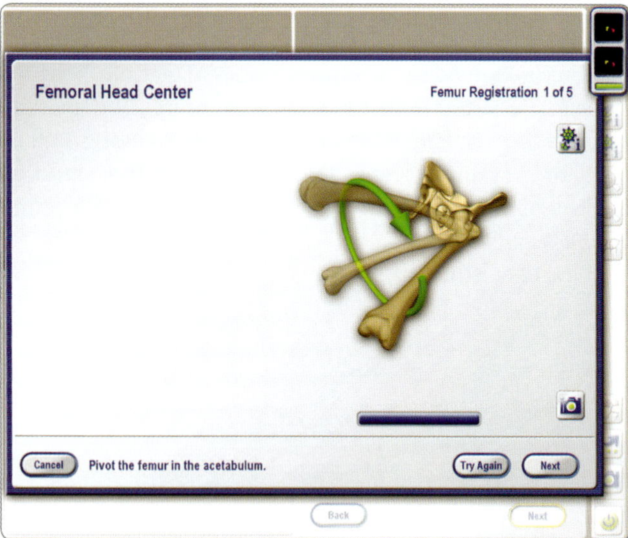

Fig. 6.3 Registering femoral head center

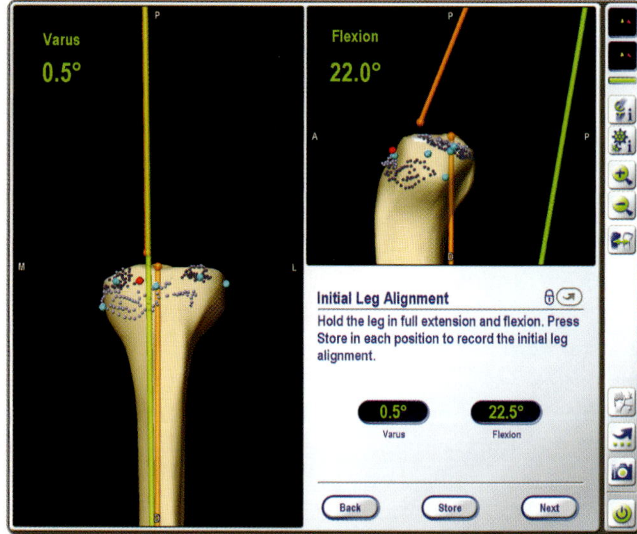

Fig. 6.4 Initial leg alignment

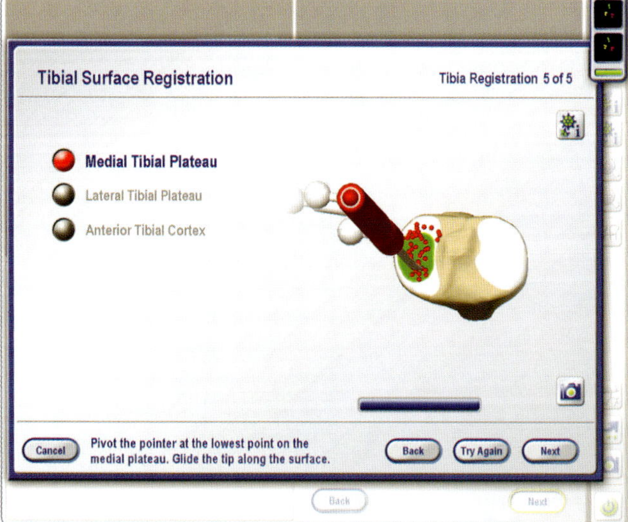

Fig. 6.5 Registration of medial tibial plateau

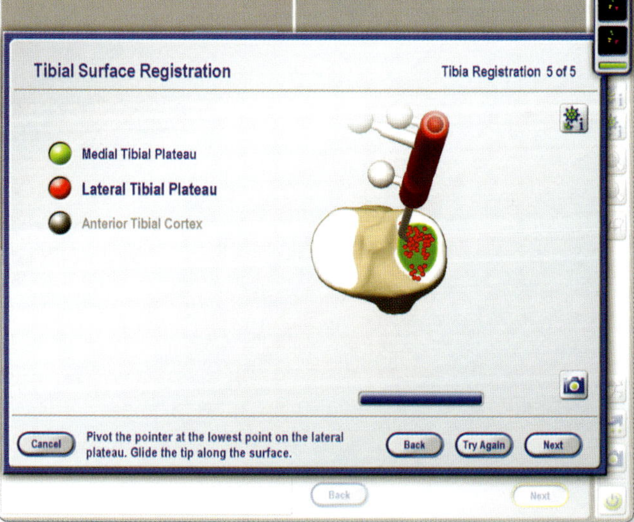

Fig. 6.6 Registration of lateral tibial plateau

iii. Anterior tibial cortex: Pivot the pointer on the anterior cortex and glide the tip along the surface till it is registered **(Fig. 6.7)**.

By these data, the computer adapt the tibial bone model to match acquired surface point.

7. *Verify tibial model*: Place the pointer on the bone surface to verify the accuracy of the tibial model. Pivot the pointer on the tibial bone surface to acquire an accuracy check point **(Fig. 6.8)**.
8. Assess the tibial resection by applying cutting block adapter on tibial cutting block and fix the cutting block by two Steinman pins (3.2 mm) through the central holes marked by squares. Put the oscillating saw in the slot of tibial cutting block and cut the tibia.
9. Verify tibial resection by putting the cutting block adapter over the resected tibia and do correction of tibial resection if any **(Fig. 6.9)**.
10. *Femoral landmark registration*:
    i. Medial epicondylar point.
    ii. Lateral epicondylar point.
    iii. Anterior cortex point.
    iv. Whiteside line.
11. Femoral surface registration **(Figs 6.10 to 6.12)**
    i. Medial condyle.
    ii. Lateral condyle.
    iii. Anterior femoral cortex.

    By these data the computer adapt the femoral bone model to match acquired surface point
12. *Verify femoral model*: Place the pointer on the bone surface to verify the accuracy of the femoral model. Pivot the pointer on the femoral bone surface to acquire an accuracy check point **(Fig. 6.13)**.
13. Assess the distal femoral resection by applying cutting block adapter on distal femoral cutting block and fix the

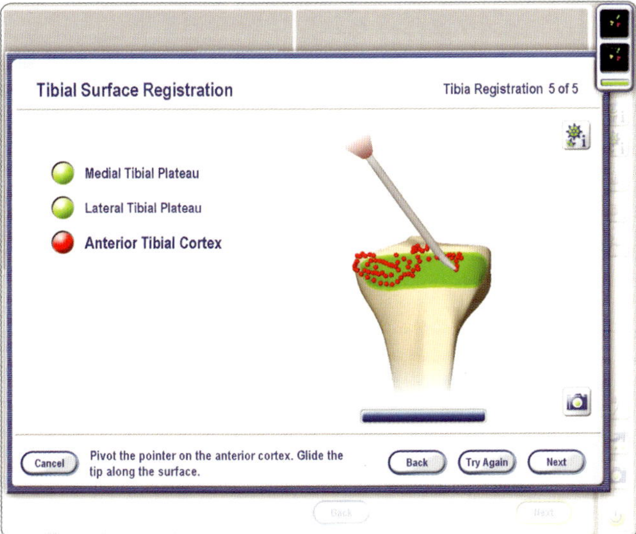

Fig. 6.7 Registration of anterior tibial cortex

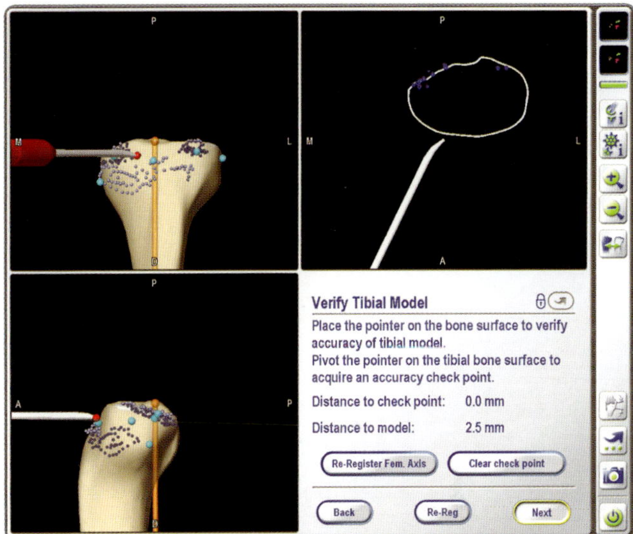

Fig. 6.8 Verification tibial model

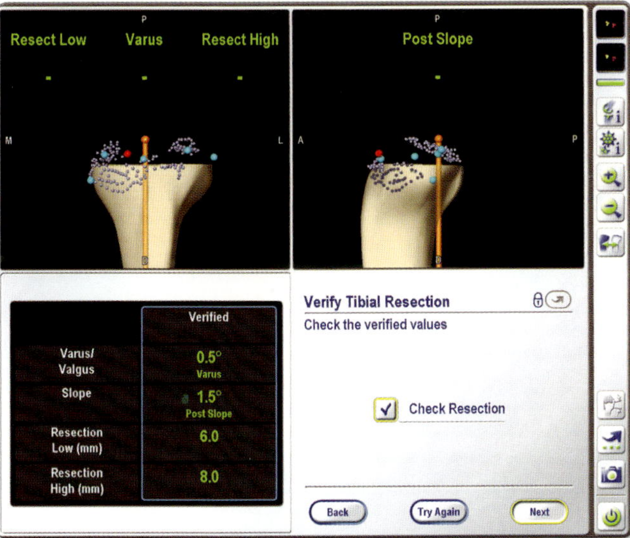

Fig. 6.9 Verification of tibial resection

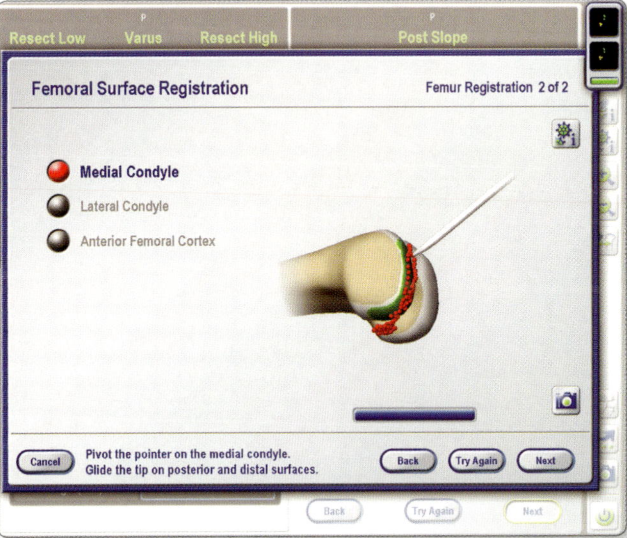

Fig. 6.10 Registration of medial femoral condyle

cutting block by two Steinmann pins (3.2 mm) through the central holes marked by squares. Put the oscillating saw in the slot of distal femoral cutting block and make the distal cut.

14. Verify the distal femoral resection by putting the cutting block adapter over the resected distal femoral surface **(Fig. 6.14)** and do correction if any.
15. Assess the anterior femoral resection by applying cutting block adapter on AP and chamfer cutting block and fix the cutting block by two Steinmann pins (3.2 mm). Put the oscillating saw in the anterior slot and make the cut.
16. Verify anterior femoral resection by cutting block adapter after putting over the resected anterior surface of femur and do the correction if any. Make posterior and chamfer cuts.
17. Box cut, components trial, patellar resection, tibial preparation and cementing technique are same as described in conventional technique.
18. Check the final leg alignment.

Resultwise, there is no difference between conventional technique and navigation system. There is theoretical chance of fat embolism in conventional technique which we have not encountered in more than 3000 TKR by conventional technique. To prevent this possible fat embolism, wash the medullary canal of femur by 100 mL normal saline just after drilling and before passing the intramedullary fluted rod and again wash the medullary

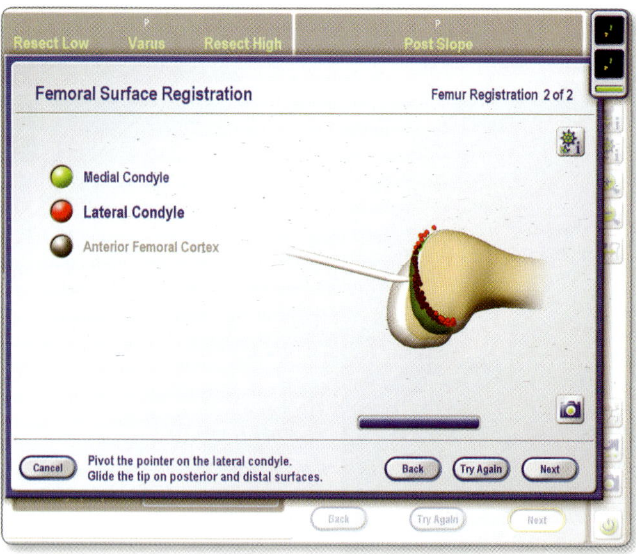

Fig. 6.11 Registration of lateral femoral condyle

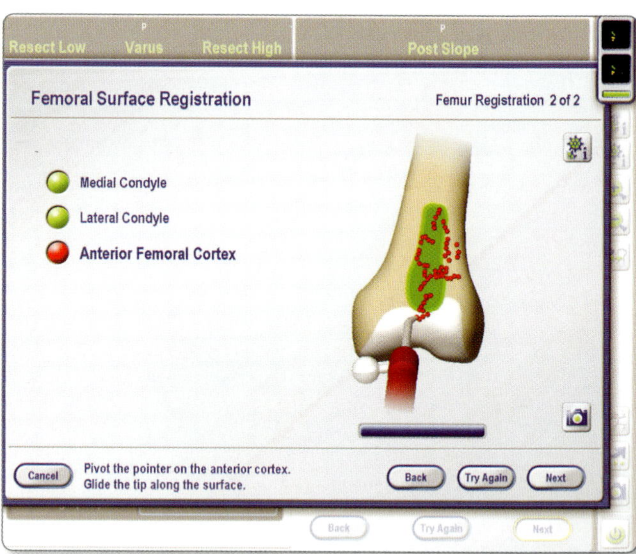

Fig. 6.12 Registration of anterior femoral cortex

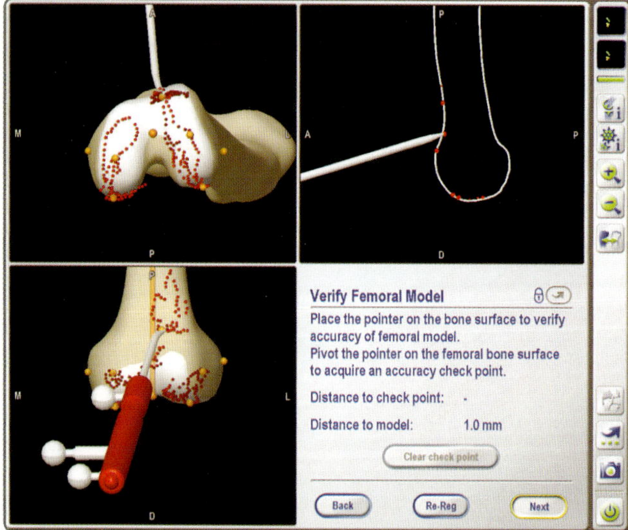

Fig. 6.13 Verification of femoral model

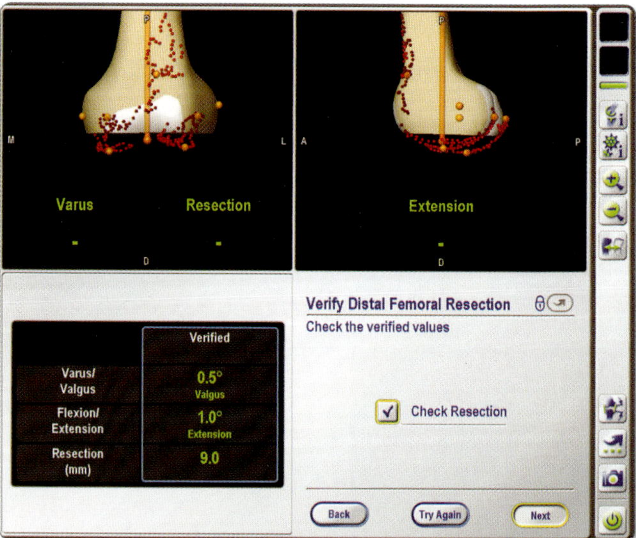

Fig. 6.14 Verification of distal femoral resection

canal by 100 mL normal saline just before blocking the canal by bone piece. Approximately 30 minutes more time is required and incision is slightly bigger in navigation system to accommodate the proximal Schanz screws applied for Y-femoral array. Blood loss depends upon haemostasis achieved after release of tourniquet at the end of surgery. Blocking the opening of medullary canal by resected bone piece (usually taken from box cut) prevents extra blood loss from medullary canal postoperatively in conventional technique. There is no significant difference in blood loss. Both techniques are equally accurate. Mistake can occur in both the techniques if minute details of the procedures and assessment of tibial, femoral resection and ligament balancing are not followed.

TKR with navigation system is more useful in patients with arthritis of the knee and extra-articular femoral and/or tibial deformity, retained hardware or intramedullary implants.

Additional Instruments Required during TKR by Naviagation System (Fig. 6.15)

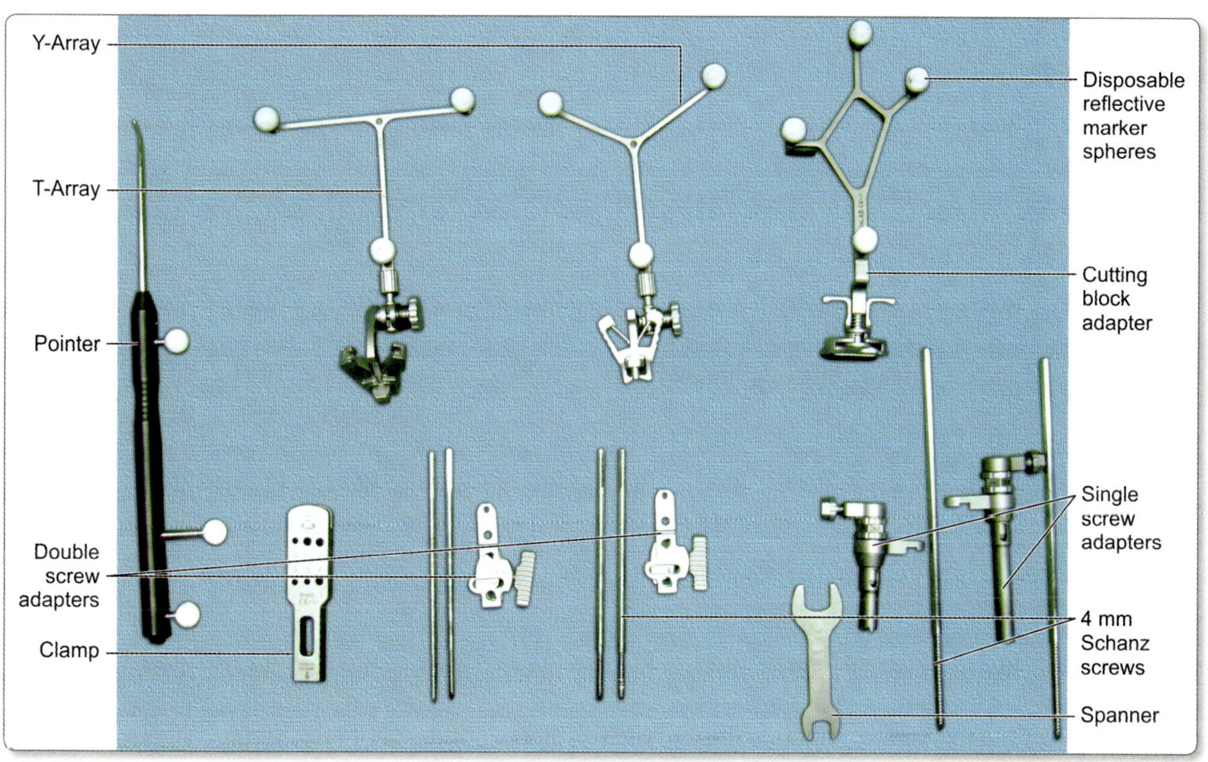

Fig. 6.15 Additional instruments during navigation system

Total Hip Replacement

7

CHAPTER

CHAPTER OUTLINE

Preoperative Planning

This enables the surgeon to prepare for the case and anticipate situations that may arise during surgery.

Goals

1. Determine preoperative limb length discrepancy.
2. Assess acetabular component size and placement.
3. Determine femoral component size, position and fit.
4. Assess femoral offset.

Preoperative templating is helpful for accurate implant sizing, placement and alignment.

X-ray hip with upper 2/3rd thigh—AP view with 15° internal rotation provides the most important information:

1. A level for the neck resection which will restore leg length.
2. The appropriate neck offset for an anatomical position of femoral head.
3. The medial-lateral dimensions of the femoral canal which determine the overall size of the implant.
4. Bony landmark of the pelvis and the correct anatomical position of the acetabular component relative to landmarks such as the tear drop.

X-ray hip with upper 2/3rd thigh—lateral view confirms the diameter of the femoral canal and reveals any abnormalities in this plane.

Determine the Limb Length Discrepancy Radiographically

Draw a reference line through the most inferior part of the ischial tuberosity (bottom of the obturator foramen) on proper AP view X-ray of both hip joints **(Fig. 7.1)**. Measure the distance from the lesser trochanter landmark or the tip of the greater trochanter to the reference line on each side. The difference between the two is the radiographic limb length discrepancy **(Fig. 7.2)**.

The reference line passes through the lesser trochanter (same level) in normal hip and the distance between the reference line and the tip of greater trochanter is equal on both sides **(Fig. 7.1)**.

In proper AP view of normal hip, the reference line usually passes through the lesser trochanter. The reference line passing below the lesser trochanter indicates the radiological shortening of the limb as shown in **Figure 7.3**.

The distance between the reference line and the lesser trochanter is the approximate shortening which has to be compensated when both hips are involved.

Alternatively, the radiological assessment of limb length discrepancy can also be done by drawing an inter-teardrop line and a line at the level of lesser trochanters. Compare the distance between the inter-teardrop line and a line at the level of lesser trochanters as shown in **Figure 7.4**.

There is shortening of the left lower limb as the distance between the inter-teardrop line and a line passing through the lesser trochanter is less on left side.

The limb length discrepancy is corrected peroperatively as shown on the X-ray in **Figure 7.5** where shortening of both lower limbs has been compensated.

After THR, the reference line is passing above the lesser trochanters indicating that there is lengthening of both lower limbs, left > right **(Fig. 7.6)**.

"Thus, the reference line passing through lesser trochanter indicates that both lower limbs are equal.

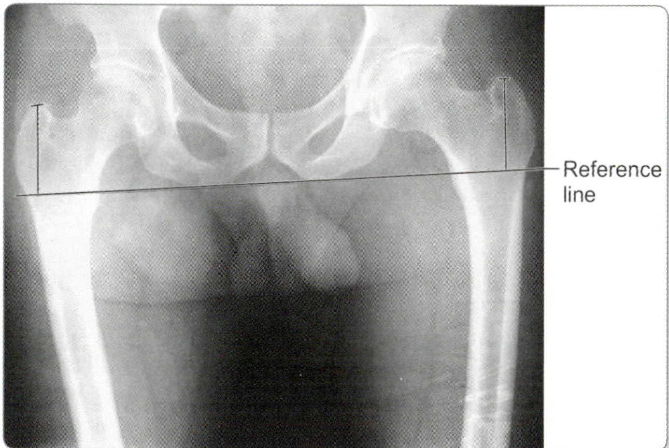

Fig. 7.1 Normal hip

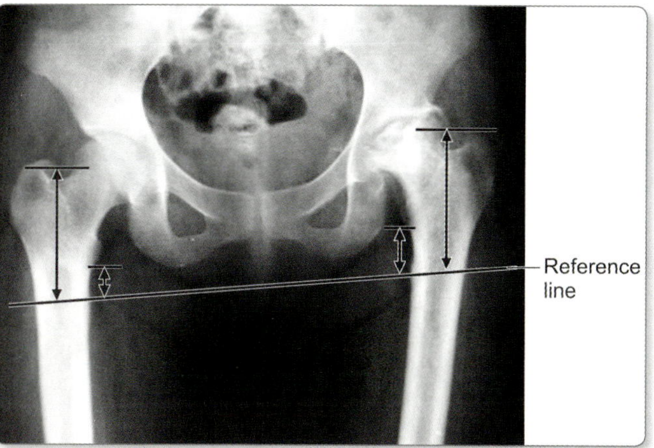

Fig. 7.2 Difference between the reference line and the lesser trochanter landmark or the tip of the greater trochanter on each side shows leg length discrepancy which can be measured

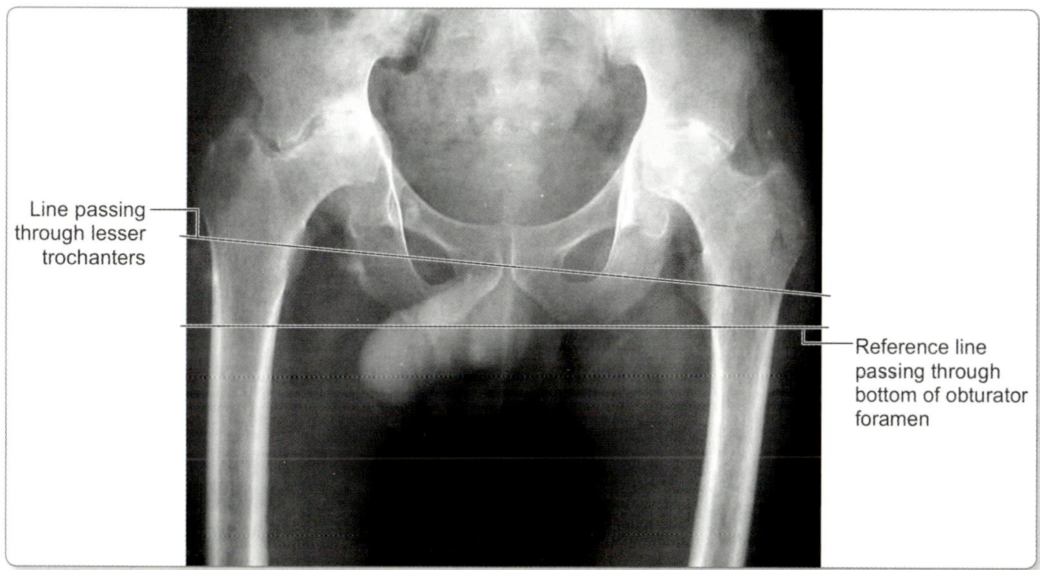

Fig. 7.3 Both lower limbs are shortened (R>L) as the reference line is passing below the lesser trochanter

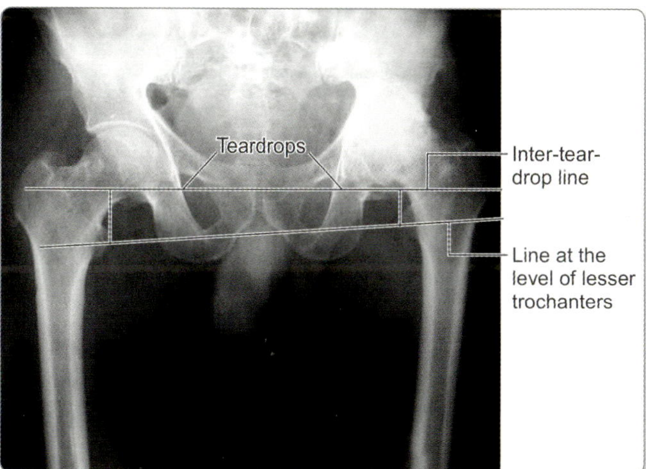

Fig. 7.4 AVN with severe arthritis of left hip and normal right hip

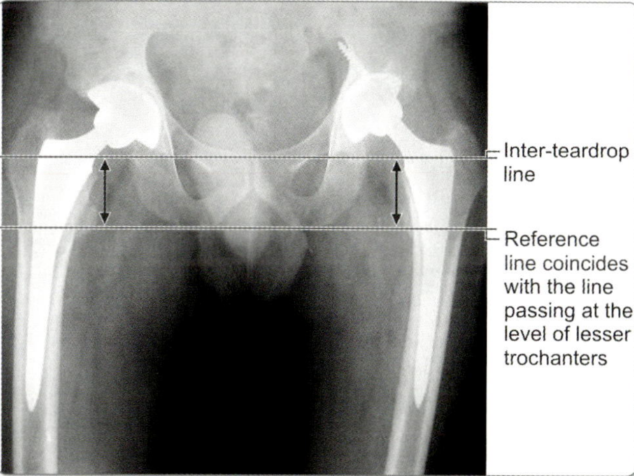

Fig. 7.5 After THR, the reference line is passing at the level of the lesser trochanters. Shortening of both lower limbs compensated. The distance between the inter-tear drop line and the line passing at the level of lesser trochanter is equal on both sides

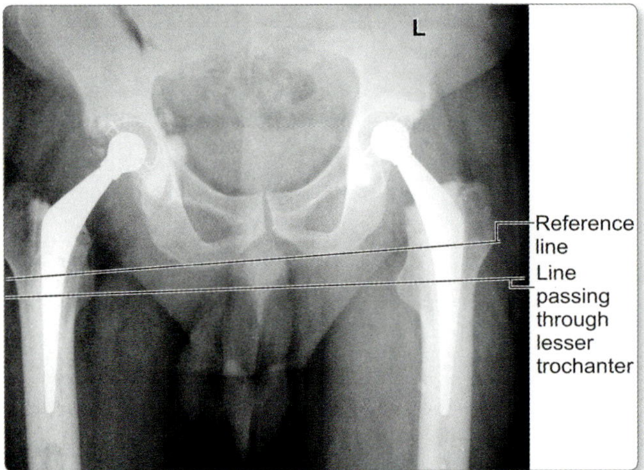

Fig. 7.6 Postoperative lengthening of both lower limbs

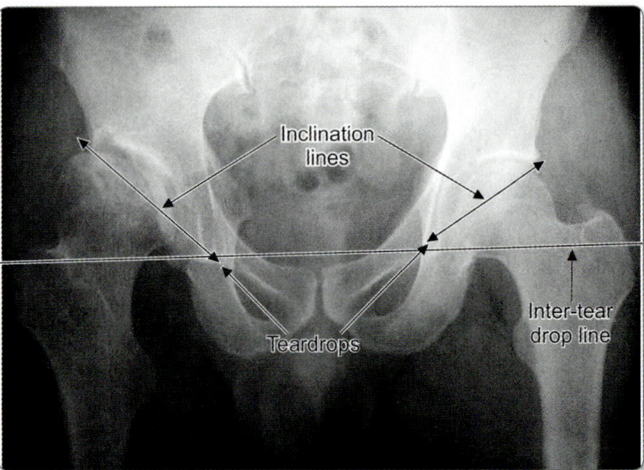

Fig. 7.7 Larger inclination line indicates proximal migration of acetabulum which requires reconstruction so that the acetabular cup can be implanted at the level of teardrop

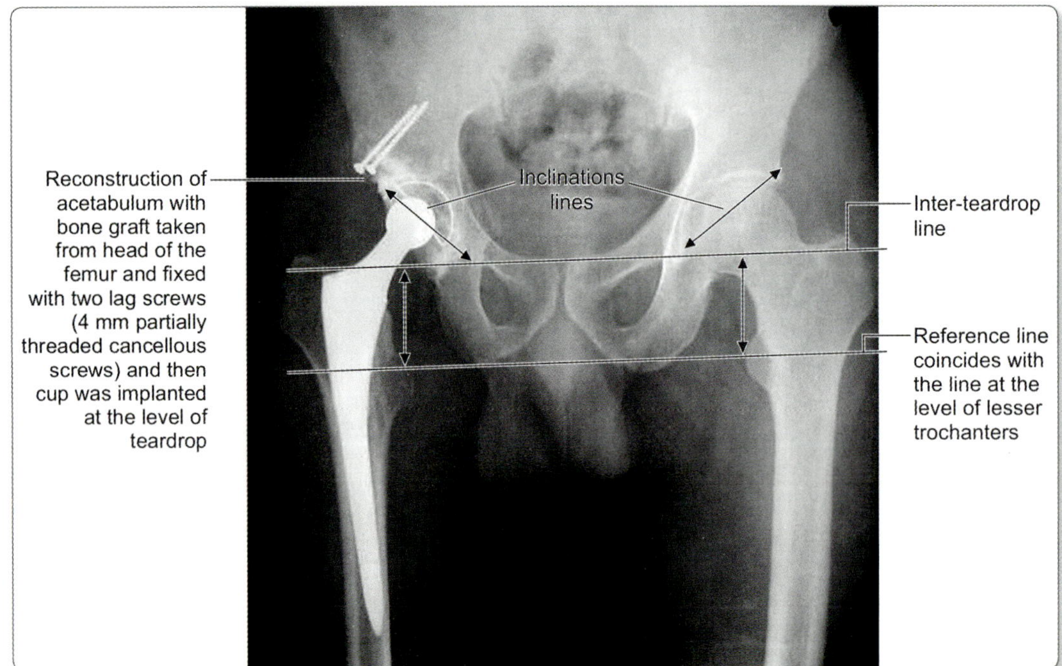

Fig. 7.8 Inclination lines are equal on both sides after reconstruction of the acetabulum and both lower limbs are equal as reference line coincides with the line at the level of lesser trochanter or the distance between inter-teardrop line and line at the level of lesser trochanter are equal on both sides

The reference line passing below the lesser trochanter indicates shortening. The reference line passing above the lesser trochanter indicates lengthening."

Determine the proximal migration of acetabulum radiologically:
Draw a line joining the teardrops which is known as inter-teardrop line. Draw an inclination line from the teardrop to the superior margin of the acetabulum. Determine the length of inclination line and compare with the normal side, if possible. This will tell the approximate amount of migration of acetabulum and possibility of reconstruction of the acetabulum **(Figs 7.7 and 7.8)**.

Templating

Templates include 20% magnification to compensate for the X-ray magnification.

Templating for Uncemented Acetabular Cup (Duraloc Shell)

The templates allow assessment of most likely size of cup to be implanted. Aim is to maximize bone contact on structurally sound bone for optimal bone ingrowth. Take the X-ray hip AP view. Mark the bottom of the teardrop and

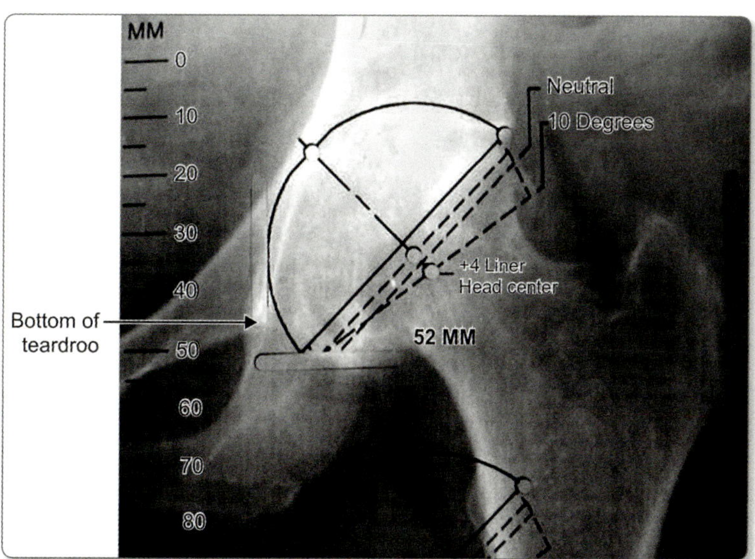

Fig. 7.9 Templating for Duraloc shell

intended center of rotation of the bearing surface. Place the template over X-ray of hip keeping three points in mind:

1. Bottom of teardrop.
2. Intended center of rotation of bearing surface.
3. Structurally sound bone.

The most inferior part of the cup should lie at the level of the bottom of the teardrop and cup should cover the optimal position of the acetabulum. Thus, the most likely size of cup is determined as shown in **Figure 7.9**.

Templating for Summit Stem (Uncemented Femoral Component)

Templating on AP View of X-ray Hip

Put the femoral template along the long-axis of the femur and select the template size that will fit the proximal femur and equalize the leg length **(Fig. 7.10)**. Draw the neck resection line at the point where the selected stem provides the desired amount of leg length.

Templating on Lateral View X-ray of Hip

The selected femoral template should fit in the lateral plane **(Fig. 7.11)**. There will be three-point fixation as shown in **Figure 7.12**.

Templating for C-stem (Cemented Femoral Component)

Take proper AP view X-ray of hip with upper 2/3rd thigh in 15° internal rotation. Draw a line along the long-axis of the femur and long-axis of neck (femoral neck axis). Mark the center of rotation. The template is placed over the X-ray so that the center line of implant is in line with the long-axis of the femur, the neck along the femoral neck axis and the center of the femoral head over the center of rotation. The "bow tie mark" is in the neutral position. The center of the bow tie mark is the proposed neck resection. The cement mantle outline should fill the proximal femoral canal **(Figs 7.13 and 7.14)**. The level of neck resection, the appropriate neck offset and the medial-lateral dimension of the femoral canal will determine the overall size of the implant. If the opposite hip is normal then it can be used as reference.

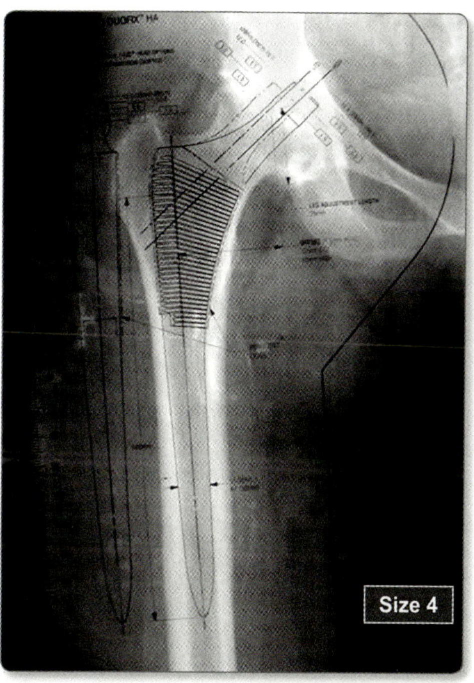

Fig. 7.10 Templating on AP view

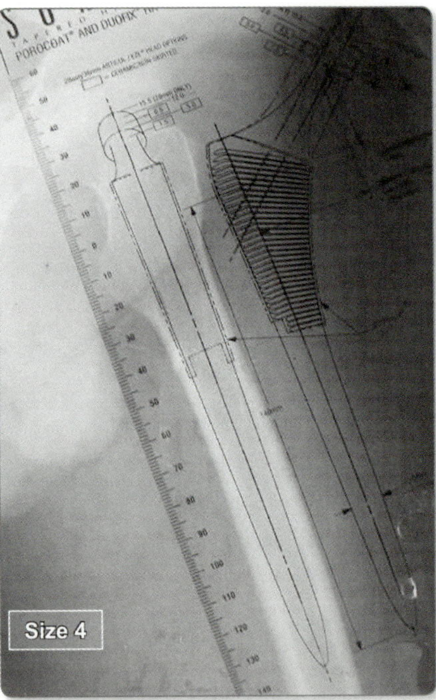

Fig. 7.11 Templating on lateral view

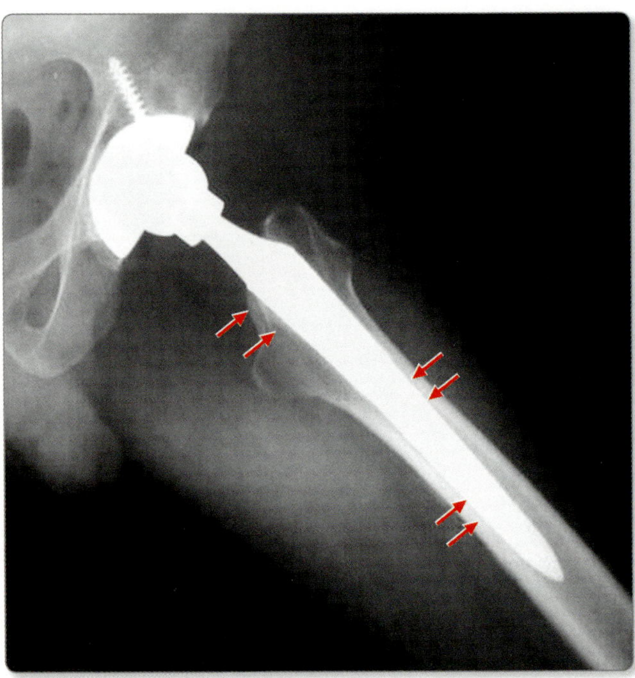

Fig. 7.12 Postoperative lateral view X-ray with three-point fixation as marked by arrows

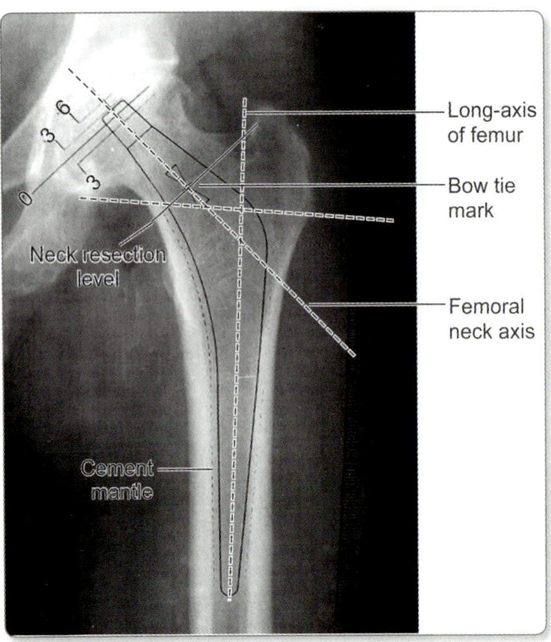

Fig. 7.13 Templating in AP view (size 2)

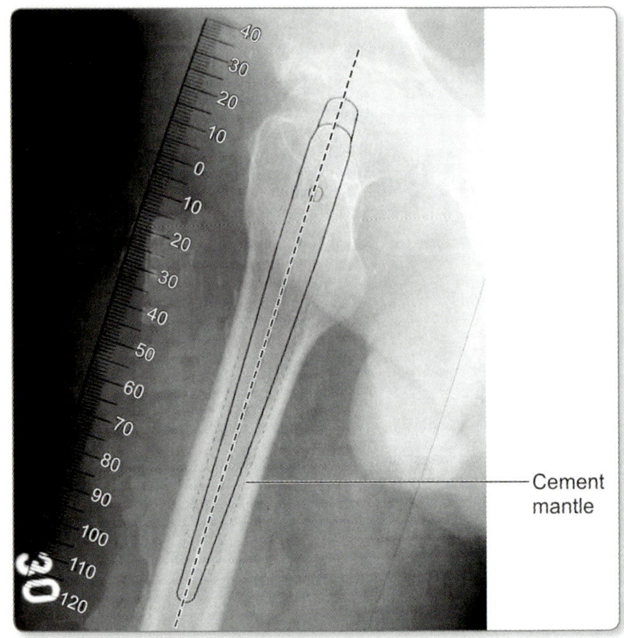

Fig. 7.14 Templating in lateral view (size 2)

Template for Cemented Acetabular Cup

The template is placed over the AP view X-ray of hip relative to the bottom of teardrop and intended center of rotation of hip and find out the approximate size of the cup with cement mantle outline as in **Figure 7.15**.

Investigations, consent for surgery, physiotherapy, education and training, risk-benefit ratio, preparation of the patient for surgery and arranging blood are similar to TKR.

Anesthesia

Preferably spinal and epidural. In some cases of ankylosing spondylitis where spinal anesthesia is not possible due to stiff spine (calcified ligamentum flavum) and intubation is difficult due to stiff cervical spine, fiberoptic flexible laryngoscope may be required for intubation.

Bladder is catheterized.

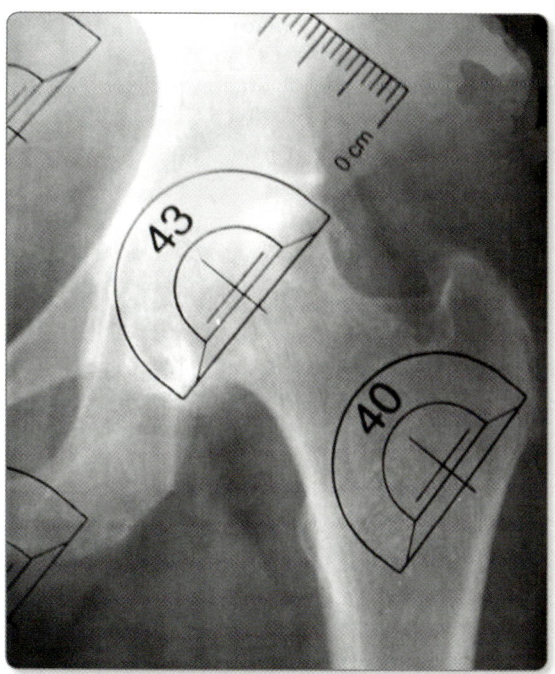

Fig. 7.15 Templating for Elite plus LPW cup

Positioning—Lateral Position

Apply cotton pad on the lower part of opposite leg and loose bandage. Apply electrocautery pad on the upper part of opposite leg. Turn the patient so that the operative side is above. Apply back support over the lumbar region so that it does not interfere with access during surgery and anterior support over the pubic symphysis slightly toward the abdominal side so that it will not prevent the hip flexion during surgery and should not press the femoral vessels of the opposite limb. Two more supports are applied over the chest and the back to keep the patient in absolutely lateral position **(Figs 7.16 and 7.17)**. Tie the loose bandage of opposite limb over the side bar of the table to keep the opposite hip and knee flexed. With the patient in this position, the pelvis tends to flex approximately 20° into an anteverted position. Appreciation of this will allow correct orientation of the cup during cementing. Well-padded support is used to support the upper arm. Keep the operating table at lowermost level. One attendant will hold the leg. Put polyethylene drape under the leg. Another attendant will scrub the limb from loin at the level of umbilicus to toes. Make it dry by sponges and pour spirit over the limb.

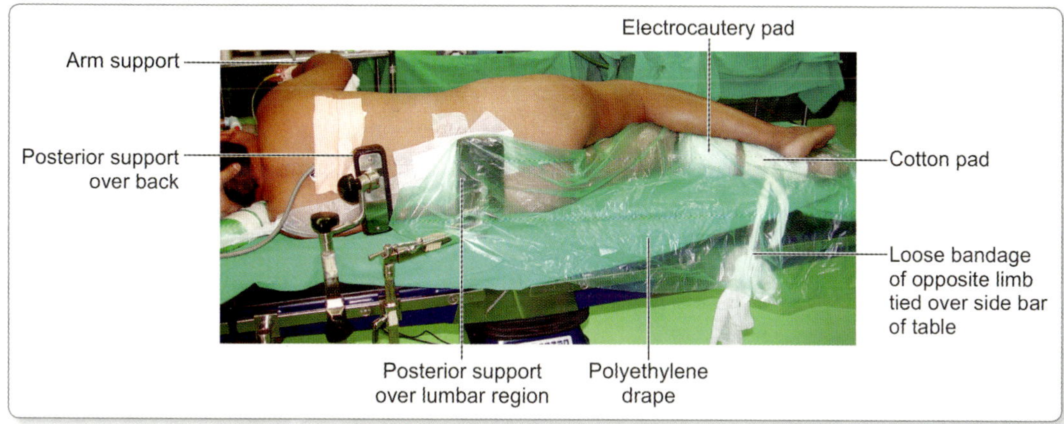

Fig. 7.16 Lateral position (posterior aspect)

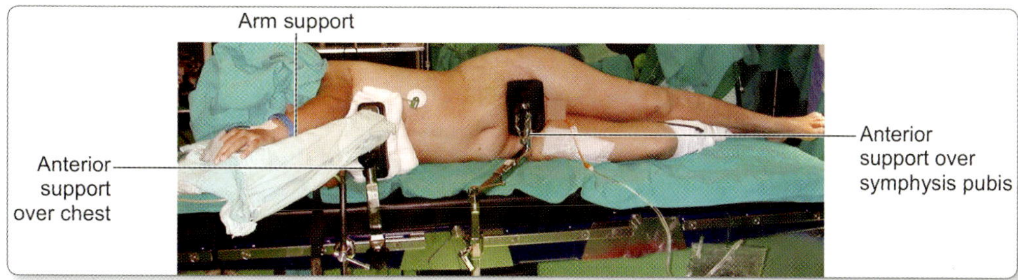

Fig. 7.17 Lateral position (anterior aspect)

Draping

The surgeons get prepared by wearing body exhaust system. Apply betadine solution from loin to toes. Remove the polyethylene drape. Apply one sterile polyethylene drape beneath the limb near groin, 2nd under limb and 3rd above loin exposing the ASIS (anterior superior iliac spine) and PSIS (posterior superior iliac spine). Apply one large sheet under the limb and another sheet over the loin and spread above. Hold these two sheets by towel clips anteriorly and posteriorly fixing with skin to avoid slip. Hold the leg with sponge and apply betadine solution over lower leg and foot. Dry the lower leg and foot by gauze piece. Apply two 8.5 number gloves over foot to cover it. Apply double layered stockinet from foot to loin and fix it proximally with sheets by multiple towel clips. Hold the leg and foot in a towel, fix it by one small towel clip and apply bandage preferably self-sticking bandage. Apply one curtain on proximal part. Apply U-drape and two side sheets from anterior and posterior, fix them with towel clips above and below the thigh. Apply one hole-towel and fix with two towel clips proximally. Keep two suctions and electrocautery on proximal part anteriorly in a towel bag. Keep the limb in 30° flexion at hip. Cut the stockinet in the straight line of femur from mid-thigh to just distal to PSIS. Apply betadine solution and make it dry with dry gauze piece. Apply InteguSeal (sterile, film-forming cyanoacrylate liquid, provided in a ready-to-use applicator) microbial sealant to the operative field to lock the skin pathogens and thus prevent contamination of the incision site. Assistant will abduct the hip. Palpate the tip of greater trochanter and mark the greater trochanter with sterile marking pencil or methylene blue and draw a line 4 fingers breadth proximal and distal to the base of greater trochanter, proximal line towards the PSIS. In 30° flexion of hip, this line is straight **(Fig. 7.18)**. Apply the large Ioban over the operating field. Every member of surgical team will wear 2nd pair of gloves.

Posterior Approach

Incision

Anesthetist is asked to keep the BP of patient at 100–90/60 to avoid excessive oozing of blood. Keeping the hip in 30° flexion, give incision as per skin marking. Cut the skin and superficial fascia (with BP blade No. 22). Assistant will abduct the hip, make a small longitudinal cut (nick) in deep fascia (tensor fascia lata) with 2nd knife (BP blade No.24).

Exposure and Dislocation of Hip

Cut the deep fascia with curved scissors and proximally split the gluteus maximum muscle in the line of incision. Apply Charnley's retractor. Split the trochanteric bursa with Kocher and electrocautery. Apply 90° narrow blade retractor or Hohmann in the proximal part of incision to retract the posterior border of gluteus medius. Ask the assistant to keep the hip in extended position. Define the insertion of short external rotators of hip (piriformis, superior gemellus, obturator internus, inferior gemellus, obturator externus and quadratus femoris) **(Fig. 7.19)** by sponge. The superior and inferior gemelli join together along with the obturator internus to form the conjoined tendon. Take the electrocautery and cut the short external rotators of hip and capsule starting from the piriformis fossa and along the intertrochanteric crest. The gemelli protect the sciatic nerve. Give T-shaped incision in the capsule along the neck of femur up to the head at 10 O' clock position for right hip

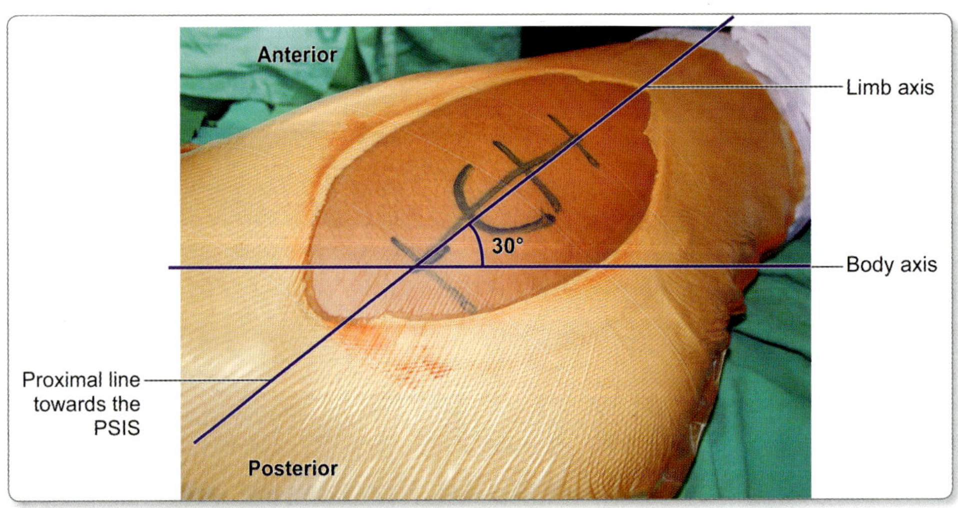

Fig. 7.18 After draping and marking for skin incision (Straight line of incision on 30° flexion at hip)

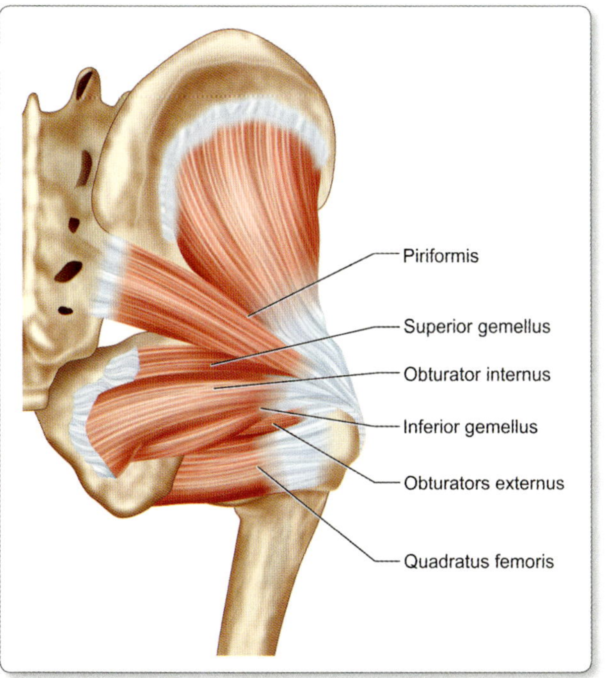

Fig. 7.19 Diagrammatic picture showing the short external rotator muscles of hip

or 2 O' clock position for left and another incision at 12 O' clock position **(Fig. 7.20)**. Expose the lesser trochanter by cutting the insertion of iliopsoas by electrocautery.

Retract the soft tissue in distal part of incision and expose the insertion of gluteus maximus tendon. Cut the insertion of gluteus maximus tendon near femoral attachment and tensor fascia lata. However, cutting the insertion of gluteus maximus tendon is not required in all cases but it is recommended in long standing cases with marked shortening. Sometimes, little release of the posterior border of vastus lateralis at the origin is required. The assistant will extend and gradually internally rotate the hip by holding the leg and knee flexed at 90°. Release the capsule by electrocautery from the neck of the femur. The assistant will use the suction to suck the smoke and blood. Dislocate the hip gently by flexion, adduction, internal rotation and by **pump handle technique** (up and down movement of thigh by holding the leg with knee flexed at 90°, adducted and internally rotated position of hip) **(Fig. 7.21)**. The hip dislocation should be done by the surgeon and not by the assistant to avoid undue force which may lead to fracture of femur or acetabulum. If dislocation is difficult, then look

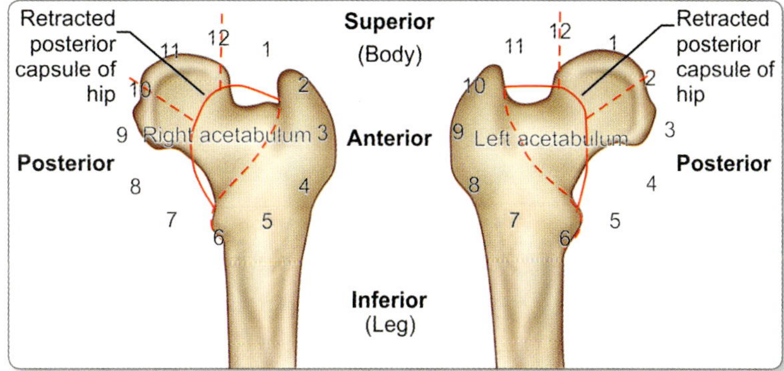

Fig. 7.20 Dotted red lines on face of a clock indicate the line of incision along the intertrochanteric crest, lesser trochanter and in the capsule (solid red line) after retraction

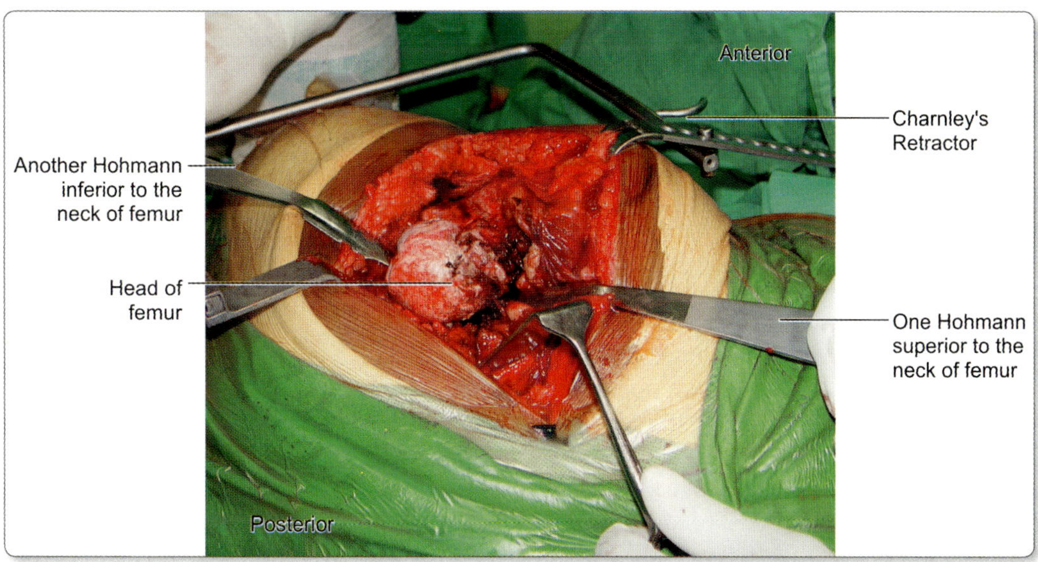

Fig. 7.21 Posterior exposure of the Hip

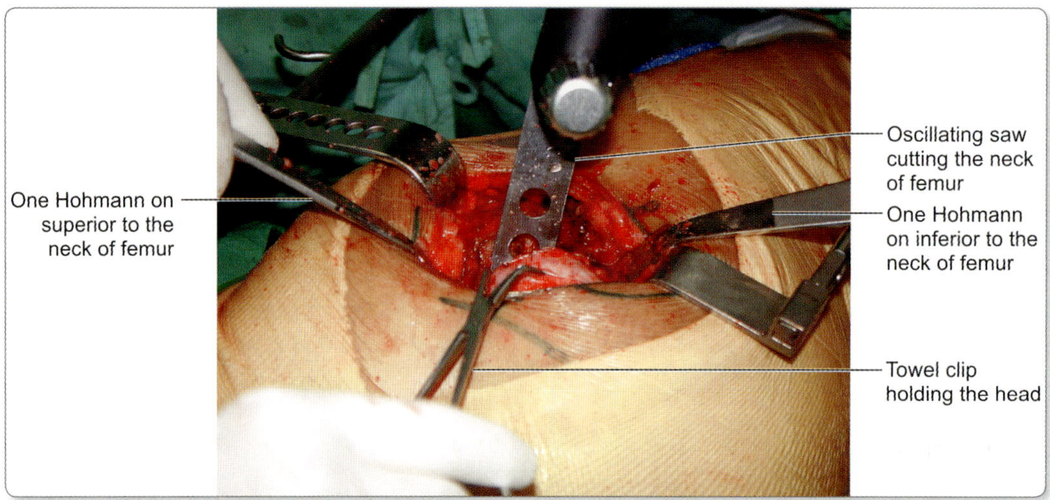

Fig. 7.22 Femoral neck resection by oscillating saw

for the causes like posterior osteophytes (most common), fibrous or bony ankylosis, protrusio acetabuli, coxa magna and thickened ligamentum teres. Remove the posterior osteophytes if any by nibbler or curved osteotome and hammer (posterior acetabuloplasty) and dislocate the hip gently. For other causes, first release between the head and acetabulum by electrocautery and retry gentle dislocation of hip if not then do neck resection in situ to avoid undue force during dislocation which may lead to fracture of femur or acetabulum (*See* the technique of neck resection in situ in chapter eight).

Uncemented THR (Summit Stem)

Femoral Neck Resection

One assistant will hold the limb with knee flexed at 90° and hip at 45°, adducted and internally rotated so that sole of the foot will face the ceiling. Apply the neck resection guide along the shaft of the femur so that proximal tip of guide is at the level of tip of the greater trochanter and cut is along the inclination of neck of guide which is 10–15 mm (one finger breadth) from the lesser trochanter. Before cutting, mark the level of neck resection with electrocautery. The neck resection line is perpendicular to the femoral neck axis starting from the calcar one finger breadth away from the lesser trochanter and ending near the piriform fossa **(Fig. 8.3A, Chapter 8)**. Apply two Hohmanns, one over the superior aspect and another over the inferior aspect of femoral neck to protect the soft tissues. The assistant will lift the thigh to keep the neck of femur parallel to the ground to avoid oblique cut. Another assistant will hold the femoral head with towel clip or head holding forceps to avoid accidental fall. Cut the neck with oscillating saw as per mark **(Fig. 7.22)**. Pass the straight osteotome through the neck resection and lever out the femoral head. Cut the ligamentum teres with curved scissors or electrocautery and remove the head. Keep the hip in extension.

Exposure of Acetabulum

Assistant will retract the femoral neck by Kocher against posterior wall of acetabulum and posterior border of gluteus medius by 90° narrow blade retractor. Remove the overhanging tissues from anterosuperior aspect of acetabulum. Apply pins on chain, 1st pin anterosuperiorly at 1 O' clock position for right hip and 11 O' clock position for left hip and 2nd pin posterosuperiorly at 11 O' clock position for right hip and 1 O' clock postion for left hip. Fix the chain with Kocher. Remove the labrum from acetabular margin and ligamentum teres from the acetabulum. Retract the soft tissues inferiorly by 90° blade deep retractor. Apply 3rd pin posteroinferiorly at 8 O'clock position for right hip and 4 O' clock position for left hip to retract the soft tissues. Apply 45° curve Hohmann on the anterior margin of the acetabulum at 2 O' clock position for right hip and 10 O' clock position for left hip to retract the femur anteriorly. Make a small nick in the transverse ligament of acetabular notch by electrocautery and apply Wroblewski retractor in the acetabular notch at 6 O'clock position. Thus 360° of acetabulum is exposed **(Figs 7.23 to 7.25)**. Keep the limb straight on the table in neutral rotation.

Insertion of Acetabular Cup

Remove the soft tissues from the acetabular rim. Remove the cartilage by ring curette. Start reaming the acetabulum with 40 mm size acetabular reamer in 45° abduction and 20° anteversion **(Fig. 7.26)**. Gradually increase the size

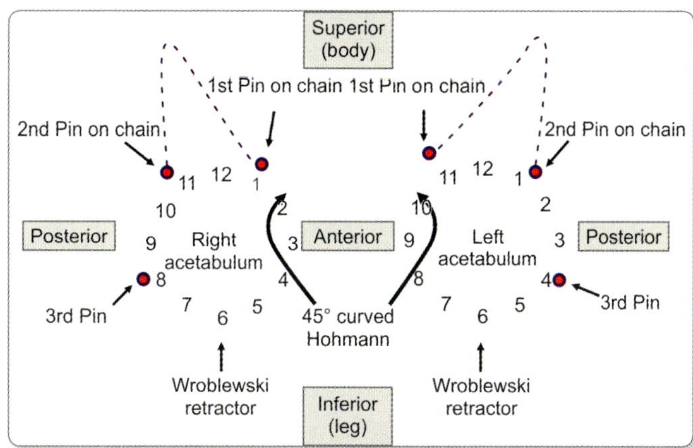

Fig. 7.23 Diagrammatic picture showing positions of different retractors on face of a clock while exposure of 360° of acetabulum

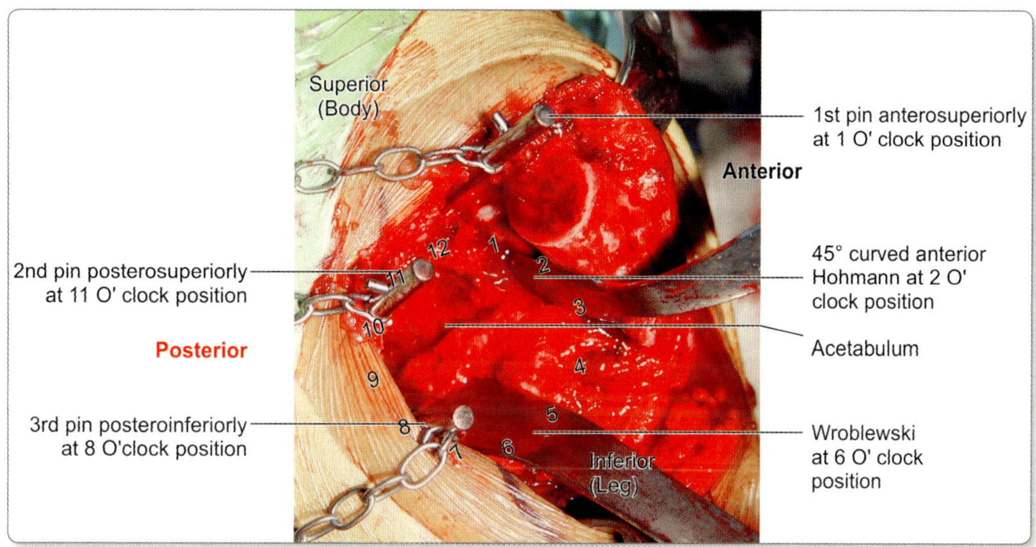

Fig. 7.24 Position of different retractors while exposure of right acetabulum

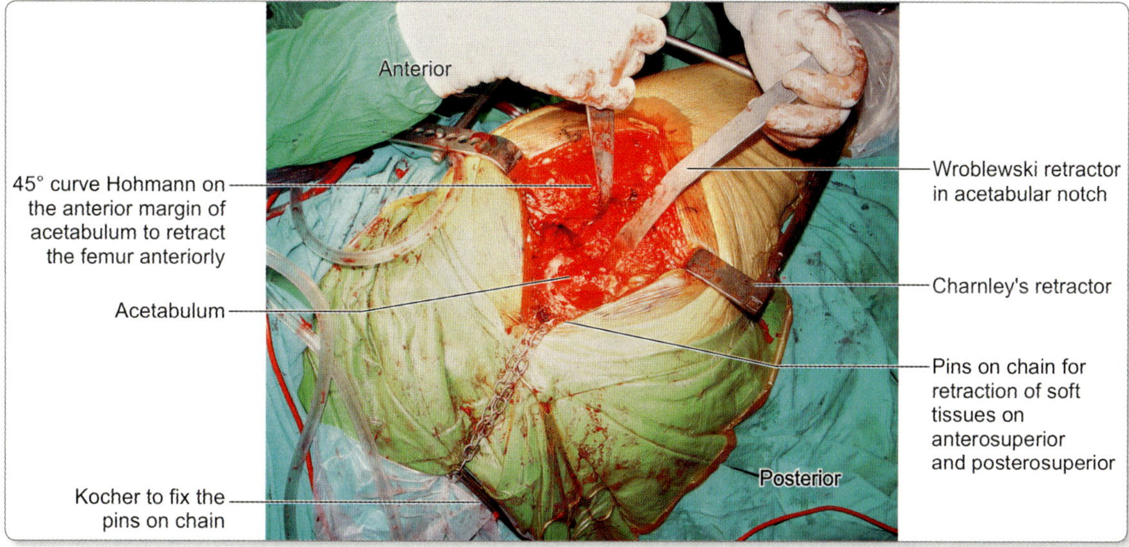

Fig. 7.25 360° of acetabulum is exposed

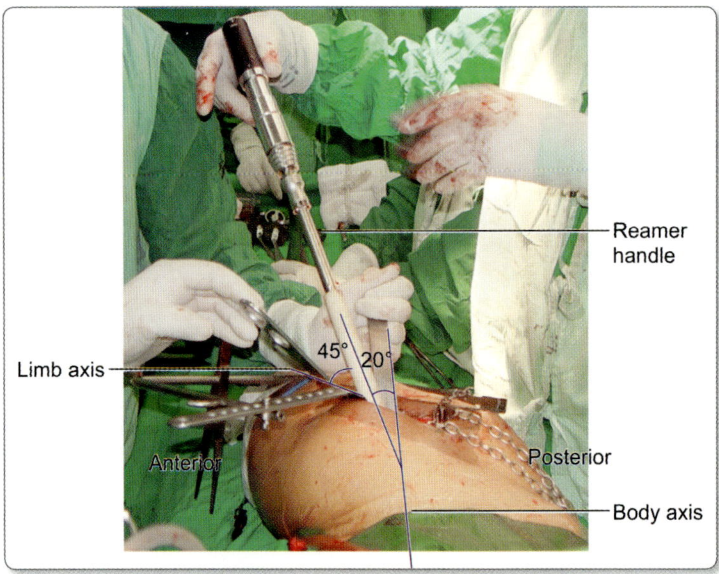

Fig. 7.26 Reaming in 20° anteversion and 45° abduction

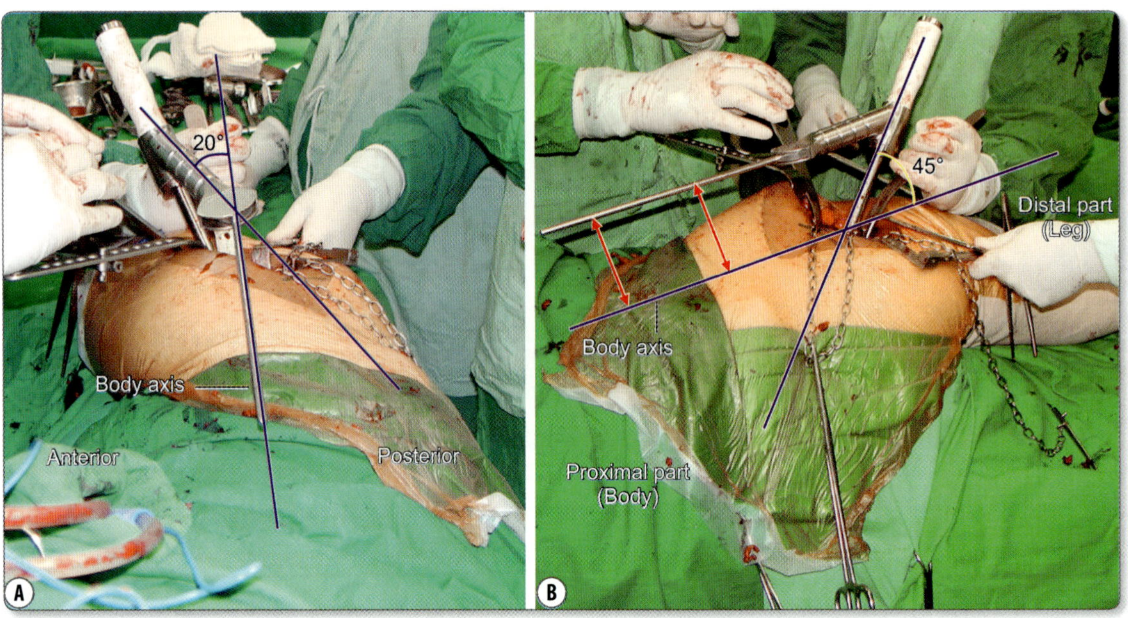

Figs 7.27A and B Acetabular angle guide set at 20° anteversion and 45° abduction during insertion of acetabular cup

of reamer (40, 42, 44, 46, 48, 50, 52, 54, 56 and 58 mm) till acetabulum is freshly bleeding and a hemispherical dome is achieved, i.e. all cartilage is removed and minimum size up to 46 mm is achieved so that the smallest acetabular cup (Duraloc shell) of size 48 mm can be applied (size of Duraloc shell is 48, 50, 52, 54, 56, 58 and 60 mm).

Final tuning of acetabular floor can be done by reaming with 40 mm or 44 mm acetabular reamer. Attach the appropriate size trial cup with acetabular cup holder (one size higher than the final reamer, i.e. if reaming is done with 52 mm size reamer then trial cup and hence the Duraloc shell is of 54 mm size). Set the acetabular angle guide at 20° anteversion. Apply over the handle of the cup holder. Keeping handle of cup holder at 45° abduction, give several gentle blows over the cup holder till the trial cup snuggly fits in the acetabulum **(Figs 7.27A and B)**.

In between the blows of hammer, allow the acetabulum to expand. Proper fitting of trial cup is assessed by its position, cortical bone contact and gently moving the cup holder. Snuggly fitted trial cup will not move. The inferior rim of the trial cup should be in level with the bottom of the teardrop. Remove the trial cup with cup holder. Bone graft from femoral head may be applied in acetabulum if the acetabular floor is thin or cysts are present. Apply

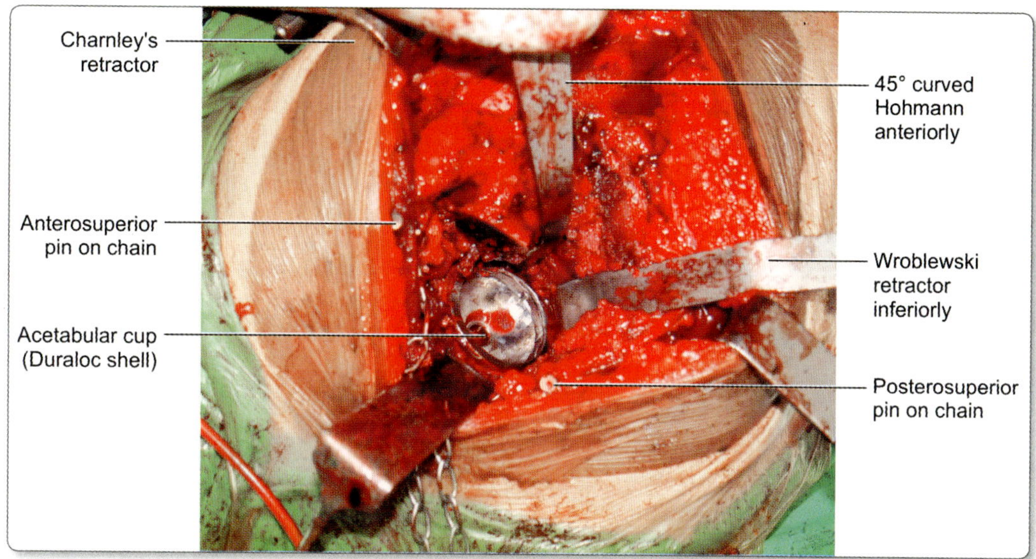

Fig. 7.28 Implanted uncemented cup (Duraloc shell)

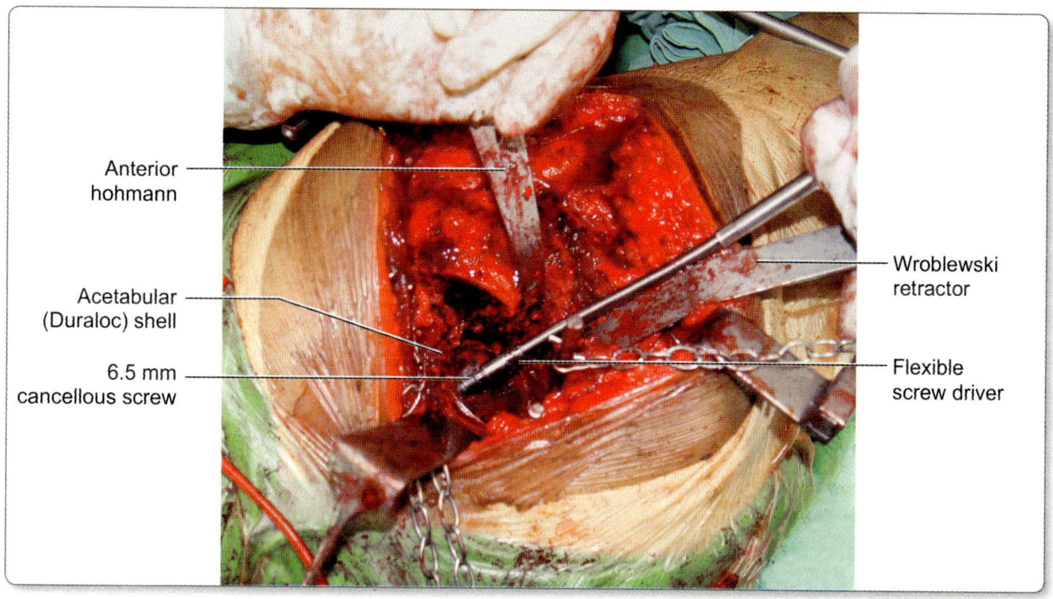

Fig. 7.29 Passing screw in the hole of acetabular shell

the selected Duraloc shell on acetabular cup holder. Put it in the acetabulum in such a way that the screw holes of acetabular cup are aligned with the roof of the acetabulum. Set the acetabular angle guide at 20° anteversion and apply over the handle of acetabular cup holder. Keeping the angle guide parallel to the body in 20° anteversion and handle of cup holder at 45° abduction, give several gentle blows with hammer over the handle of the cup holder till the Duraloc shell is snugly fitted in the acetabulum **(Fig. 7.28)**. Check the stability by moving the cup holder.

Wash the cup with normal saline. If required, 4.5 mm drill hole is made with angled drill through drill guide in one or two holes of Duraloc shell. Take the measurement with depth gauge and apply appropriate size screws (usually 25 or 30 mm long, 6.5 mm cancellous screws) **(Fig. 7.29)**. If the screw is applied, the head of screw should be appropriately fitted in the hole of acetabular cup (Duraloc shell), otherwise the head of screw will interfere with the proper sitting of acetabular liner. Proper fitting of acetabular liner (polyethylene liner) is confirmed by trial acetabular liner.

Apply the angled or hooded polyethylene liner (10° lip Duraloc Marathon liner) of appropriate size. The hood of the liner is placed in posterosuperior position and pressed firmly by the hand. Final impaction into the shell

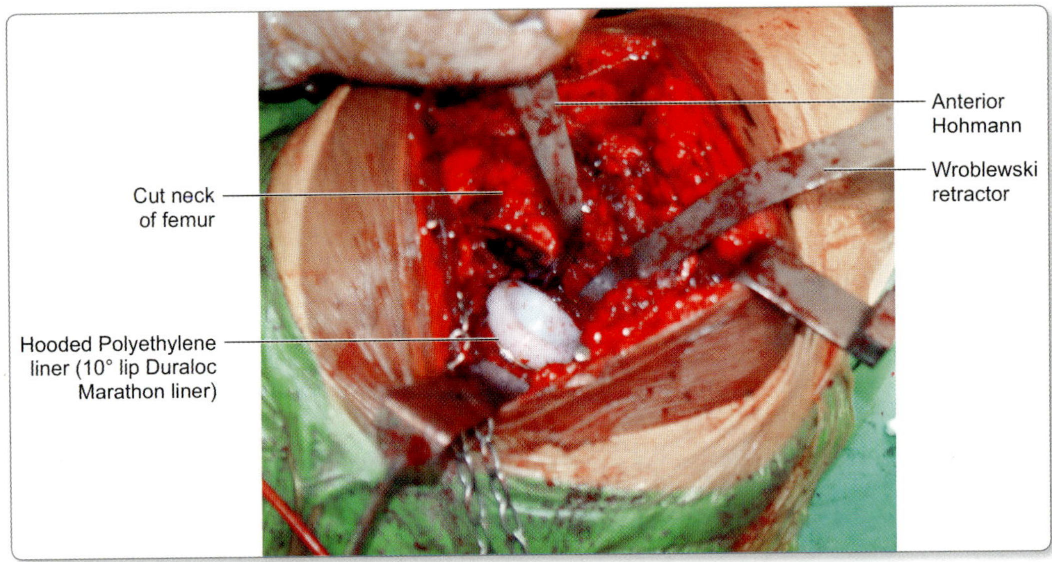

Fig. 7.30 After implantation of acetabular cup and acetabular liner

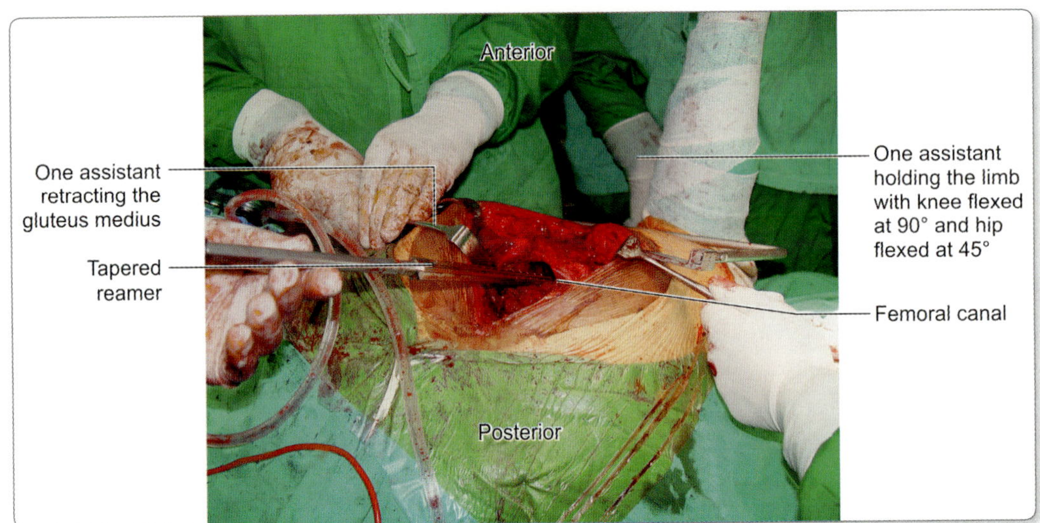

Fig. 7.31 Reaming of femoral canal

is completed using the polyethylene headed liner impactor until the liner locks into place **(Fig.7.30)**. Cover the liner with betadine soaked gauze piece. Remove the pins on chain, anterior Hohmann and Wroblewski retractor.

Insertion of Femoral Component

One assistant will hold the limb with knee flexed at 90° and hip at 45°, adducted and internally rotated so that sole of the foot will face the ceiling. Other assistant will retract the posterior border of gluteus medius to expose the piriformis fossa. Clean the area of piriformis fossa by electrocautery and curette. Find out the entry point for femoral canal over the piriformis fossa **(Figs 8.3A and B, chapter 8)**. Take the Excel IM initiator attached with T-handle and make the entry hole in the femoral canal by advancing till full circumference. Remove excel IM initiator. Attach the T-handle with excel canal probe and pass in the medullary canal of the femur till the superior margin of the cutting flutes meets the neck resection. The canal probe should pass easily if proper alignment has been achieved. It is important to have circumferential clearance with the canal probe to avoid reaming in varus (i.e. neutral alignment of the canal). Attach the trochanteric reamer (lateralizer) to the T- handle and insert it into the canal. Advance the trochanteric reamer until the cutting region of the reamer is aligned with the greater trochanter. This will lateralize the proximal entry point for the subsequent reamers and broaches. Fine tuning of lateralization may be done by femoral rasp. Then pass the tapered reamers to prepare the distal femur starting from size 0–1 as per mark GT (greater trochanter referencing) till it is snugly fitting in the femoral canal **(Fig. 7.31)**. The

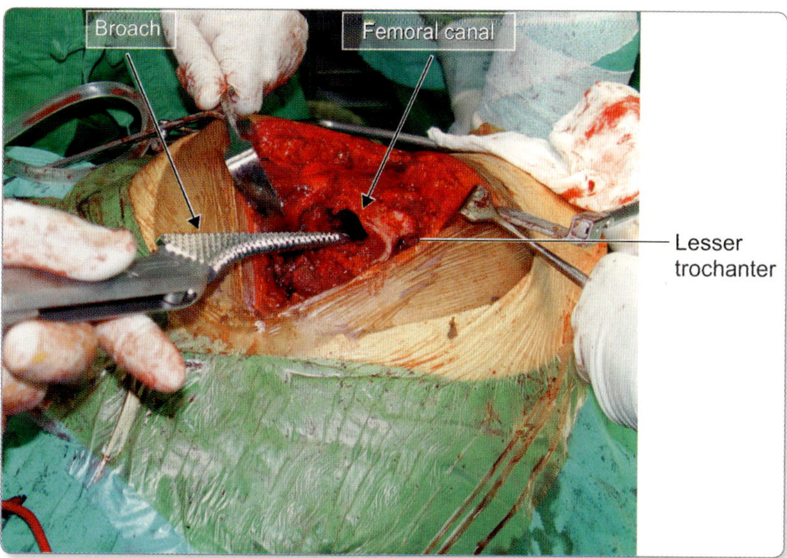

Fig. 7.32 Broaching in 20° anteversion in relation to lesser trochanter

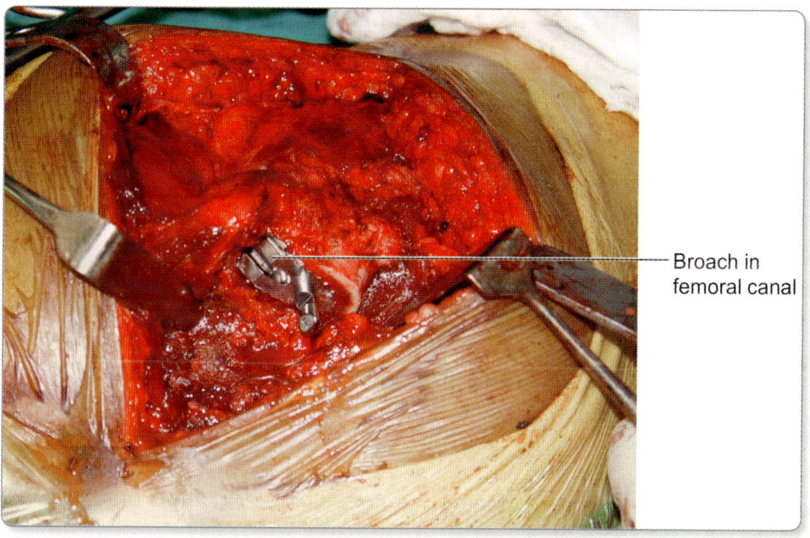

Fig. 7.33 Broach in place for trial reduction

sizes of tapered reamers are 0–1, 2–3, 4–5, 6–7 and 8–9. Use a nibbler to remove the bone bridge, if any, between the entry hole in femoral canal and resected neck of femur. Alternatively, use a box osteotome (anteversion osteotome) to enter the femoral canal at the junction of the femoral neck and the greater trochanter.

Attach size 0 femoral broach to broach handle. Advance the broach down the medullary canal first by manual pressure and then by hammer in proper alignment and 20° anteversion **(Fig. 7.32)**. Check the anteversion in relation to lesser trochanter. Gradually increase the size of broach till the appropriate size broach snugly fits in the canal up to the neck. The sizes of broach are 0 to 8. The final broach should fit and fill the proximal femur with the top of the cutting teeth resting at the level of neck resection and rotationally stable **(Fig. 7.33)**. In between the hammering, allow the femoral canal to expand and carefully hear the sound of hammering to notice any change in the tone of sound.

Remove the broach handle. Remove the betadine soaked gauze piece from the implanted cup. Select either the small or large calcar planer and attach it to power reamer. Place the planer over the broach stud and mill the calcar to the broach face **(Fig. 7.34)**. Make certain that the planer is rotating before engaging the calcar. This will prevent the planer from binding on the calcar.

Apply the trial neck and +1.5 head trial over the broach. Apply one gauze piece around the trial neck. Loosen the Charnley's retractor. For reduction, the assistant will apply the traction in extended position of hip with knee flexed at 90 degree. Another assistant will hold the gauze piece around the trial neck and apply gentle traction along the long-axis of femur. The surgeon will gently push the head in

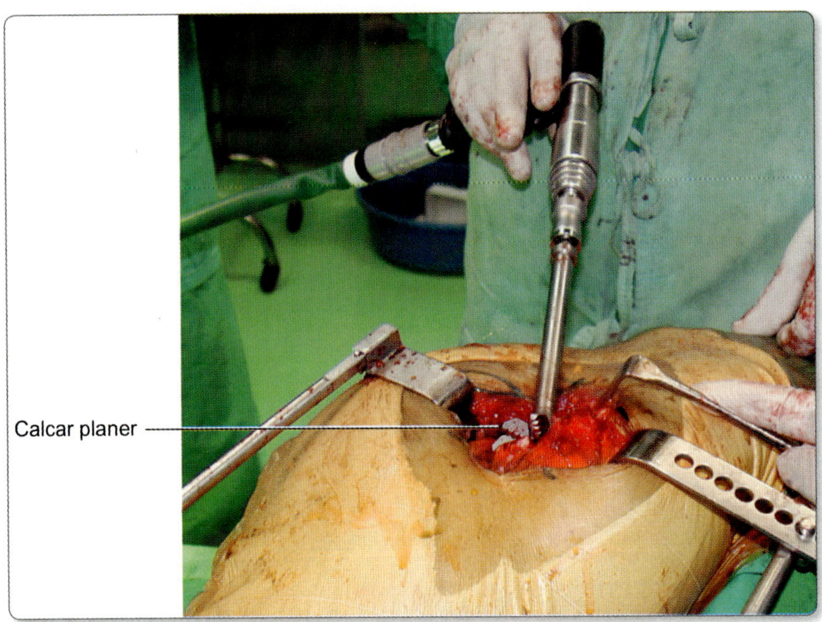

Fig. 7.34 Use of calcar planer to mill the calcar to the broach face

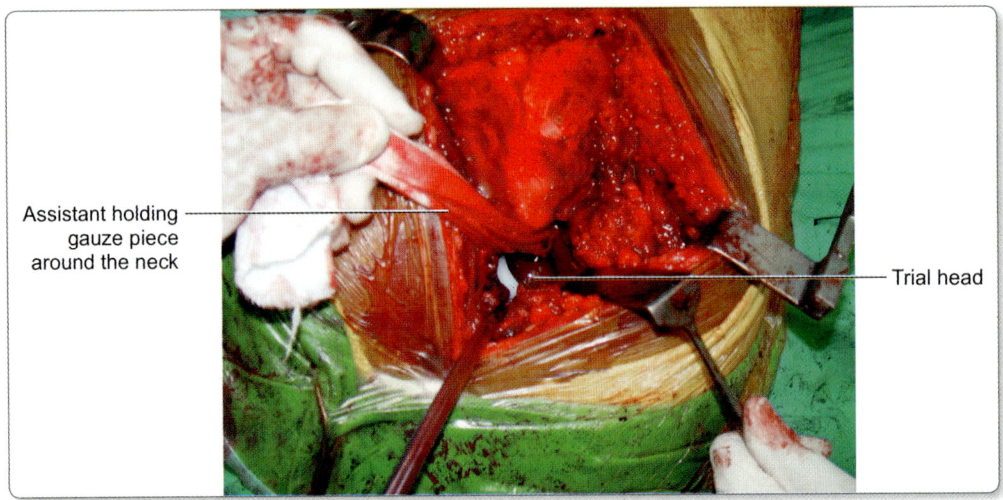

Fig. 7.35 Trial reduction with broach and trial head

acetabulum while retracting the soft tissues by fingers. Head impactor is helpful for pushing the head during reduction. When the head is near the margin of acetabulum, the assistant will gently externally rotate the limb and the hip is reduced **(Fig. 7.35)**.

Tighten the Charnley's retractor. Check the movement and stability of hip. Flex the hip at 90°. Check the adduction and internal rotation. Extend the hip. Check the abduction, external rotation, internal rotation and suck test (pull the leg in extension to see the amount of opening between head and acetabulum and opening should not be more than 2 mm). Check the amount of tension in abductor muscles (palpate the anterior border of gluteus medius). Check that the center of trial head is at the level of tip of greater trochanter. Finally check the limb length by comparing the level of lower poles of patella in identical position of both limbs. With the hip in 90° of flexion and 0° of abduction, internal rotation should be at least 45° with no tendency to dislocate. In extension, there should be full external rotation with no tendency to dislocate or impinge.

Trial may be done with the higher size of the trial head (+5, +8.5, +12, +15.5) as per the requirement after assessment of movements, stability, tension in abductor muscles and limb length. Loosen the Charnley's retractor and dislocate the hip by pulling the neck with gauze piece already applied around trial neck while assistant is giving traction, flexion, adduction and internal rotation. Remove the trial head and neck. But final selection of the head should be done after

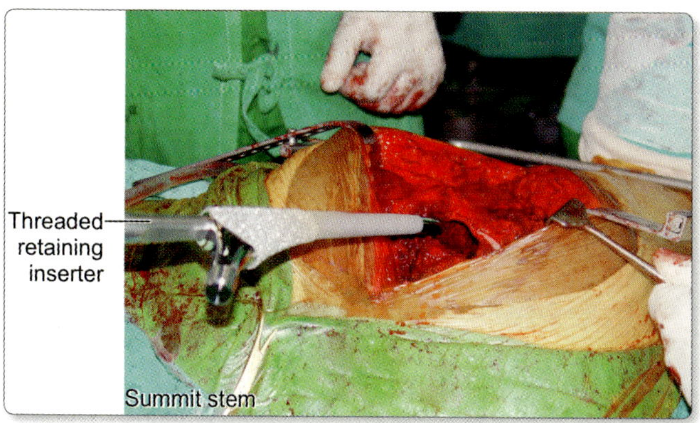

Fig. 7.36 Summit uncemented stem being applied in 20° anteversion

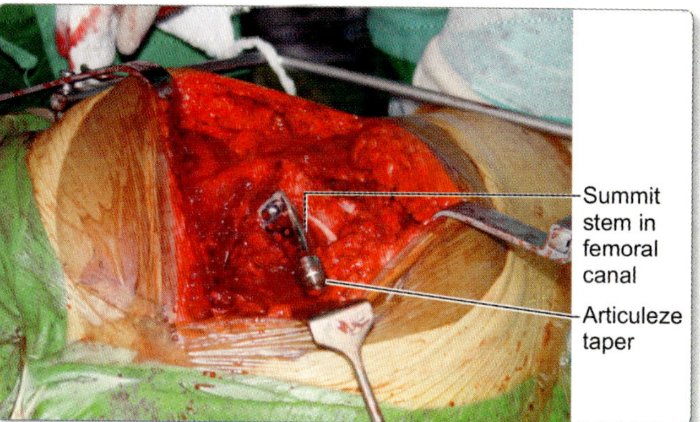

Figs 7.37 Summit uncemented stem fixed in 20° anteversion as compared with lesser trochanter

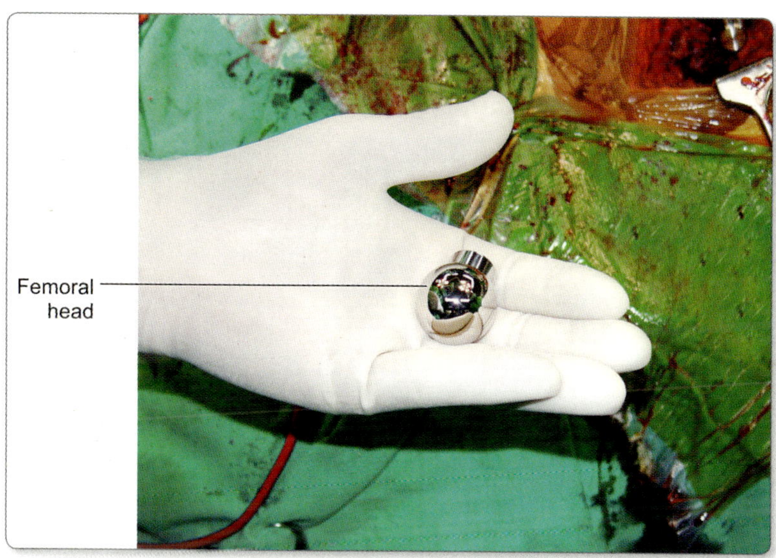

Fig. 7.38 Determined size of head

the final trial following final implantation of the femoral component. Remove the broach by attaching the broach handle and retrograde hammering. Take the appropriate size summit tapered proximally coated femoral implant (the porous-coated region of the femoral component is oversized by 0.375 mm per side relative to the instrumentation). The size available for summit stem is from 1 to 8. The final size of summit stem is same as the final size of the broach. Attach it on the threaded retaining inserter to control rotation and apply it in the femoral canal in 20° anteversion in relation to lesser trochanter. First push the stem by manual pressure and then gently hammer it **(Figs 7.36 and 7.37)**. Carefully hear the sound of hammering to notice any change. In between the hammering, allow the femoral canal to expand.

Once the threaded retaining inserter reaches at the level of greater trochanter, exchange with non-threaded retaining inserter and hammer till the neck of the implant is at the level of cut surface of the femur. Exchange of inserter is to avoid sometimes engaging in proximal femur and removal of threaded retaining inserter becomes difficult.

Apply the trial head of size +1.5 over the neck of the femoral implant, reduce the hip and assess the stability, movements, suck test, abductor tension and limb length. Accordingly determine the size of the head **(Fig. 7.38)**. Clean and dry the articuleze taper. Introduce the appropriate femoral head (12/14 cone) by firmly pushing and twisting the femoral head into place on the taper. Keep the head impactor over the head and give three gentle blows

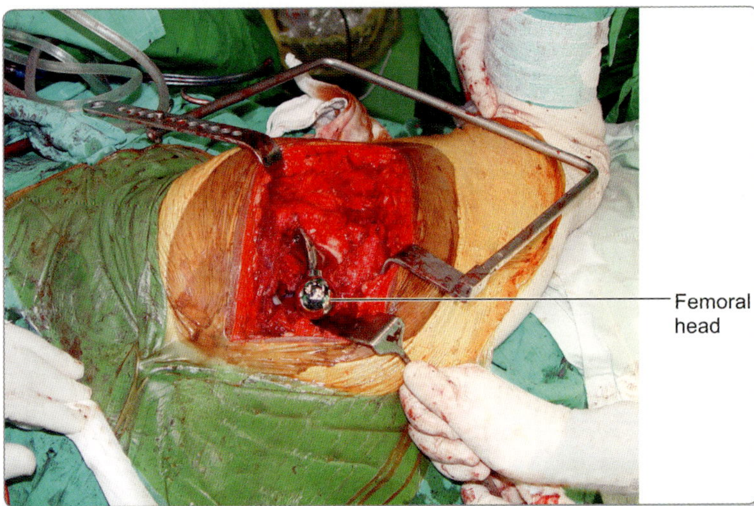

Fig. 7.39 Head applied on summit stem

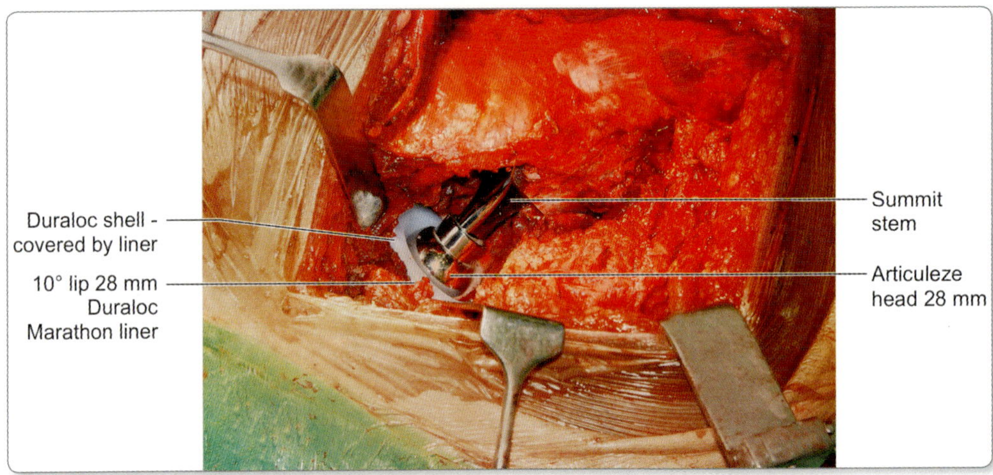

Fig. 7.40 After Implantation of all four components of uncemented THR

by mallet. Fixation of head is confirmed by pulling the head **(Fig. 7.39)**.

Loosen the Charnley's retractor and reduce the head **(Fig. 7.40)** as described. Recheck the stability, movements, suck test, abductor tension (palpate the anterior border of gluteus medius) and limb length. Clean the wound with gentamicin mixed normal saline by pulse lavage. Load two vials of gentamicin in a syringe and pour it in the wound.

Closure of the Wound

Take No.1 vicryl and apply 4 sutures in the short external rotator muscles (piriformis, superior gemellus, obturator internus, inferior gemellus, obturator externus and quadratus femoris) after protecting the sciatic nerve. Suture one for piriformis tendon, suture two for conjoined tendon of superior gemellus, obturator internus and inferior gamellus, suture 3 and 4 for obturator externus and quadratus femoris. Make 4 drill holes by 2.5 mm drill bit one-by-one in the intertrochanteric crest and pass the sutures in each hole **(Fig. 7.41)**. For passing the suture in each hole, pass the straight needle with nylon thread in reverse direction. Pass the suture of external rotator muscle through the loop of nylon thread of the straight needle and pull the straight needle out from the hole. Similarly pass the other sutures of external rotator muscles one-by-one

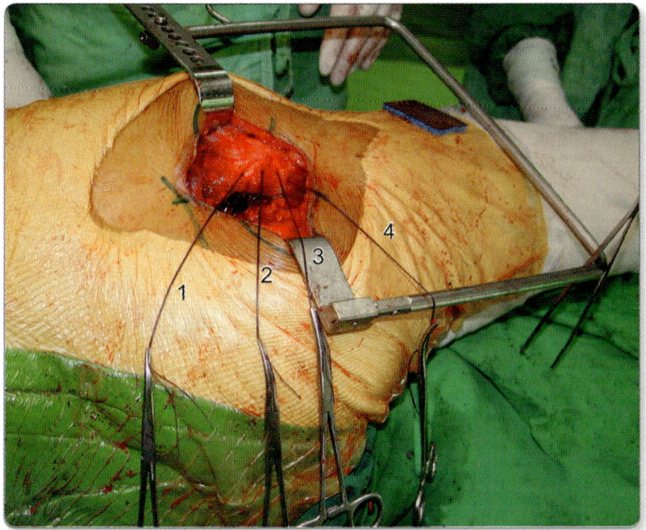

Fig. 7.41 Anchoring of external rotator muscles by four sutures (1, 2, 3 and 4) passed through the drill holes in the intertrochanteric crest

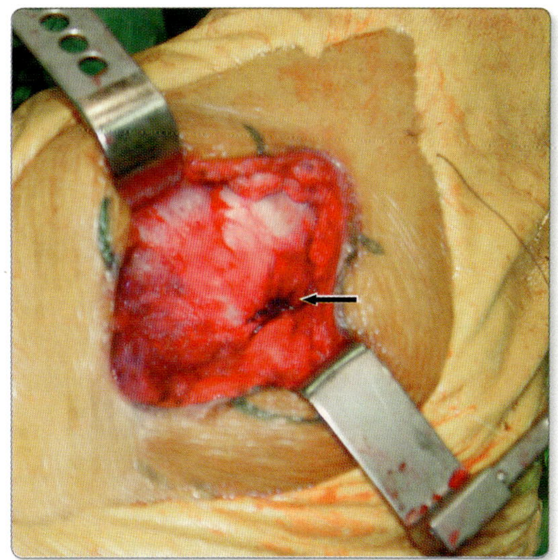

Fig. 7.42 After ligation of the four sutures together (i.e. repair of the short external rotator muscles)

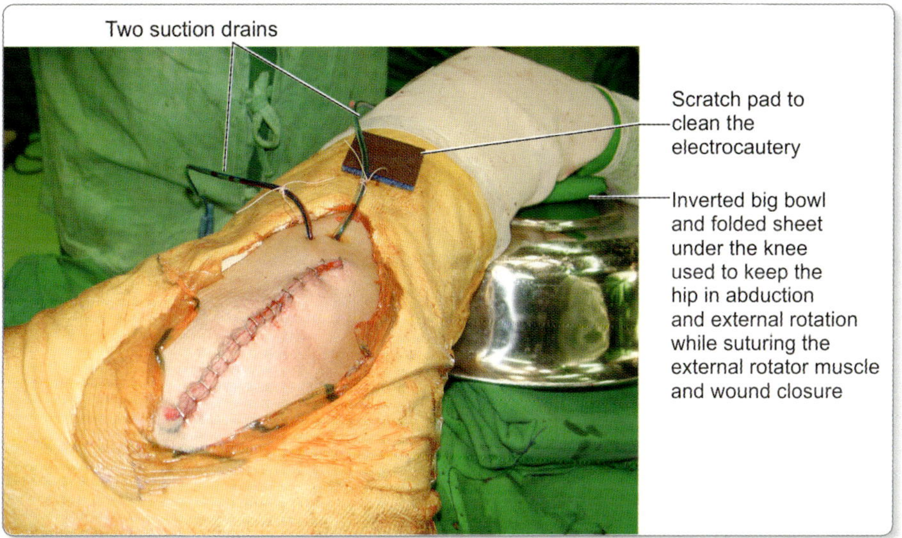

Fig. 7.43 Two suction drains and wound closure by staples

(Fig. 7.42). Loosen the Charnley's retractor. Keep the hip in abduction and external rotation. Inverted big bowl and folded sheet **(Fig. 7.43)** under the knee can be used to keep the hip in abduction and external rotation which facilitates the suturing of external rotator muscles and wound closure. Ligate the sutures one-by-one and cut the extra thread **(Fig. 7.42)**. Remove the Charnley's retractor. Retract the inferior part of wound and suture the insertion of gluteus maximus by two interrupted sutures with No.1 vicryl, if it is cut. Put 2 suction drains (No. 14). Close the tensor fascia lata in lower part of wound and gluteus maximus in upper part by interlocking continuous suture with No.1 vicryl. Apply interrupted subcutaneous sutures with No.1 vicryl. Apply staples to close the wound. Fix the suction drains by thread. Clean the wound and adjacent area with betadine.

Apply betadine gauze piece, dressing pad and seal the wound by elastoplast. Remove the supports and make the patient supine. Shift the patient in ICU. Keep the limb in abduction with one pillow in between two limbs and neutral rotation with derotation bar.

Give IV antibiotic (1 g Cefotaxime)

The postoperative advice, physiotherapy (See physiotherapy for THR in chapter twelve) and follow-up schedule are similar to TKR.

Preoperative and Postoperative X-rays (Figs 7.44 to 7.58)

Implantation of pinnacle cup or Delta motion is similar to Duraloc shell as described. For pinnacle cup, minimum reaming is 42 mm for smallest size (44 mm) cup while for

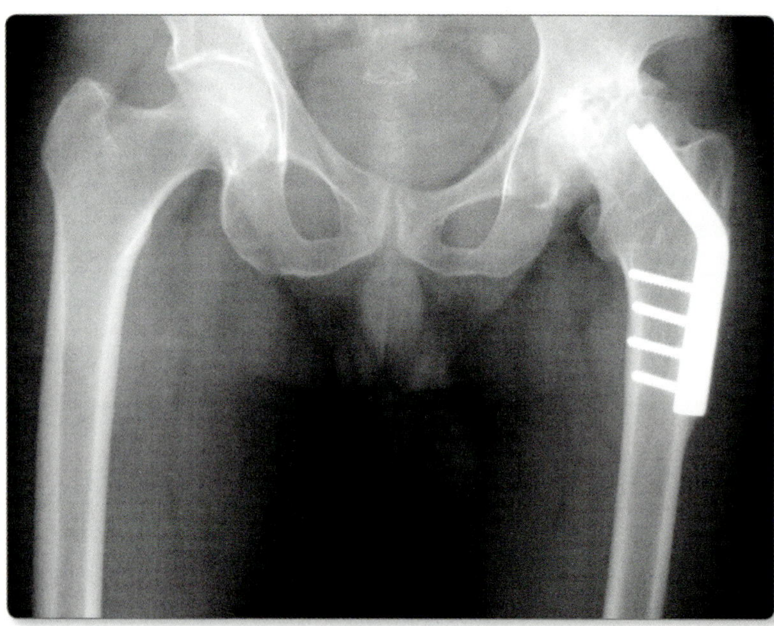

Fig. 7.44 Post-traumatic AVN left hip

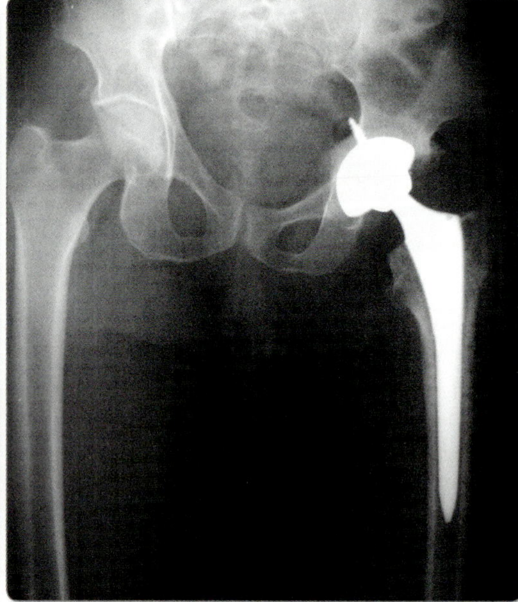

Fig. 7.45 Postoperative

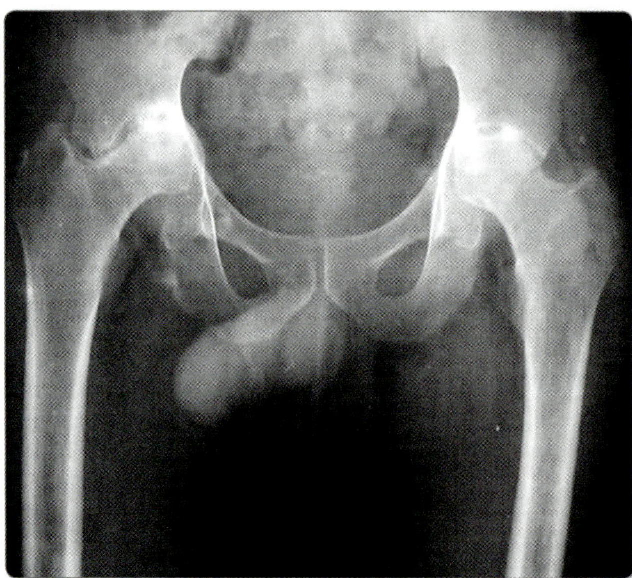

Fig. 7.46 Arthritis both hip joints

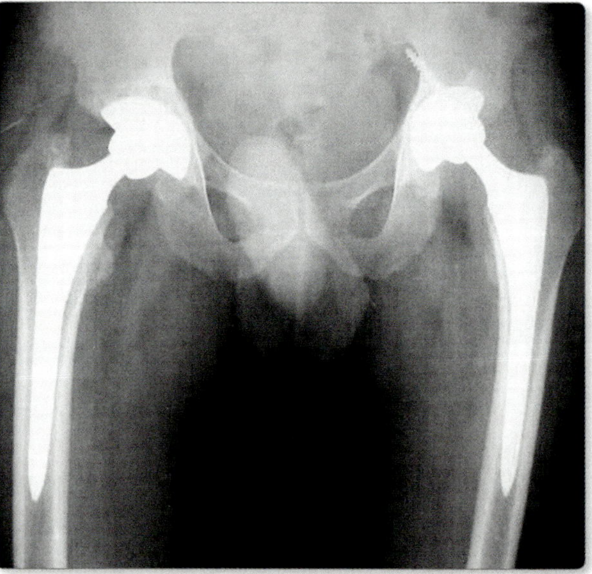

Fig. 7.47 Both hips—Summit stem, Duraloc shell, plastic liner and 28 mm head

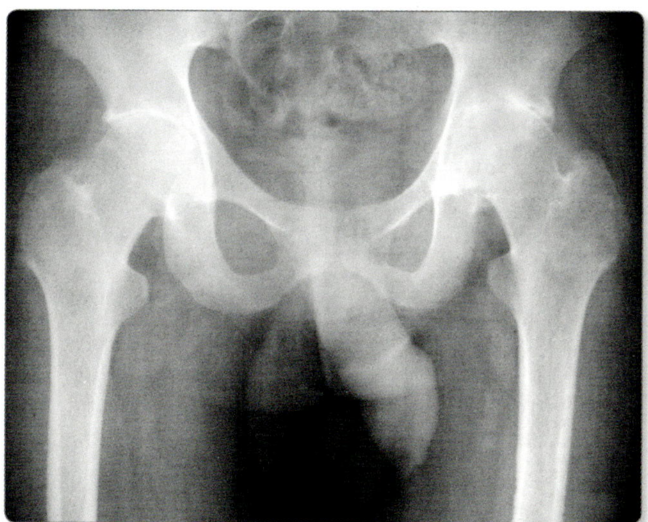

Fig. 7.48 Ankylosing spondylitis with arthritis both hips

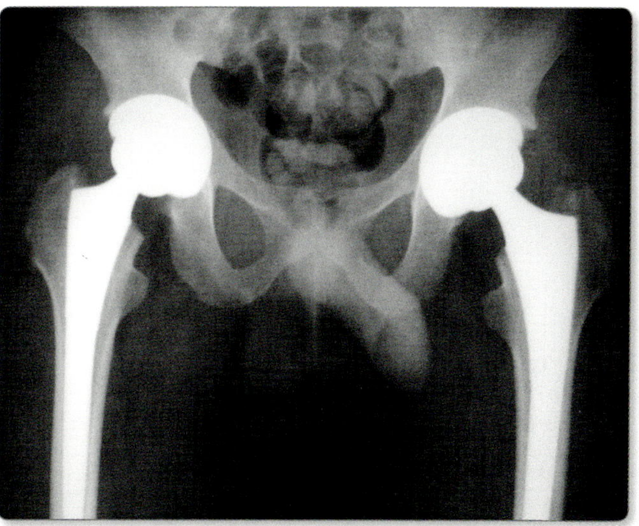

Fig. 7.49 Uncemented (Summit) stem with pinnacle cups and metal on ceramic 36 mm heads to both hips

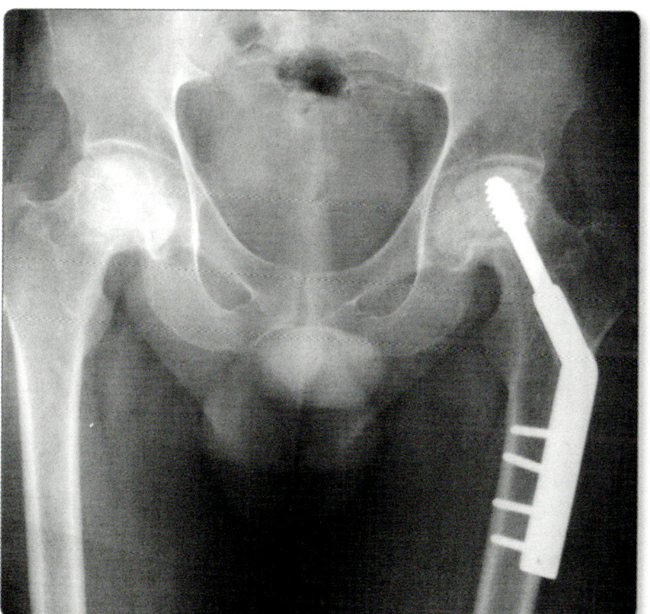

Fig. 7.50 AVN both hip joints

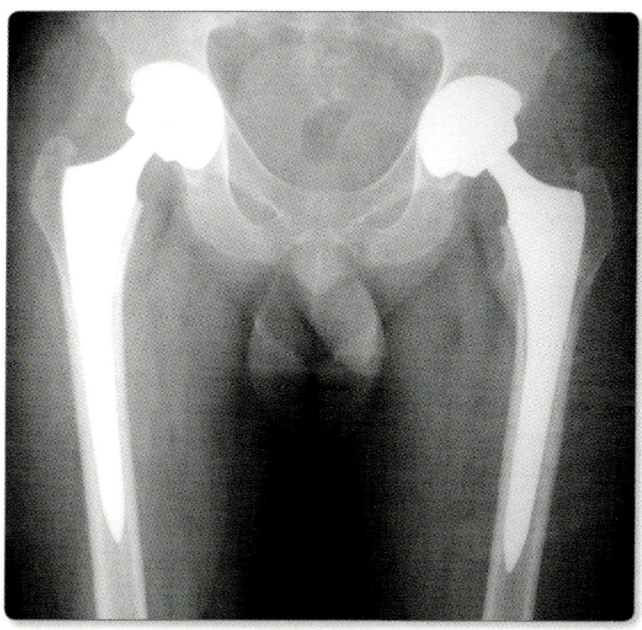

Fig. 7.51 Uncemented (summit) stem with pinnacle cups and ceramic on ceramic 36 mm heads to both hips

Duraloc cup, minimum reaming is 46 mm for smallest size (48 mm) cup.

Duraloc shell is more suitable for relatively shallow acetabular socket and pinnacle cup or Delta motion cup is suitable for deep acetabular socket. Multiholes Duraloc or pinnacle shell is more suitable where reconstruction of acetabulum is required as multiple holes provide space in different directions for application of cancellous screws in the sound part of acetabulum.

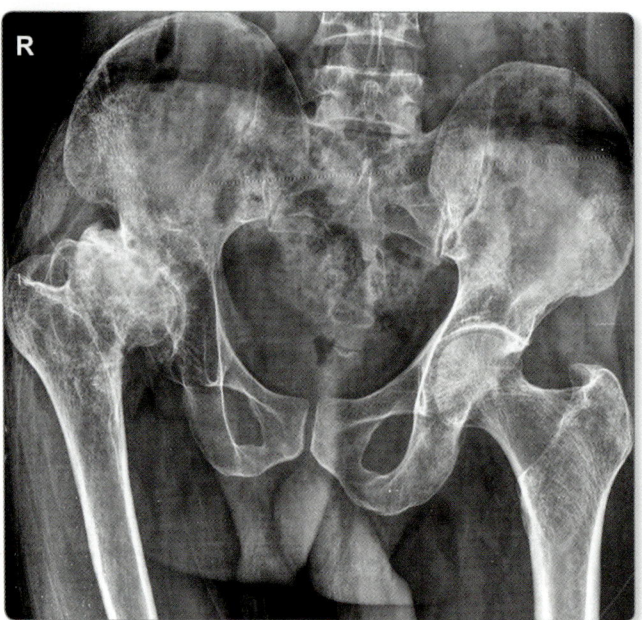

Fig. 7.52 Preoperative AVN with arthritis in dysplastic hip following hip injury in childhood

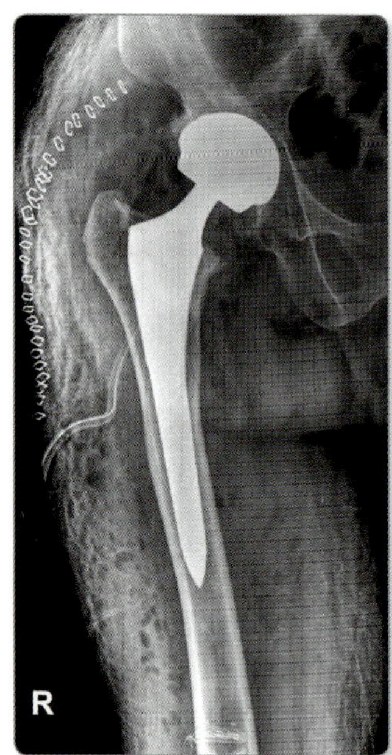

Fig. 7.53 Postoperative with delta motion implant

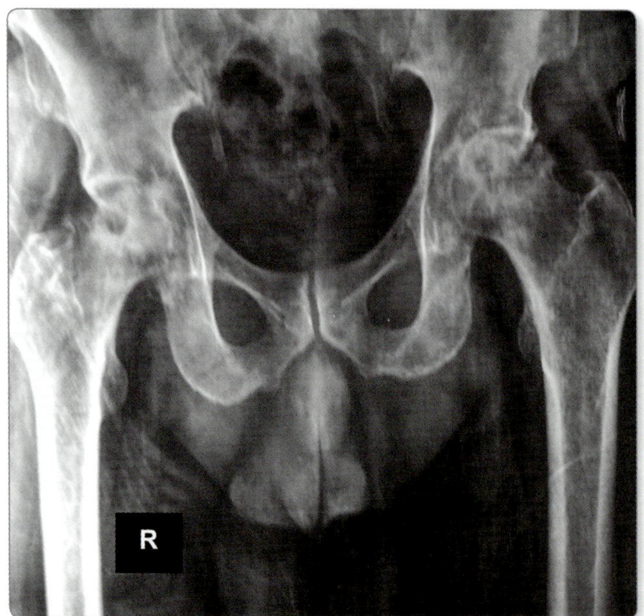

Fig. 7.54 Preoperative AVN in both hips

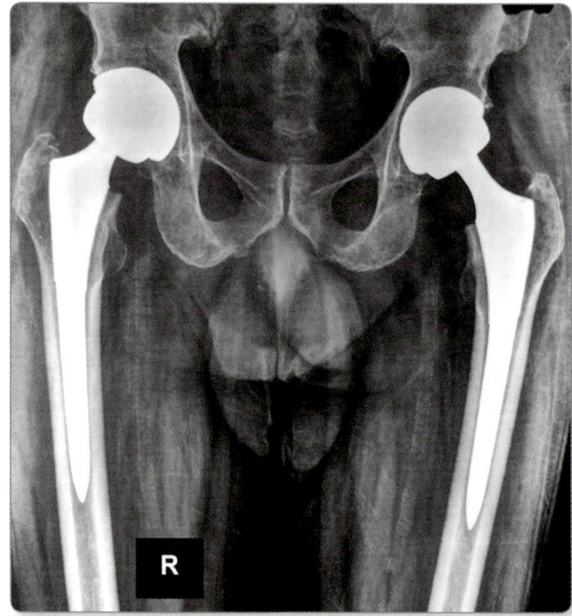

Fig. 7.55 Postoperative with delta motion

Self-centering bipolar head with 28 mm articuleze with uncemented Summit stem **(Figs 7.56 to 7.58)**. (Younger patient with failed fixation of fractured neck of femur).

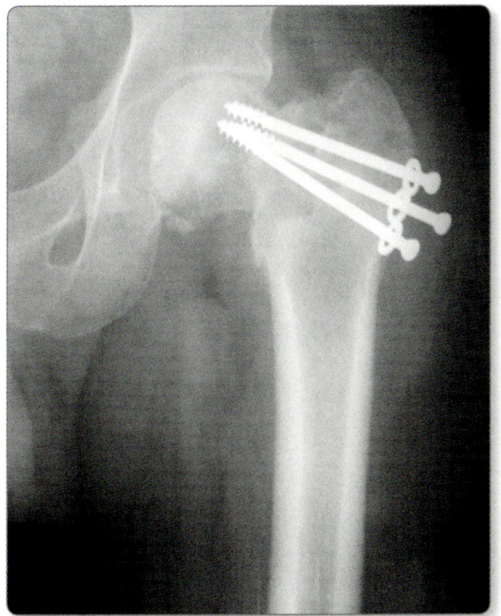
Fig. 7.56 Non-union fracture neck femur head (AP view)

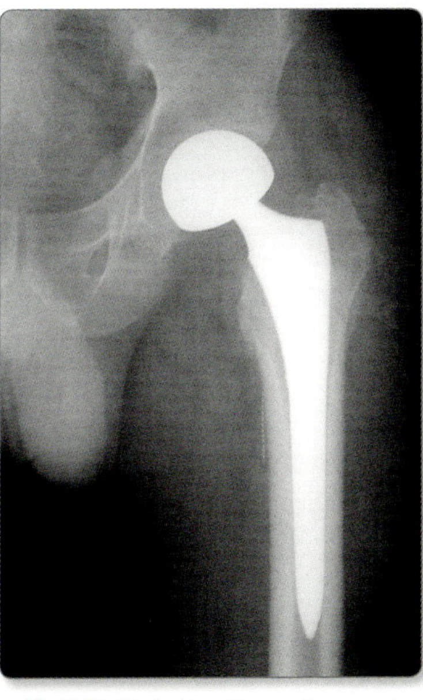
Fig. 7.57 Bipolar hip with summit stem and self-centering bipolar head

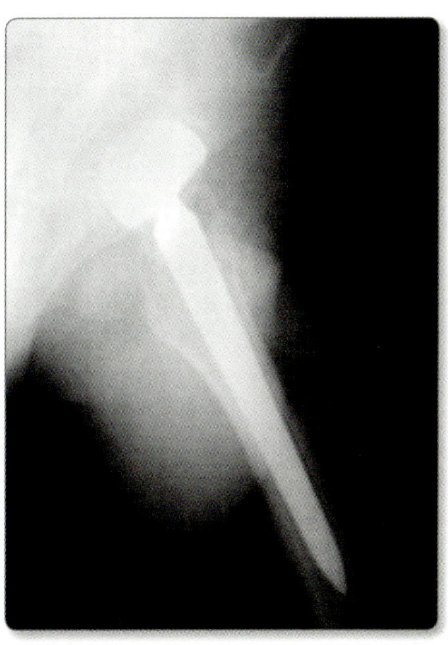
Fig. 7.58 Lateral view

Instruments Required for Uncemented THR (Summit stem) (Figs 7.59 and 7.60)

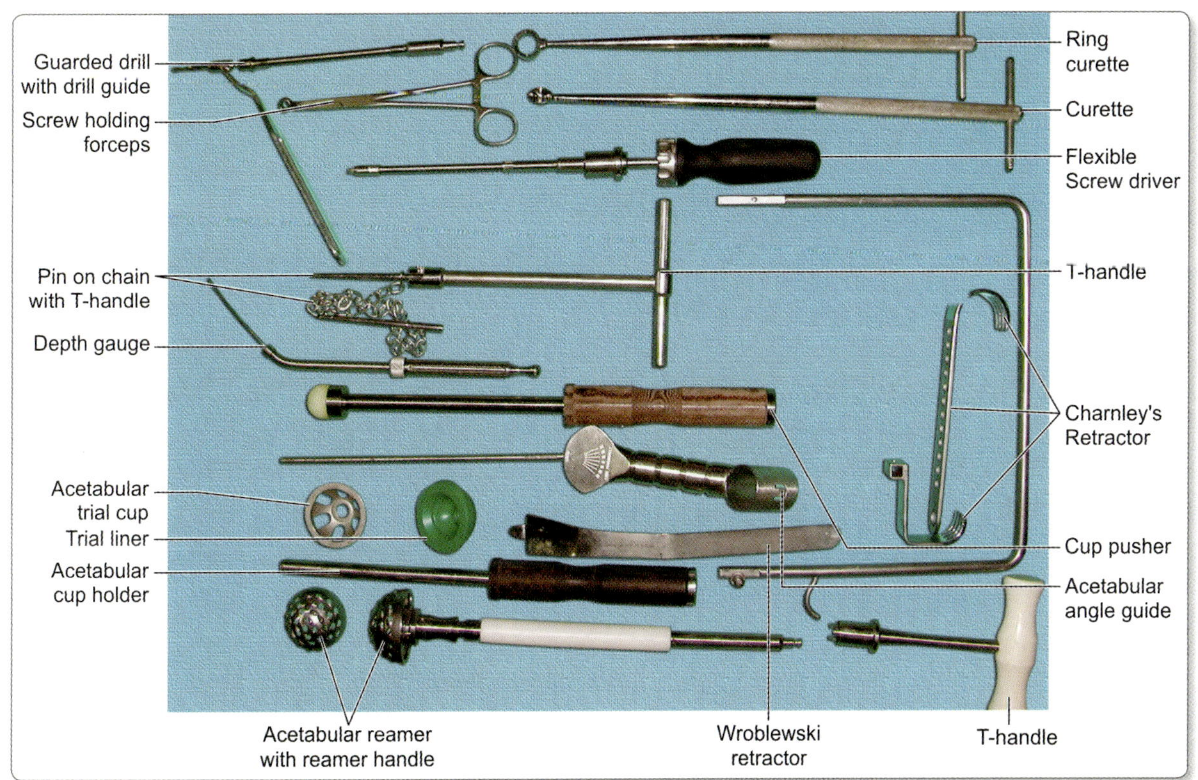

Fig. 7.59 Instruments for implantation of uncemented cup (Duraloc shell)

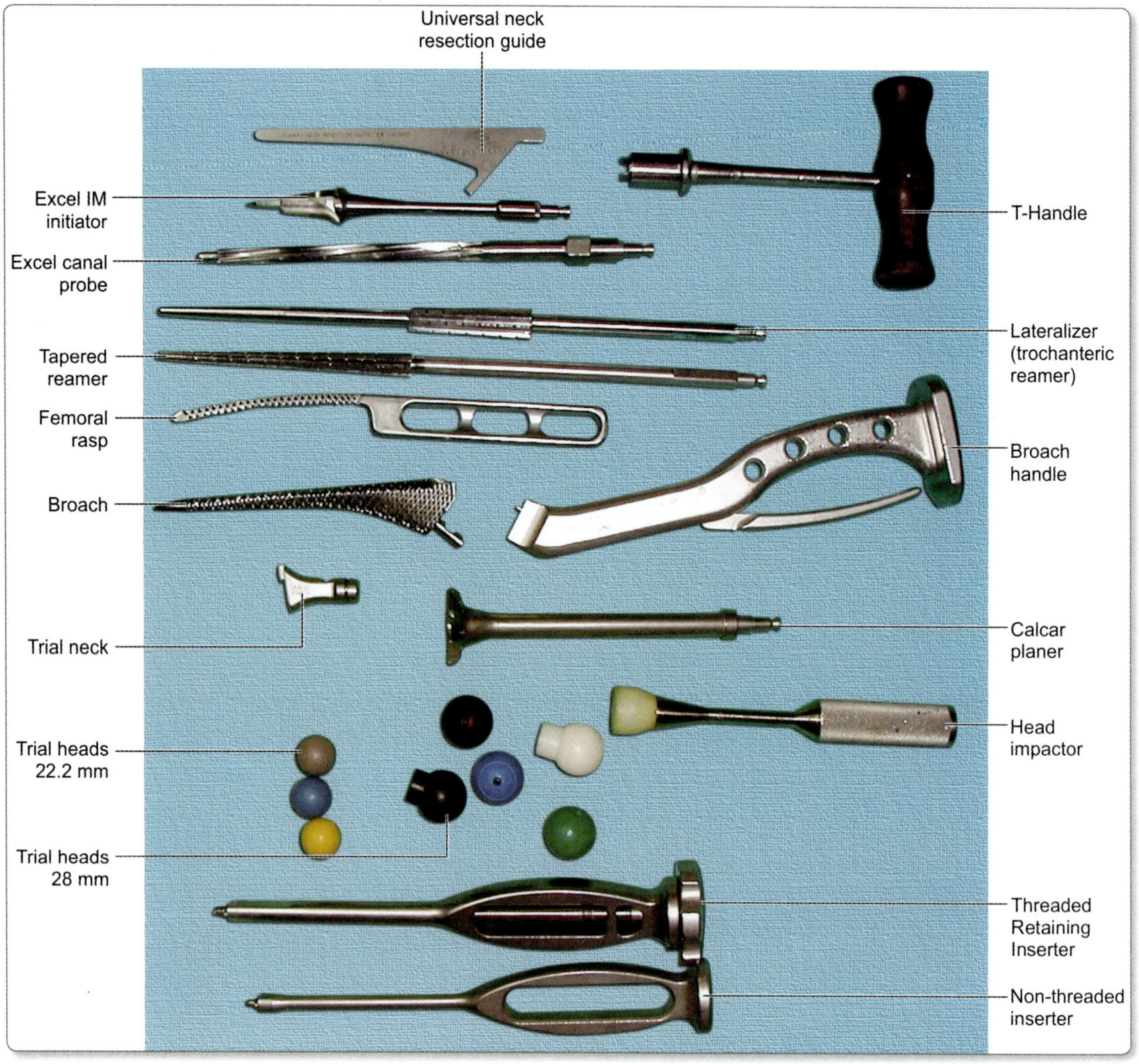

Universal neck resection guide
Excel IM initiator
Excel canal probe
Tapered reamer
Femoral rasp
Broach
Trial neck
Trial heads 22.2 mm
Trial heads 28 mm
T-Handle
Lateralizer (trochanteric reamer)
Broach handle
Calcar planer
Head impactor
Threaded Retaining Inserter
Non-threaded inserter

Fig. 7.60 Instruments for implantation of uncemented femoral stem (Summit stem)

Instruments Required for Pinnacle Cup and Head (Fig. 7.61)

Pinnacle trial cup
Pinnacle trial liner
Pinnacle trial head, 36 mm

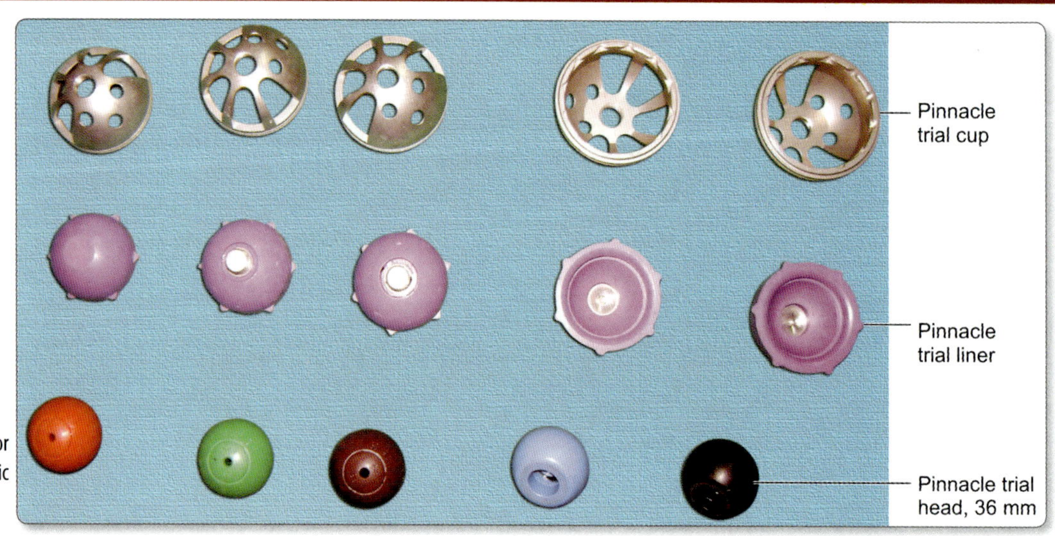

Fig. 7.61 Instruments for metal or ceramic on ceramic (Pinnacle)

Instruments Required for Delta Motion Cup and Head (Fig. 7.62)

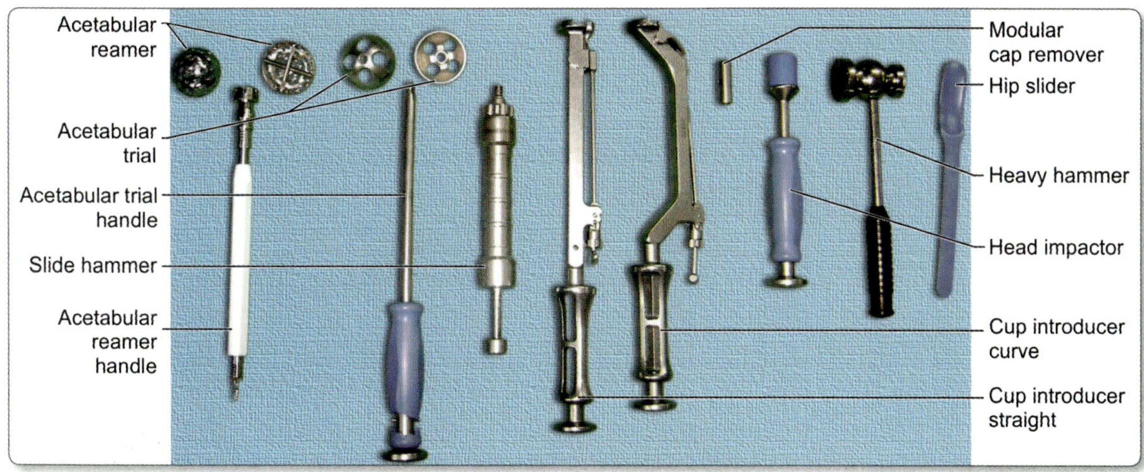

Fig. 7.62 Instruments for delta motion THR

Implants Required for Uncemented THR (Summit stem)

1. Acetabular shell (Duraloc shell or sector)
   Duraloc shell (3 holes)—48, 50, 52, 54, 56, 58, 60, 62, 64 and 66 mm OD
2. Cancellous bone screws 6.5 mm—15, 20, 25, 30, 35, 40 and 45 mm
3. Liner—hooded acetabular liner
   Duraloc marathon liner (10° lip 28 mm ID) - 48, 50, 52, 54, 56, 58, 60, 62, 64 and 66 mm OD
4. Summit tapered hip stem porocoat (standard)—12/14 cone, neck angle—130°

Size	Stem length	Base offset	Neck length	Leg adjustment length
1	125 mm	36 mm	31 mm	27 mm
2	130 mm	38 mm	32 mm	28 mm
3	135 mm	38 mm	32 mm	29 mm
4	140 mm	40 mm	34 mm	30 mm
5	145 mm	40 mm	34 mm	31 mm
6	150 mm	42 mm	36 mm	32 mm
7	155 mm	42 mm	36 mm	33 mm
8	160 mm	44 mm	38 mm	34 mm

5. Articuleze—Femoral head (28 mm, 12/14 cone) - +1.5, + 5, + 8.5, + 12.
   (22.2 mm cobalt chrome, 12/14 cone)— -2, 0, +2
6. Self-centering Bipolar heads for 28 mm articuleze—sizes—39, 40, 41, 42, 43, 44, 45, 46, 47, 48, 49, 50, 51, 52, 53, 54, 55, 56 and 57 mm.

Implants Required For Pinnacle Cup and Head (Ceramic on Ceramic or Ceramic on Polyethylene Liner)

Pinnacle cup (3 holes and multi holes) sizes:
- 44 and 46 mm (for 28 mm liner and head)
- 48 and 50 mm (for 32 mm liner and head
- 52, 54, 56, 58, 60, 62, 64 and 66 mm (for 36 mm liner and head)

Pinnacle liner—
- Ceramic or polyethylene sizes:
- 44, 46 mm (ID 28 mm)
- 48, 50 mm (ID 32 mm)
- 52, 54, 56, 58, 60, 62, 64, 66 mm (ID 36 mm)

Pinnacle head (metal, 28 mm, 12/14 cone): +1.5, +5, +8.5, +12
Pinnacle head (metal, 32 mm, 12/14 cone): +1, +5, +9
Pinnacle head (metal, 36 mm, 12/14 cone): -2, +1.5, +5, +8.5, +12
Pinnacle head (Ceramic, 28mm, 12/14 cone): +1.5, +5, +8.5
Pinnacle head (Ceramic, 32 mm, 12/14 cone): +1, +5, +9
Pinnacle head (Ceramic, 36 mm, 12/14 cone): +1.5, +5, +8.5, +12.

Implants Required for Delta Motion Cup and Head

Delta motion cup - 42, 44, 46, 48, 50, 52, 54, 56, 58 and 60 mm OD
Delta modular sleeve—small (+1.5), medium (+5), large (+8.5), X-large (+12).

Delta motion modular head—
32 mm head for 42 and 44 mm cup
36 mm haed for 46 and 48 mm cup
40 mm head for 50 and 52 mm cup
44 mm head for 54 and 56 mm cup
48 mm head for 58 and 60 mm cup.

Different Measurements of Femoral Stem (Fig. 7.63)

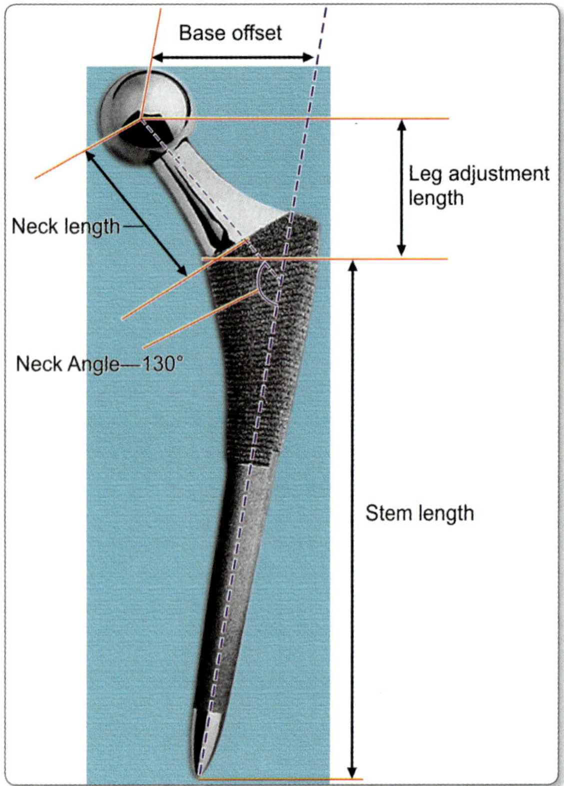

Fig. 7.63 Summit tapered hip stem porocoat with 28 mm head

Features of Summit Tapered Hip System (Fig. 7.64)

1. It is made up of biocompatible high-strength, low-stiffness, forged titanium alloy combined with proximal porocoat porous coating and hydroxyapatite (HA) coating. The porocoat porous coating process results in a strong bond of proud, randomly arranged beads that form interconnecting pores for bone ingrowth (see chapter 8, **Fig. 8.10**). Porocoat porous coating exhibits a pore size in the optimal range for bony ingrowth, resulting in a more efficient and uniform transmission of stresses. The precision controlled, 35 micron HA does not occlude the pores in porocoat porous coating.

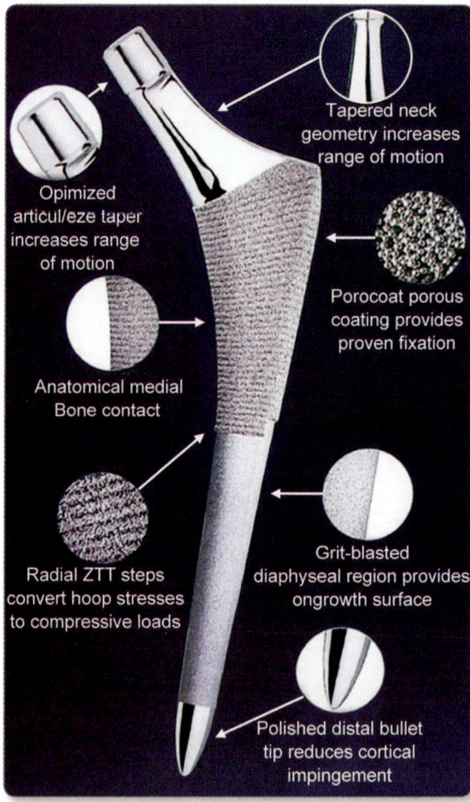

Fig. 7.64 Summit tapered hip system (standard offset)

2. The 3° proximal to distal taper creates a stem geometry with proven stability.
3. The medially rounded, laterally flared proximal cross-sectional geometry provides rotational stability and fit most femora.
4. The length of the stem provides immediate three-point fixation **(Fig. 7.12)** while the conical contact created by 3° taper results in proximal stress transfer.
5. The radial ZTT structure provides internal collars perpendicular to the trabeculae of the proximal femur. This transmits the vertical forces created by the tapered implant to the host bone in compression rather than in shear.
6. The grit-blasted diaphyseal region provides a roughened surface that enables the potential for bony ingrowth.
7. Polished distal bullet tip reduces cortical impingement.
8. A 130° neck shaft angle enables femoral offset restoration and soft tissue tensioning without affecting leg length.
9. The neck geometry has been optimized for increased range of motion. Enhancements include narrowed anteroposterior neck flats and an optimized articuleze taper (12/14 taper). The polished neck is designed to reduce wear debris generation secondary to prosthetic impingement.

Cemented THR (C-Stem)

Anesthesia, positioning, draping, approach, exposure and dislocation of hip are similar to uncemented THR as described earlier.

Femoral Neck Resection

One assistant will hold the limb with knee flexed at 90° and hip at 45°, adducted and internally rotated so that sole of the foot will face the ceiling. Another assistant will retract the posterior border of gluteus medius and expose the piriformis fossa. Clean this area by electrocautery and curette. Find out the entry point for femoral canal over the piriformis fossa (See **Figs 8.3A and B** in chapter 8). Take the Excel™ IM initiator attached with T-handle and make the entry hole in the femoral canal by advancing it till full circumference. Accurate positioning of the entry point will avoid implant malalignment. Remove the Excel™ IM initiator. Attach the Excel canal probe to the T-handle and introduce the probe into the medullary canal of the femur at piriformis fossa. Ensure that the entry point is positioned in line with the long-axis of the femur. If the entry hole is positioned correctly, the probe should pass down the femur easily. Ream the medullary canal starting from size 8 reamer (smallest size) till snugly fitting (8, 9, 10, 11, 12, 13, 14, 15). The depth marks along the reamer shaft correspond to stem size, and reaming should stop when the appropriate depth mark is in level with the center of the femoral head which generally corresponds with tip of the greater trochanter. Keep the reamer in place and apply the neck resection guide so that the guide touches the femoral head and the greater trochanter. After checking the amount of neck cut (about 10–15 mm, i.e. one finger breadth from the lesser trochanter) with saw blade passed through standard slot (at 135°), fix the neck resection guide with two pins. Apply two Hohmann, one over the superior aspect and another over the inferior aspect of femoral neck to protect the soft tissues. The assistant will hold the limb in such a way that knee is flexed at 90° and sole of the foot is facing the ceiling and lifting the thigh to keep the neck of femur parallel to the ground to avoid oblique cut. Hold the femoral head with head holding clamp or towel clip to avoid accidental fall. Cut the neck of femur with oscillating saw. Pass a straight osteotome through the neck resection and lever out the femoral head. Cut the ligamentum teres with scissors or electrocautery and remove the head. Pack the femoral canal with small ribbon gauze to avoid bleeding from femoral canal. Keep the hip in extension.

Exposure of Acetabulum as described for uncemented THR.

Insertion of Acetabular Cup

By the help of ring curette, remove the cartilage from acetabulum. Do trial with size 40 and 43 trial cup for containment of cup in 20° anteversion. The inferior rim of the cup trial should be in level with the bottom of the tear drop. Ream the acetabulum with gradually increasing size of acetabular reamer starting from 40 to 48 for 40 or 43 size cup (for cement layer of 3–5 mm), keeping the angle of inclination (abduction) of 45° and 20° anteversion. Reaming is done till the cartilage is removed and there is fresh bleeding acetabular floor. Remove all remaining articular cartilage and any medial osteophytes until healthy, bleeding subchondral bone is exposed and a symmetrical, hemispherical dome is achieved. After each curettage and reaming, clean the acetabulum by gauze piece lollypop. Check the size of acetabulum and do trial with appropriate size planned cup and if any adjustment is required, do it by acetabular reamer. Make multiple drill holes in the superior, anterior and posterior acetabular floor with guarded drill. Avoid drilling of the medial wall of acetabulum. Pour normal saline in the acetabulum and wash with acetabular brush. Suck the fluid from acetabulum by suction. Pack the acetabulum with hydrogen peroxide soaked gauze piece to avoid bleeding. Take out one packet of 40 g CMW1 (high viscosity bone cement) and 2 packets of 40 g CMW3 (medium viscosity bone cement) from refrigerator 1/2 hour before cementing and keep them at 20°–22° room temperature. Mix 40 g bone cement (CMW1) in bowl with spoon slowly to avoid mixing of air. Start the timer to note the time passed. Take the appropriate size acetabular cup and attach to the cup introducer in such a way that operative side (R or L) is visible. Sizes of cups are 40, 43, 47, 50 and 53. Remove the hydrogen peroxide soaked gauge piece from acetabulum. Wash it with normal saline. Make it dry with gauze piece. Anesthetist gives injection Efcorlin (hydrocortisone succinate) 100 mg IV just before cementing and IV antibiotic (1 g cefotaxime). At about 3 minutes when wrinkling starts in cement, put some cement in acetabulum and pressurize it by cement pressurizer. Put rest of the cement in acetabulum and insert the selected cup keeping the vertical stem of cup introducer vertical and horizontal handle rotated 20° posteriorly in relation to the anterior superior iliac spine for 20° anteversion of acetabular cup. Locate the cup pusher on the back of cup introducer and pressurize the cement. Hold this position till cement is setting. The assistant will remove the extruded cement by curved artery forceps. When bone cement is almost half set, remove the cup introducer and pressurize the cup directly with cup pusher till the bone cement is set (in about 10 minutes). Pour normal saline to avoid thermal necrosis. Remove the extruded bone cement by curved osteotome and gentle blow of mallet. Check the stability of the cup. For checking stability, engage the threaded part of cup tester in the side hole of the cup. Pour normal saline in the acetabulum and try to move the cup with the help of cup tester. If there are no bubbles, it means cup is well-fixed. Suck the normal saline by suction. Remove the cup tester. Remove the pins on chain, anterior Hohmann and Wroblewski retractor. Put betadine soaked gauze piece in implanted cup. Remove the small ribbon gauze pack from the opening of femoral canal.

Insertion of Femoral Component

One assistant will hold the limb with knee flexed at 90° and hip at 45° , adducted and internally rotated so that sole of the foot will face the ceiling. Another assistant will retract the posterior border of gluteus medius and expose the piriformis fossa. Anteversion osteotome (Box osteotome) is used to remove cancellous bone from the proximal part of femur. Using the anteversion osteotome positioned laterally towards the greater trochanter, enlarge the entry point to the femoral canal to establish 20° of anteversion for broach alignment. Reverse the osteotome and extend the entry point medially towards the lesser trochanter. Remove a wedge of cancellous bone. In order to achieve a good cement mantle, the anatomical calcar is cleared using a curette, extending the medullary canal towards the lesser trochanter, but avoiding excavation of the lesser trochanter. Attach the broach over broach handle. Advance the broach down the medullary canal by gentle hammering while keeping the broach in the long axis of the femur and in 20° anteversion in relation to the lesser trochanter with broach starting from size 1 (in narrow femoral canal like in post polio, start with size CDH) till snugly fitting (sizes 1, 2, 3, 4). The level of bow string is at the level of cut surface of the neck of femur. In between the hammering, allow the femoral canal to expand and carefully hear the sound of hammering to notice any change. While the broach is in situ, attach the trial neck and head size 0. Remove the gauze piece from the implanted cup. Loosen the Charnley's retractor. Apply one gauze piece around the trial neck and reduce the hip. For reduction, the assistant will apply traction in extended position of hip. Another assistant will hold the gauze piece around the trial neck and apply gentle traction along the long axis of femur. The surgeon will gently push the head in the acetabulum while retracting the soft tissues by fingers. When the head is near the margin of acetabulum, the assistant will gently externally rotate the limb and the hip is reduced. Head impactor is helpful for pushing the head during reduction. Tighten the Charnley's retractor. Check the movement and stability of hip. Flex the hip at 90°. Check the adduction and internal rotation. Extend the hip. Check the abduction, external rotation, internal rotation, suck test (pull the leg in extension to see the amount of opening between head and acetabulum and opening should not be more than 2 mm). Check the amount of tension in abductor muscles (palpate the anterior border of gluteus medius), the limb length (see the level of lower pole of patella in both lower limbs in identical position). Check that the center of trial head is at the level of tip of greater trochanter. With the hip in 90° of flexion and 0° of abduction, internal rotation should be at least 45° with no tendency to dislocate. In extension, there should be full external rotation with no tendency to dislocate or impinge. If the trial reduction of head in acetabulum is very tight, do trial with head size –3. Similarly if loose then do trial with either size +3 or +6 accordingly and appropriate size of head is selected. However, final trial of head is done after implantation of the C-stem. Make any adjustments, if necessary, by changing the neck length or by using high offset neck option. Leg length may be increased or reduced by 5 mm without adjusting the femoral head, by raising or lowering the implant. Loosen the Charnley's retractor. Dislocate the hip by flexing, adducting, internally rotating and pulling it out with help of gauze piece around the neck. Tighten the Charnley's retractor. Remove the trial head and neck. Re-attach the broach handle on broach and remove the broach from the femur by lightly tapping the underside of the broach handle, keeping it in the line with the axis of the femur. The trial reduction can also be done by trial stem. Irrigate the femoral canal with normal saline to remove the blood and loose debris. Take the Hardinge cement restrictor and fix it with cement restrictor inserter. Apply it in femoral canal at the level of 13–15 cm deep in canal from neck resection level after measuring the length of broach. Depth for cement restrictor is 2 cm distal to the tip of stem. Wash the femoral canal with gentamicin mixed normal saline. Pack the femoral canal with hydrogen peroxide mixed ribbon gauze. Change gloves. The circulating nurse will open the packets of implants and bone cement. Take the appropriate size C-stem on the same trolley on which the bone cement has been taken. Apply appropriate size centralizer according to the diameter of the femoral canal. Apply the end cap. The end cap should not be used if the smallest diameter of the femoral canal is less than 10 mm at the level of the tip of the stem. The end cap should not be used without the centralizer, or a distal bone plug has been used. The centralizer is placed with fins distally. Take two packets of 40 g CMW3 (medium viscosity) bone cement in a stainless steel bowl and mix with liquid cement with the help of spoon slowly to avoid mixing of air. Start timer to note the time. At about 3 minutes when wrinkling starts, pour the CMW3 bone cement in cement syringe and load on cement gun. Apply rubber pressurizer over the base of the nozzle of cement syringe. The assistant will remove the ribbon gauze piece from the femoral canal and wash the canal with normal saline. Make the femoral canal dry by packing dry ribbon gauze piece. Remove the dry ribbon gauze piece. Put the nozzle of cement syringe deep to the canal and close the opening of canal by rubber pressurizer which has already been applied at the base of the nozzle of cement syringe. Inject the bone cement in the femoral canal retrogradely and gradually withdraw the cement gun till all cement has been injected in the canal. Just before the end of injecting the cement with some cement in the syringe, withdraw the nozzle of syringe and cut the nozzle by scissors 1 cm away from the base. Apply it in the hole of rubber pressurizer and inject the remaining cement in the femoral canal under pressure. Keep it pressurized until stem insertion. If good pressurization is achieved, fat will be extruded from the bone. Load the C-stem on the stem introducer and push it in the canal till bow string mark on the stem will tally to the level of cut surface of the neck of the femur keeping the neck in 20° anteversion in relation to the lesser trochanter and the stem in the center of the canal to avoid varus position of stem. Assistant will pressurize the cement with gauze piece near the inferior aspect of neck and remove the extruded cement by curved artery forceps. While cement is half-set, remove the inserter handle. Put index finger at inferior surface of neck of C-stem to keep it straight in the canal. When the cement sets in about 10 minutes, pour normal saline to avoid thermal necrosis. Remove gauze piece from the acetabulum. Apply the trial head size 0 (or whatever has been chosen during trial with broach or trial stem) over the neck of the C-stem. Apply one gauze piece around the neck of the C-stem. Loosen the Charnley's retractor and reduce the hip as described. Tighten the charnley's retractor. Assess the movement, stability (with the hip in 90° of flexion and 0° of abduction, internal rotation should be at least 45° with no tendency to dislocate. In extension, there should be full external rotation with no tendency to dislocate or impinge), suck test, abductor tension (palpate the anterior border of gluteus medius), limb length and finally determine the size of the head. Again loosen the Charnley's retractor and dislocate the hip. Remove the trial head. Apply the appropriate size head (9/10 cone) over the neck. Put the head impactor over the head and give three gentle blows with bell hammer. The head will be fixed over the neck of the stem which will be confirmed by pulling it. Reduce the hip, tighten the Charnley's retractor. Re-assess the movements and stability. Wash with gentamicin mixed normal saline. Load two vials of gentamicin in a syringe and pour it in the wound.

Closure of wound and application of two suction drains are similar to uncemented THR. Give IV antibiotic (1 g cefotaxime).

Postoperative advice, physiotherapy and follow-up schedule are similar to TKR. Quadriceps exercise, abduction exercise of hip, gradual knee and hip bending exercises are started (See physiotherapy for THR in chapter twelve).

Preoperative and Postoperative X-rays (Figs 7.65 to 7.74)

Both acetabulum and femoral components—cemented **(Figs 7.65 to 7.72)**.

Bipolar with cemented C-stem **(Figs 7.73 and 7.74)** (Elderly patients with fracture neck of femur).

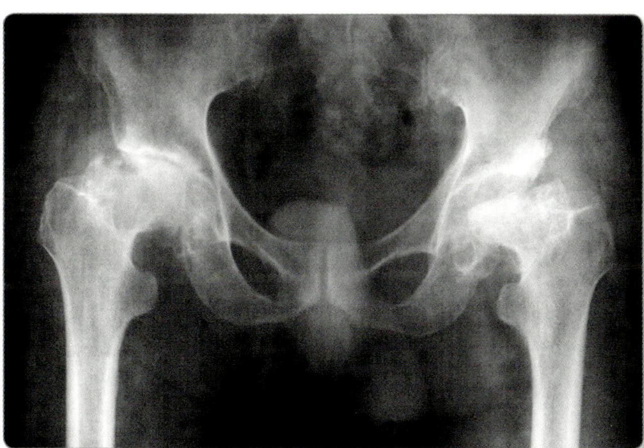

Fig. 7.65 AVN both hips with arthritis

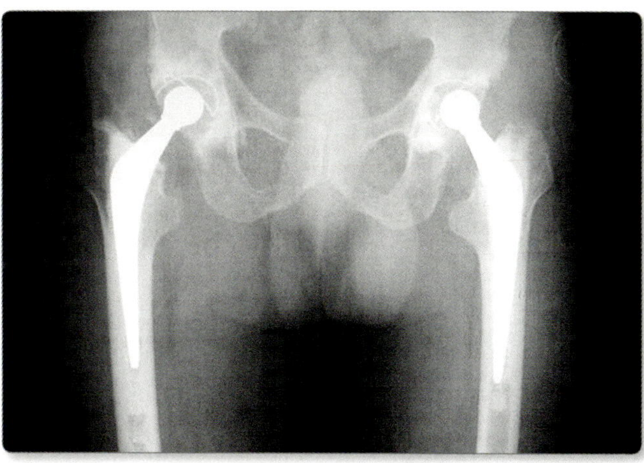

Fig. 7.66 Both hips—C-stem and acetabular cup

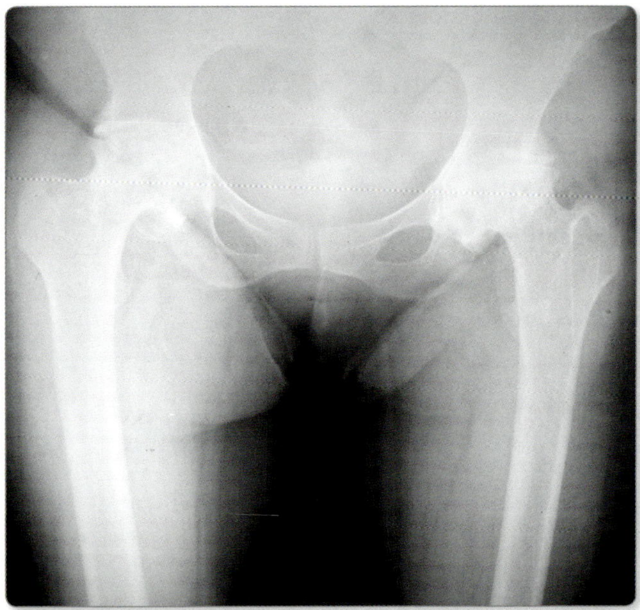

Fig. 7.67 AVN both hip joints (Preoperative)

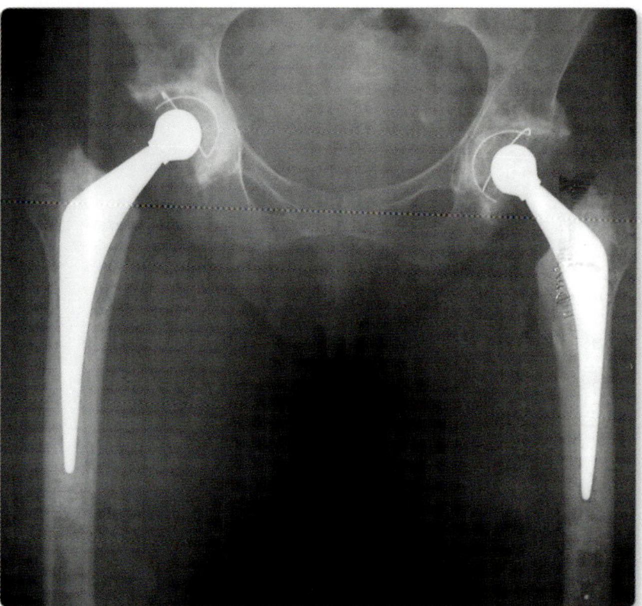

Fig. 7.68 C-stem both hip joints

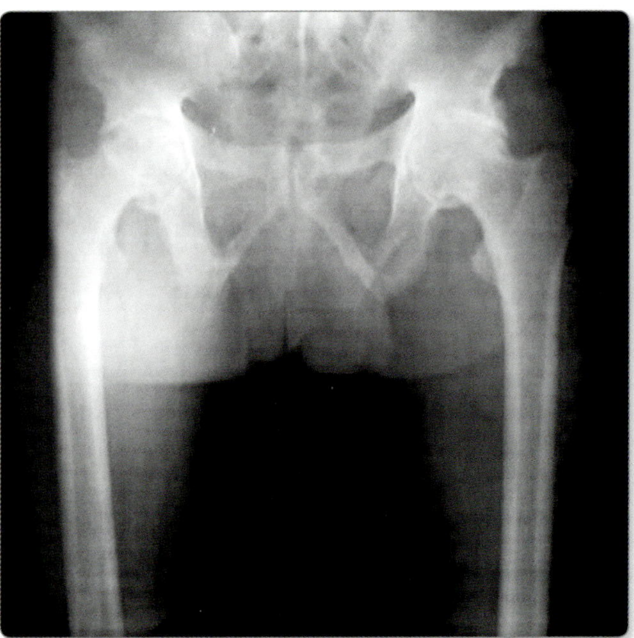

Fig. 7.69 Ankylosing spondylitis with severe arthritis both hip joints

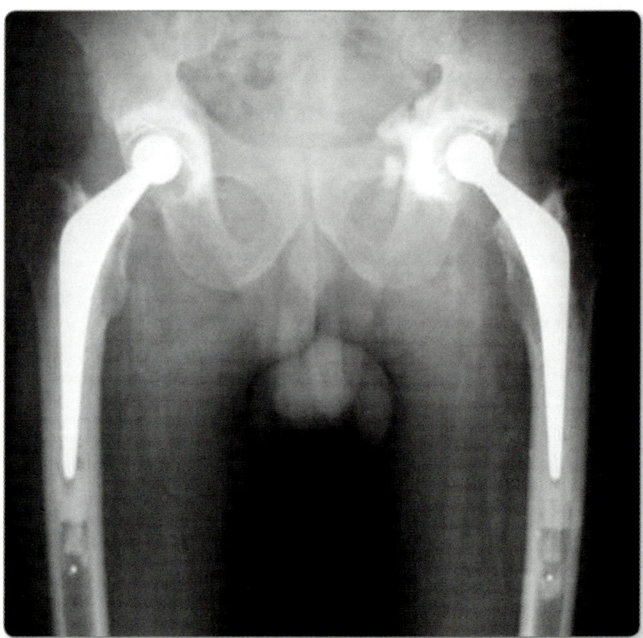

Fig. 7.70 C-Stem (Postoperative)

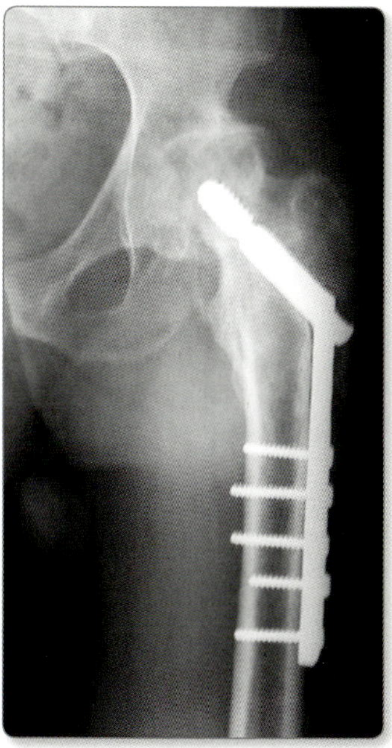

Fig. 7.71 Post traumatic AVN with arthritis

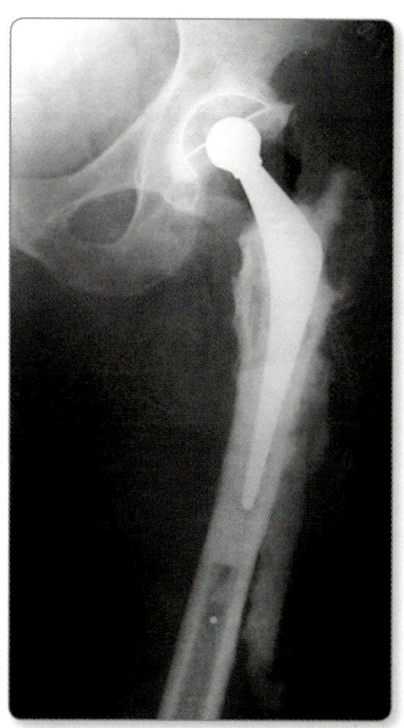

Fig. 7.72 C-stem (Postoperative)

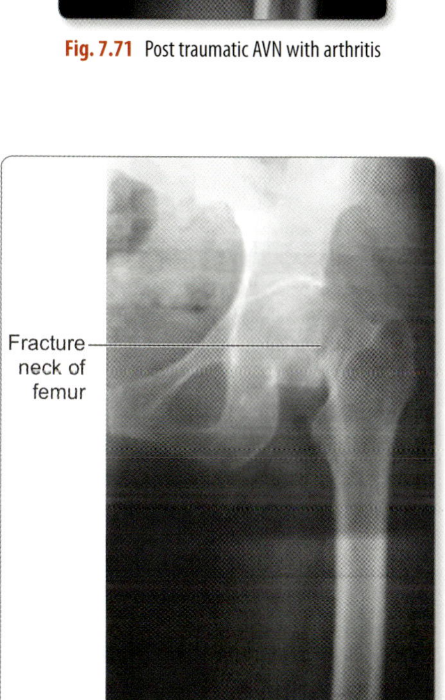

Fig. 7.73 Fracture neck of femur

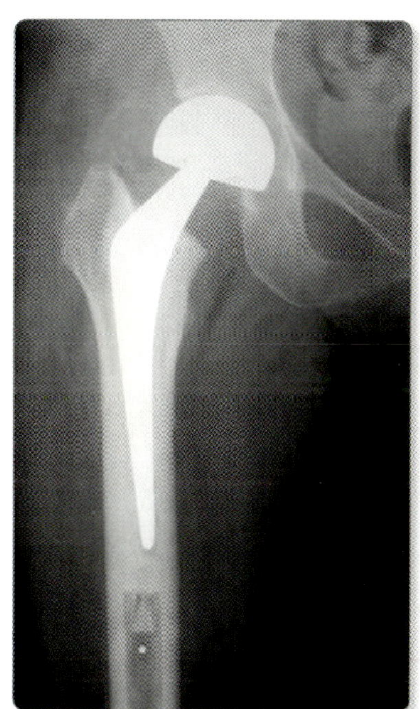

Fig. 7.74 Bipolar hip with C-stem

Instruments Required for Cemented THR (C-stem) (Figs 7.75 and 7.76)

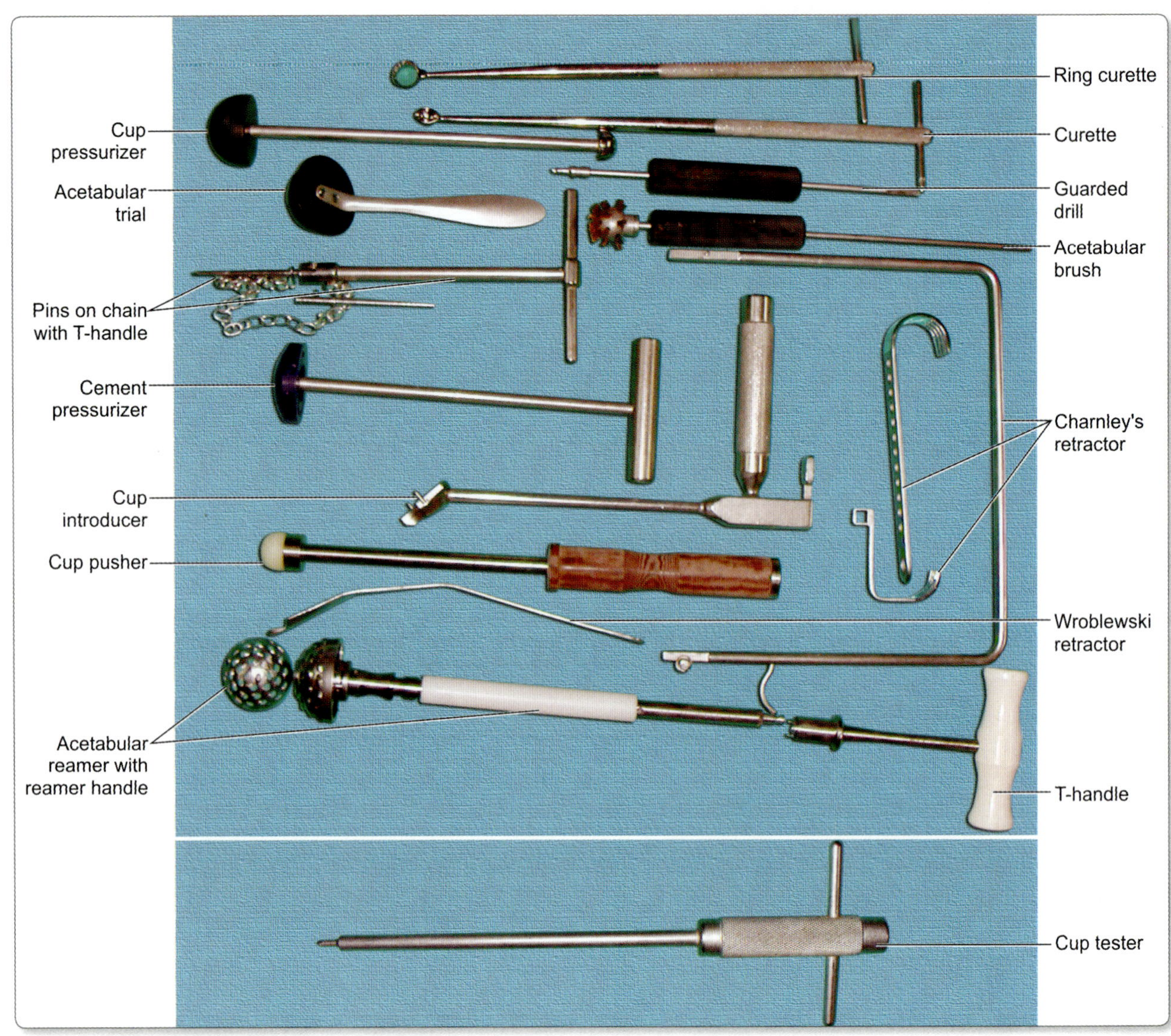

Fig.7.75 Instruments for implantation of cemented cup

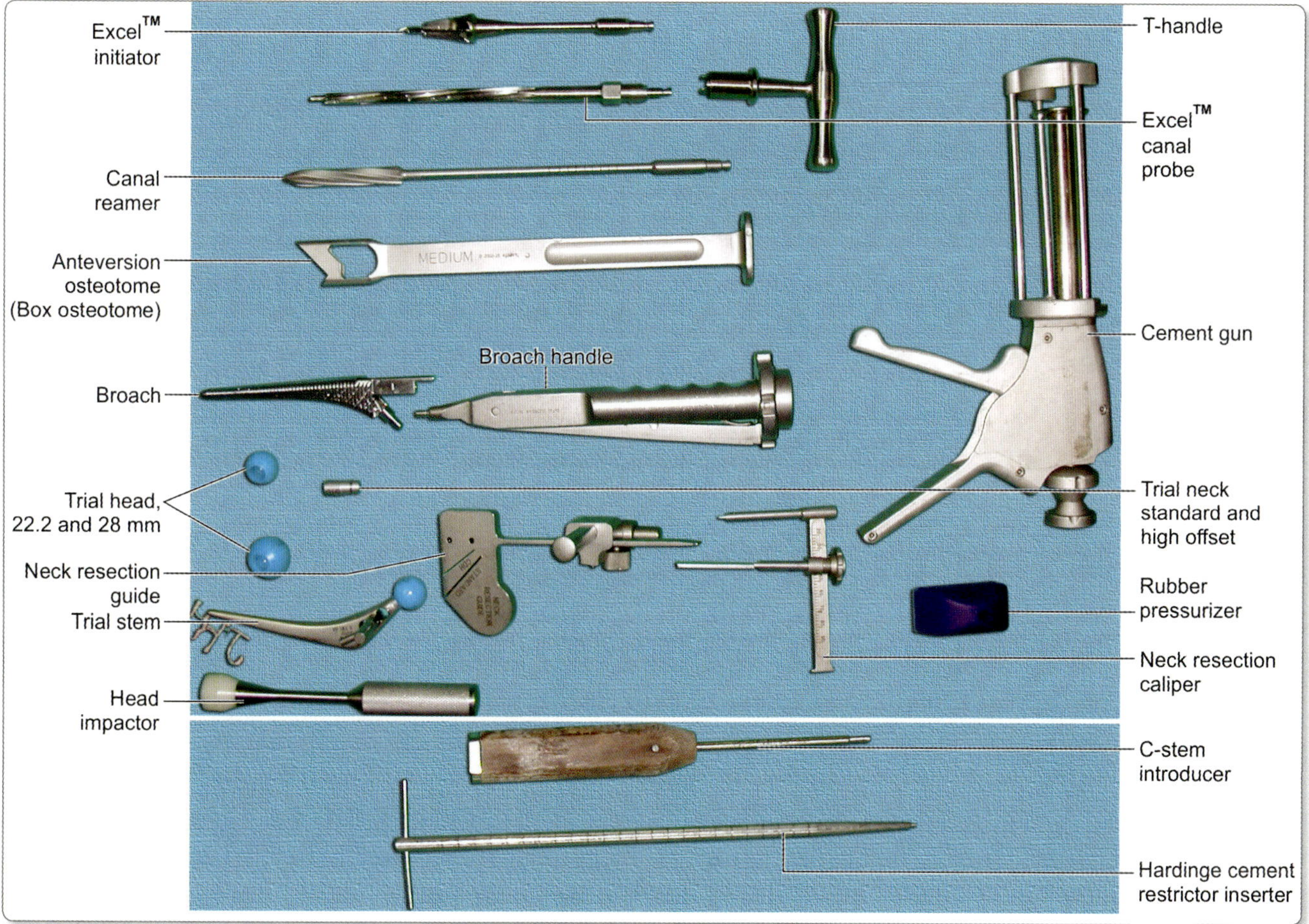

Fig. 7.76 Instruments for implantation of C-stem

Implants and Cement Required for Cemented THR (C-Stem)

1. Acetabular Cups—
   a. Elite plus LPW cup (28 mm ID)—40, 43, 47, 50, 53 mm OD
   b. Charnley LPW cup (22.2 mm ID)—40, 43, 47, 50, 53 mm OD
   (ID—Inner diameter, OD—Outer diameter)
2. Hardinge cement restrictor
3. Triple taper C-stem (9/10 cone)—neck angle - CDH - 126° and standard—135° CDH size
   Standard sizes—1, 2, 3, 4
   Size 3 high offset
   Size 4 high offset
   Size 4 long stem—200 mm and 240 mm in certain cases and revision.

Size	Stem length	Depth for cement restrictor (20 mm distal to the tip of stem)
CDH	103.0 mm	123 mm
1	106.0 mm	126 mm
2	110.5 mm	130 mm
3	115.0 mm	135 mm
4	119.5 mm	140 mm

4. End cap
5. Centralizer
6. Elite plus head (28 mm, 9/10 cone): -3, 0, +3, +6
7. Articuleze head (22.2 mm, 9/10 cone): -3, 0, +3, +6
8. CMW1 Gentamicin—40 g—1 packet
9. CMW3 Gentamicin—40 g—2 packets
10. Self - centering bipolar heads for 28 mm articuleze - sizes - 39, 40, 41, 42, 43, 44, 45, 46, 47, 48, 49, 50, 51, 52, 53, 54, 55, 56 and 57 mm.

11. Special—
Reinforcement ring— STD—50 mm ID
LG—60 mm ID.

Features of Triple Taper C-Stem (Fig. 7.77)

1. The stem begins narrow at the bottom, gradually becomes wider, and then narrows again at the top. This is called tapering and this is what is responsible for the stem's unique shape.
2. Triple tapered design secures stability within the cement.
3. Two longitudinal tapers transfer compressive load and the third taper transfers maximum load from the stem to proximal femur, minimizing the effects of stress shielding, and improving still further the prospect of long-term implant security.
4. Even distribution of the weight throughout the hip stem reduces end-bearing stresses and the risk of cement mantle fracture. The cement mantle is the wall of cement between the bone and implant. End-bearing stress is caused by too much weight being applied to the top of the stem at one time.
5. Its unique triple taper, neck shape, and profile help the implant achieve a more natural, anatomically correct distribution of weight to the thigh bone while reducing the potential for stress shielding. The system also minimizes the chances of late loosening.
6. The geometric shape of the C-stem neck allows for a high offset option designed to achieve a closer anatomical match for patients with a higher-than-normal offset or a narrow femoral canal.
7. The high offset option also reduces the risk of dislocation and impingement for patients with a high offset and to balance weak inner-thigh muscles. It also allows stability to be restored with no increase in limb length. Offset helps to counterbalance any weight difference between the leg and the center of the body.

The objective is to place the stem centrally within the medullary canal with a uniform, well-pressurized cement mantle, while avoiding distal stem support.

Assessment during Follow-up

1. Clinical assessment
   i. Pain
   ii. Limp
   iii. Support
   iv. Distance walked
   v. Stairs
   vi. Put on shoes and socks
   vii. Sitting on chair
   viii. Deformity - FFD
   ix. Limb length discrepancy
   x. Range of motion
2. Radiological assessment **(Fig. 7.78)**.

Note the grading of cement as described by Barrack et. al. and Mulroy et.al.

1. *Grade A*: Medullary canal completely filled with cement (white out).
2. *Grade B*: A slight radiolucency exists at the bone cement interface.
3. *Grade C*: A radiolucency of more than 50% at the bone cement interface.
4. *Grade D*: A radiolucency involving more than 100% of the interface between bone and cement in any projection including absence of cement distal to the stem tip.

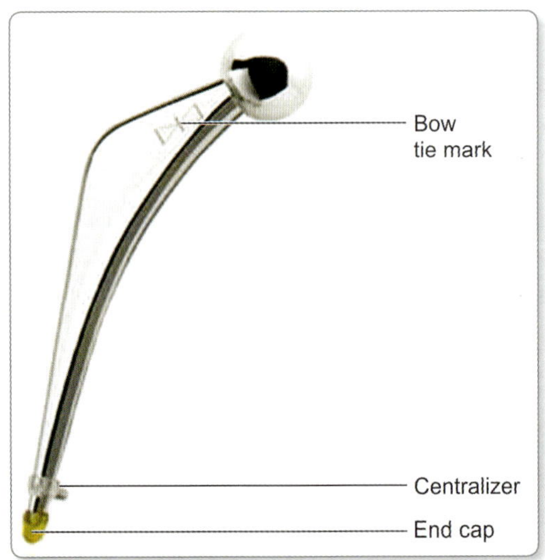

Fig. 7.77 Triple taper C-stem with 22.2 mm head

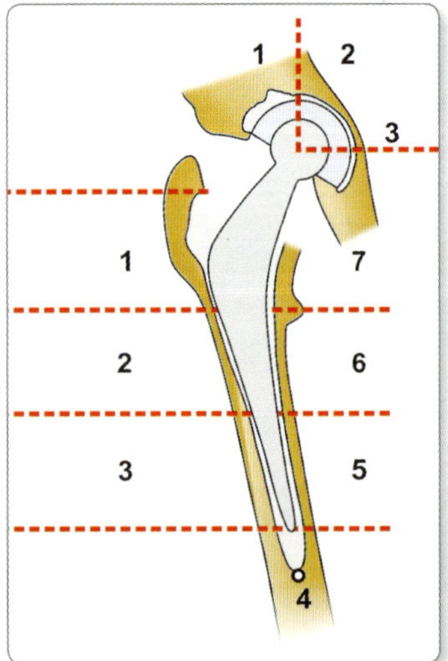

Fig. 7.78 Zones about cement mass in femur and pelvis

Radiolucent lines are commonly found in the lateral and anterior aspects of the proximal femur as these areas can be difficult to visualize and difficult to pressurize. Hence, linear radiolucencies less than 2 mm in width in the proximal 1 cm of the femur should not be considered to be indicative of loosening. Absorption of bone from the medial cortex of the femoral neck up to several milimeters is not considered abnormal. A thin (<1 mm) mantle of cement around the femoral component and defects in the mantle of cement are associated with increased loosening of the femoral component. Loosening is present if a radiolucent zone more than 2 mm wide is around the entire cement mass and increases progressively in width. Endosteal cavitation (linear osteolysis and focal osteolysis) are also suggestive of femoral loosening.

Summary of THR (Steps in Sequence)

Uncemented THR (Summit tapered Hip system)

1. Posterior approach.
2. Dislocation of hip.
3. Application of neck resection guide and mark the level of neck cut and cutting of femoral neck.
4. Exposure of acetabulum to 360°.
5. Curettage (with ring curette) and reaming of acetabulum (in proper orientation, i.e. 45° abduction, and 20° anteversion) with gradually increasing size of acetabular reamer.
6. Trial with one size higher trial cup than final reamer in proper orientation (45° abduction and 20° anteversion as guided by acetabular angle guide).
7. Bone graft from femoral head, if required.
8. Apply the appropriate size acetabular shell (Duraloc shell) in proper position (i.e. the inferior rim of cup should be at the level of bottom of teardrop) and orientation (45° abduction and 20° anteversion), keeping the screw holes of acetabular shell facing the roof of acetabulum.
9. Cancellous screws application through the screw holes of acetabulum, if required.
10. Apply the appropriate size hooded acetabular liner over the Duraloc shell in proper orientation, i.e. hood of the liner is placed in posterosuperior position.
11. Location of the femoral canal through piriformis fossa with Excel™ IM initiator and Excel™ canal probe.
12. Lateralize the proximal entry point of femoral canal by trochanteric reamer (lateralizer)—proximal reaming of femoral canal.
13. Reaming of femoral canal with gradually increasing size of tapered reamer till snugly fitting—distal reaming of femoral canal.
14. Anteversion box cut at the junction of femoral neck and greater trochanter.
15. Broaching of femoral canal in proper anteversion with gradually increasing size broach starting from size 0 till snugly fitting and rotationally stable (sizes 0, 1, 2, 3, 4, 5, 6, 7, 8).
16. Use of calcar planer.
17. Application of trial neck and +1.5 trial articuleze head over the final broach.
18. Trial reduction with trial articuleze head and determine the approximate size of head.
19. Removal of broach and insertion of appropriate size summit tapered stem (sizes 1, 2, 3, 4, 5, 6, 7, 8) in 200 anteversion.
20. Trial reduction with trial articuleze head and determine the final size of head—assess the movement, stability (with the hip in 90° of flexion and 0° of abduction, internal rotation should be at least 45° with no tendency to dislocate. In extension, there should be full external rotation with no tendency to dislocate or impinge), suck test, abductor tension (palpate the anterior border of gluteus medius), limb length and finally determine the size of the head. The center of head is at the level of tip of grater trochanter.
21. Application of appropriate size arteculeze head.
22. Reduction of hip and closure of wound with two suction drains.

Cemented THR (C-stem)

1. Posterior approach.
2. Dislocation of hip.
3. Location of femoral canal through piriformis fossa with Excel™ IM initiator and Excel™ canal probe.
4. Reaming of femoral canal with gradually increasing reamers till snugly fitting.
5. Application of neck resection guide over reamer and cutting of femoral neck.
6. Exposure of acetabulum to 360°.
7. Curettage (with ring curette), reaming in proper orientation, i.e. 45° abduction and 20° anteversion (with gradually increasing acetabular reamer), trialing (with trial cup), drilling (with guarded drill) and brushing (with acetabular brush) of acetabulum.
8. Pack the acetabulum with hydrogen peroxide soaked gauze piece, remove the pack, wash with normal saline and make the acetabulum dry.
9. Cementing of appropriate size cup in proper position (the inferior rim of cup should be at the level of bottom of teardrop) and orientation (45° abduction and 20° anteversion).
10. Anteversion box cut at the junction of femoral neck and greater trochanter.

11. Broaching of femoral canal in proper anteversion (20° anteversion in relation to lesser trochanter) with gradually increasing size of broach starting from size 1 till snugly fitting (sizes 1, 2, 3, 4).
12. Trial reduction with trial neck and size 0 trial articuleze head on final broach and determine the approximate size of head.
13. Removal of broach and application of Hardinge cement restrictor at appropriate length in femoral canal.
14. Pack the femoral canal with hydrogen peroxide soaked ribbon gauze. Remove the pack and wash with normal saline and make the canal dry with dry ribbon gauze.
15. Application of appropriate size centralizer and end cap over appropriate size C-stem.
16. Cementing of appropriate size C-stem in proper anteversion (20° anteversion) and avoid varus positioning. The "bow-tie" mark of C-stem coincides with the cut surface of the neck.
17. Trial reduction with trial articuleze head and determine the final size of head—assess the movement, stability (with the hip in 90° of flexion and 0° of abduction, internal rotation should be at least 45° with no tendency to dislocate. In extension, there should be full external rotation with no tendency to dislocate or impinge), suck test, abductor tension (palpate the anterior border of gluteus medius), limb length and finally determine the size of the head. The center of head is at the level of tip of greater trochanter.
18. Application of appropriate size articuleze head.
19. Reduction of hip and closure of wound with two suction drains.

Important Points and THR in Difficult Situations

8

CHAPTER

CHAPTER OUTLINE

- Important Points
- Total Hip Replacement (THR) in Difficult Situations

Important Points

1. Whenever planned to do uncemented total hip replacement (THR) (Summit tapered stem), set of cemented THR (C-stem) should also be kept ready in case required like in shallow acetabulum or defective acetabular wall where uncemented cup is not snuggly fitting or the largest size of summit stem is loose.
2. Maximum concentration of mind is required during insertion of acetabular cup and femoral stem in view of their orientation and anteversion (i.e. 45° abduction and 20° anteversion of acetabular cup and 20° anteversion of femoral stem and avoid varus positioning of femoral stem).

First X-ray shows poorly performed THR in which orientation of cup and femoral stem is not proper leading to unreduced hip resulting into bedridden patient and severe osteoporosis of femur **(Fig. 8.1)**. The blunder is that the inclination (abduction) of cup seems to be almost 80° and anteversion 0° while anteversion of femoral stem seems to be almost 90°. The normal inclination (abduction) of cup should be 45° and anteversion 20° and the normal anteversion of femoral stem should be 20°. These criteria have been achieved in 2nd X-ray after revision THR of the same patient leading to reduced hip **(Fig. 8.2)**. All cement from femoral canal could not be removed, hence, CDH femoral C-stem has been applied with good pressurization of bone cement. First X-ray also shows very poor cementing.

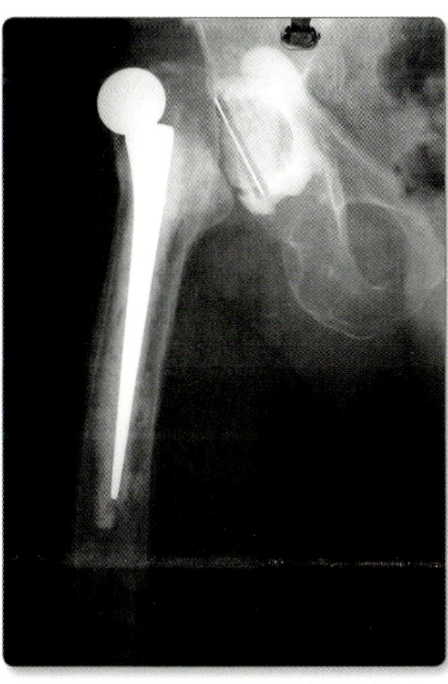

Fig. 8.1 First X-ray—failed THR from the day of surgery

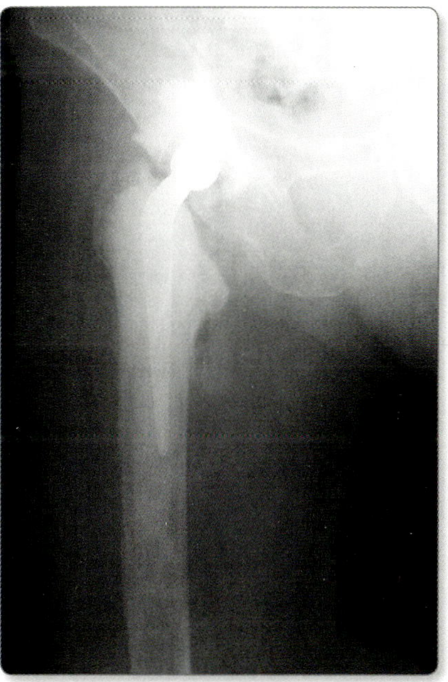

Fig. 8.2 Second X-ray of the same patient after revision THR

3. Applying the stem in varus position is a common error by the beginners which leads to failure of the replaced joint. This varus positioning of stem is due to wrong entry point. To avoid varus positioning of stem, the entry point should be over the piriformis fossa as shown in **Figures 8.3A and B** below:

   One assistant will hold the limb with knee flexed at 90° and hip at 45°, adducted and internally rotated so that sole of the foot will face the ceiling. Other assistant will retract the posterior border of gluteus medius and expose the piriformis fossa. Clean this area by electrocautery and curette. Make the entry point over the piriformis fossa **(Figs 8.3A and B)** with Excel IM initiator by advancing it till full circumference and then find out the femoral canal with Excel canal probe by passing in the medullary canal of the femur. Accurate positioning of the entry point will avoid malalignment of the stem **(Figs 8.4 to 8.12)**.

   If calcar is absent and planned for uncemented stem, then choose distal fixation stem (e.g. solution stem) **(Figs 8.6 and 8.7)**.
4. It is advisable to apply one or two screws (usually 25 or 30 mm long 6.5 mm cancellous screws) in the superior and/or posterosuperior aspect of acetabular shell for

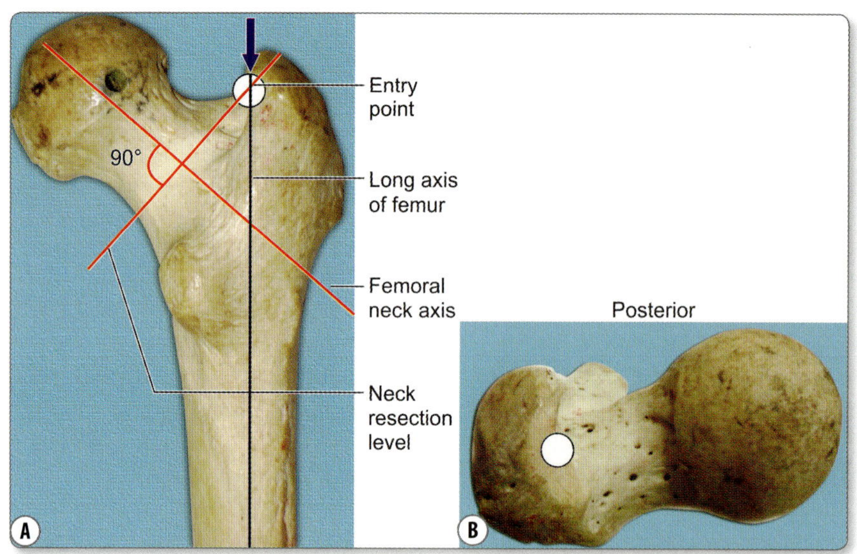

Figs 8.3A and B Correct entry point over piriformis fossa

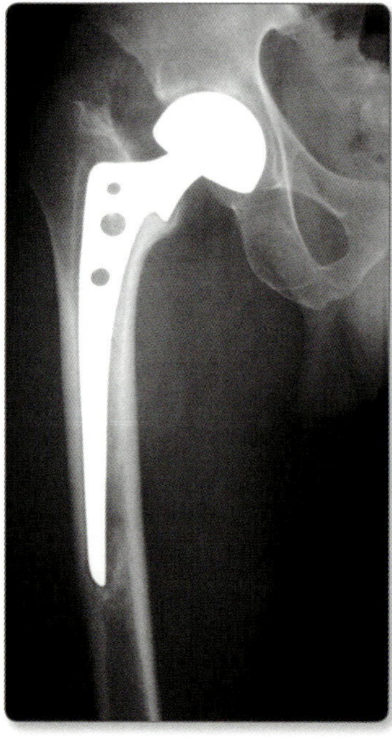

Fig. 8.4 Failed prosthesis due to wrong entry point leads to varus positioning of stem

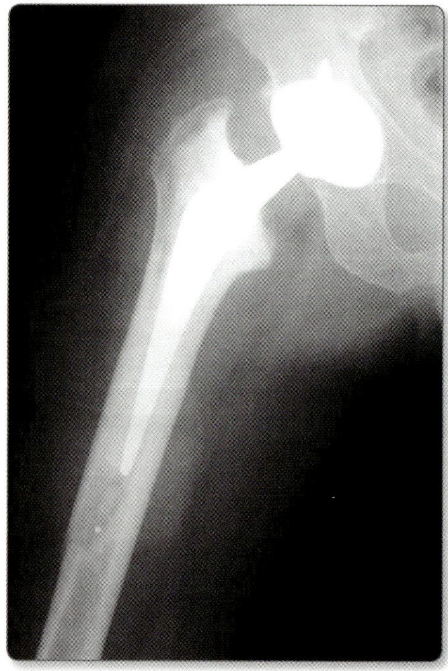

Fig. 8.5 Revision THR (Hybrid—uncemented Duraloc shell and cemented C-stem) with appropriate positioning of stem

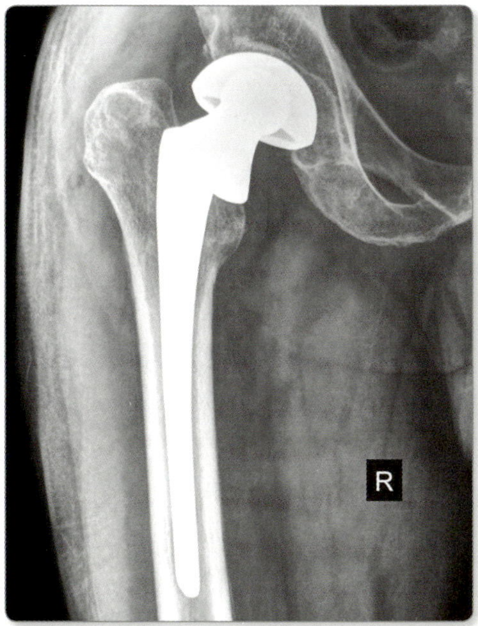

Fig. 8.6 Failed prosthesis due to wrong entry point and loose stem

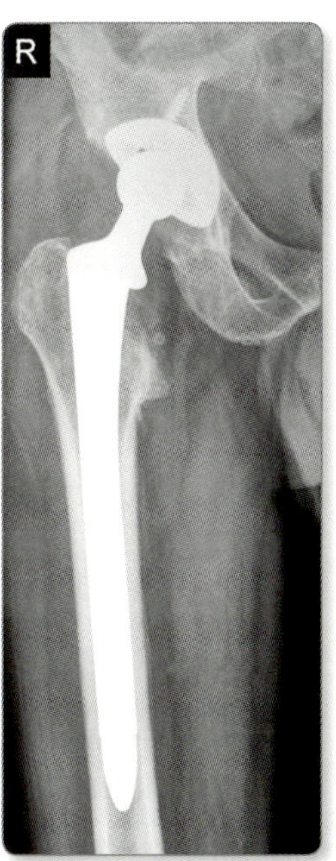

Fig. 8.7 Revision THR—uncemented Duraloc shell with appropriate positioning of uncemented distal fixation stem (e.g. solution stem)

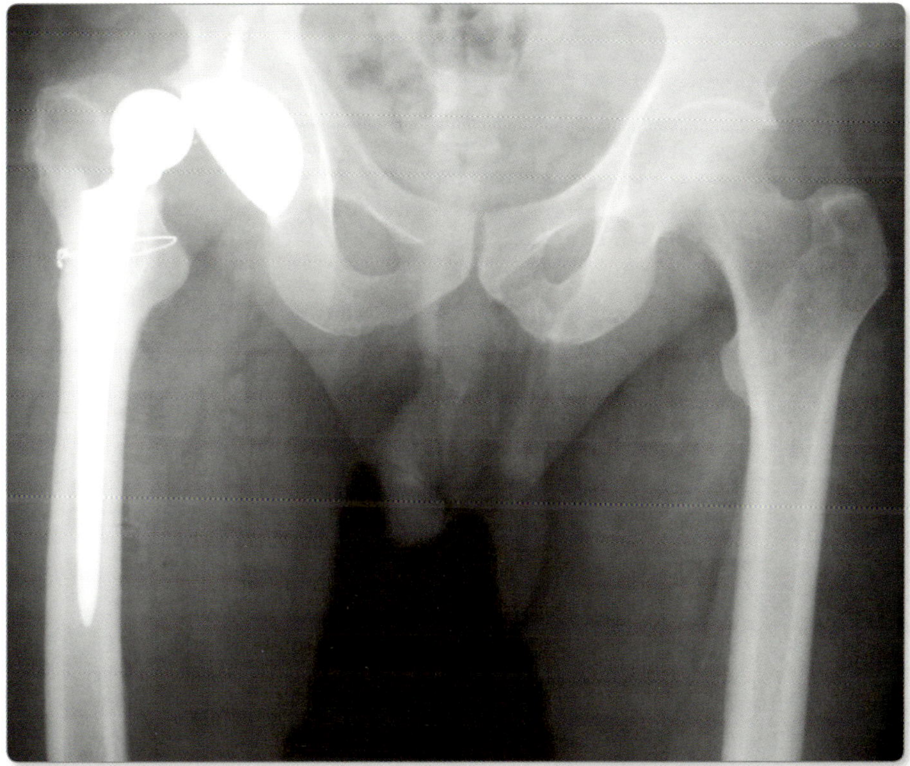

Fig. 8.8 Failed prosthesis due to wrong entry point

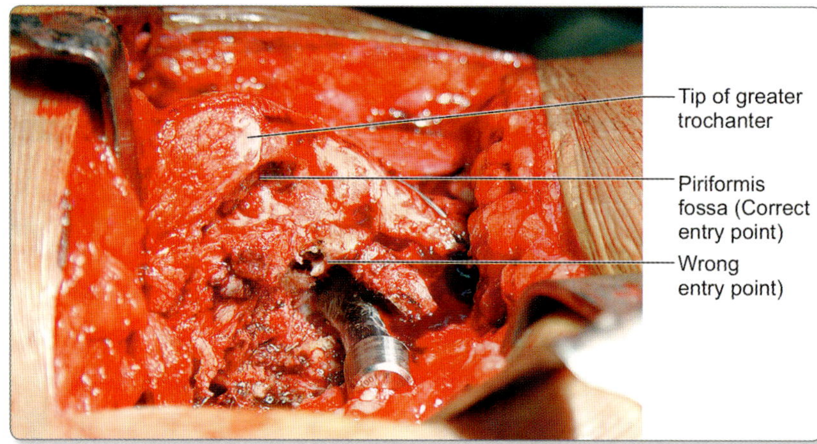

Fig. 8.9 Wrong entry point (away from piriformis fossa leads to undersize prosthesis, fracture and sinking of prosthesis leads to dislocation)

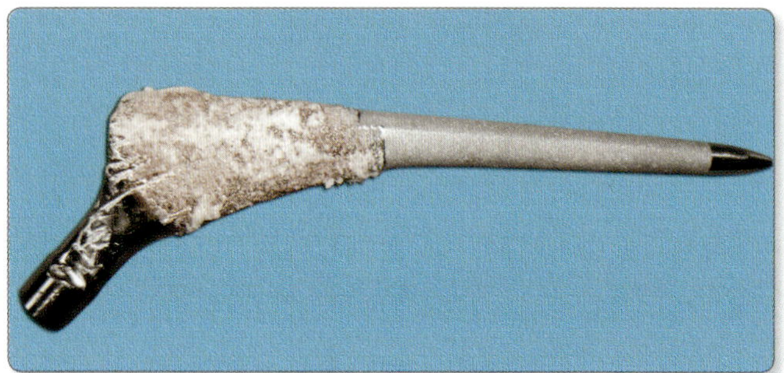

Fig. 8.10 Removed prosthesis (Summit stem size 2)

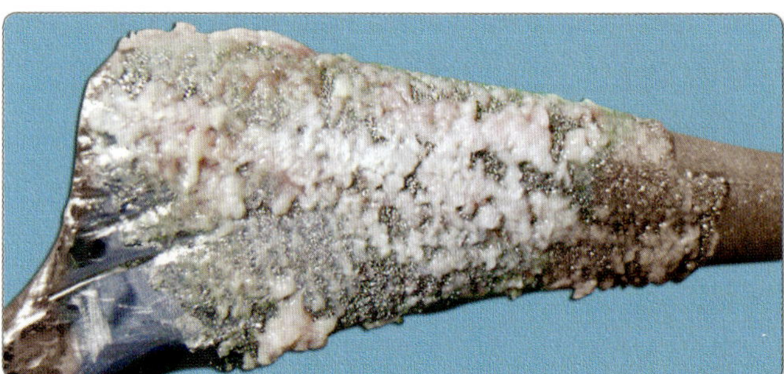

Fig. 8.11 Bone ingrowths over summit stem in 3 months duration

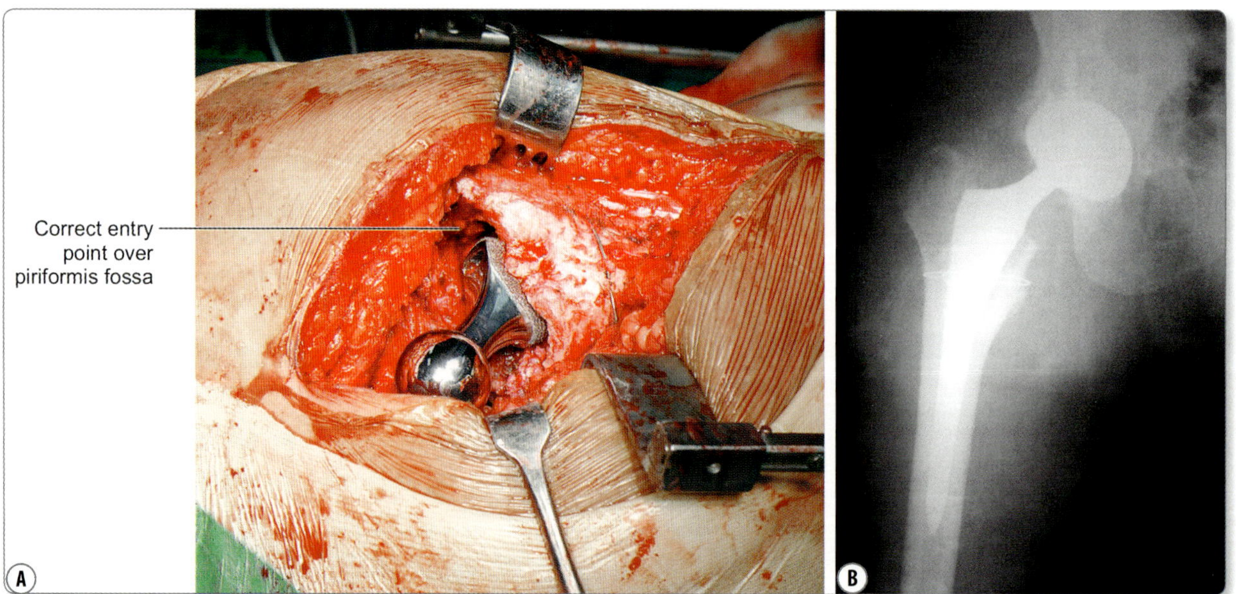

Figs 8.12A and B After revisison of stem, insertion of femoral prosthesis (Summit stem) over piriformis fossa (Summit stem size 5, the actual size)

additional fixation. This usually prevents inadvertent displacement of the acetabular shell during trial or final reduction of the hip.

Total Hip Replacement in Difficult Situations

Assess difficult situations like:

1. Protrusio acetabuli, thin acetabular wall or cysts.
2. Dysplastic hip.
3. Ankylosis of hip.
4. Fixed external rotation deformity.
5. Acetabular wall defect.
6. Proximal migration of acetabulum.
7. Associated fractures.

Difficulties may be in exposure, dislocation, reconstruction of hip or implantation of the components. Plan properly to overcome the possible difficulties during surgery. If required, take 3D-CT scan of both hip joints to assess the type of additional procedures required. Procedures like posterior acetabuloplasty (removal of posterior osteophytes), in situ femoral neck resection and establishment of acetabular cavity are required. Other procedures like building up the wall defect by bone graft taken from resected femoral head, lateralization or medialization of cup may be required to restore the center of rotation of hip to its anatomic location to establish normal joint mechanics. Release of insertion of gluteus maximum tendon is usually required during exposure of hip joint in the above situations. Special attention is given over postoperative physiotherapy like hip abduction exercise, quadriceps exercise, gradual knee and hip bending exercises under supervision of physiotherapist. Gluteal muscle function improves whenever movement is achieved.

Additional Procedures

1. Bone graft from femoral head is applied in acetabulum if protrusio acetabuli, thin acetabular wall or cysts are present before putting the cemented cup **(Figs 8.13 and 8.14)** or acetabular shell in uncemented hip **(Figs 8.15 to 8.18)**. Lateralization of hip center is required for restoration of hip joint lateral and inferior. Cancellous bone graft is harvested from the cut femoral head. For harvesting the graft, one assistant will hold the cut femoral head with help of two towel clips and keep on the instrument trolley. Remove the remnant neck from the subcapital region. Take 40 size acetabular reamer on reamer handle and ream the head so that cancellous bone graft is being collected in the acetabular reamer. Collect sufficient amount of bone graft and put it in the acetabulum and compact the graft by pressing with cup trial or with size 40 acetabular reamer by moving in reverse direction in the floor of acetabulum. The graft should not be too much otherwise that will cause loosening of the acetabular shell. Cup is rim fit and not medial wall fit.

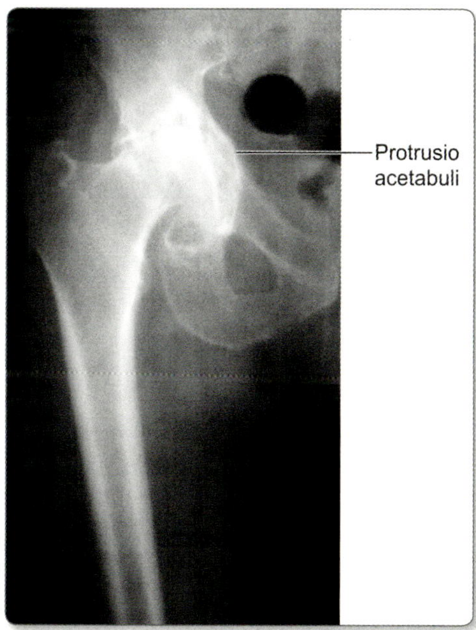

Fig. 8.13 AVN with protrusio acetabuli

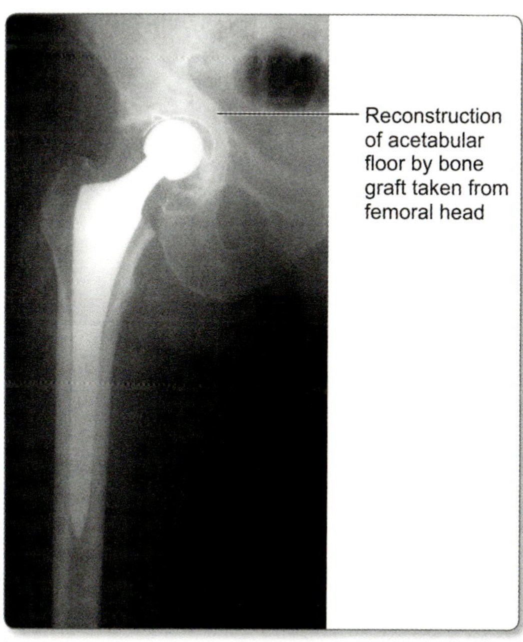

Fig. 8.14 Cemented cup and uncemented stem (Hybrid)

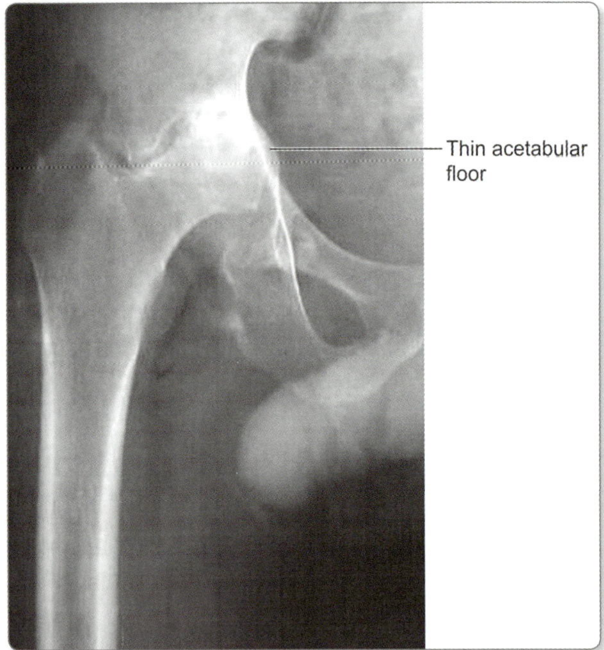

Fig. 8.15 Arthritis hip with thin acetabular floor

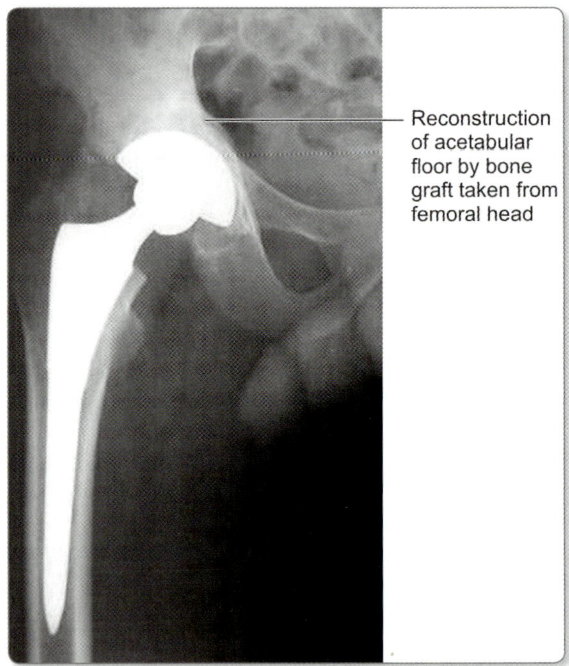

Fig. 8.16 Uncemented cup and uncemented stem

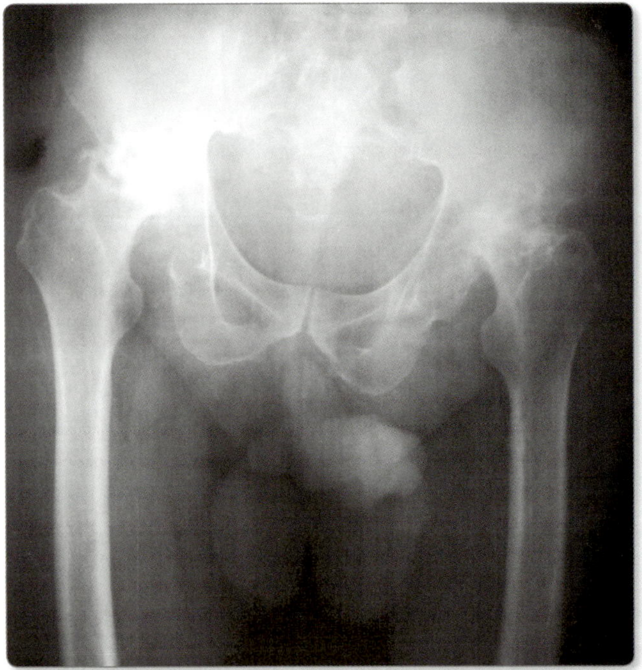

Fig. 8.17 AVN with arthritis and thin acetabular wall and cysts

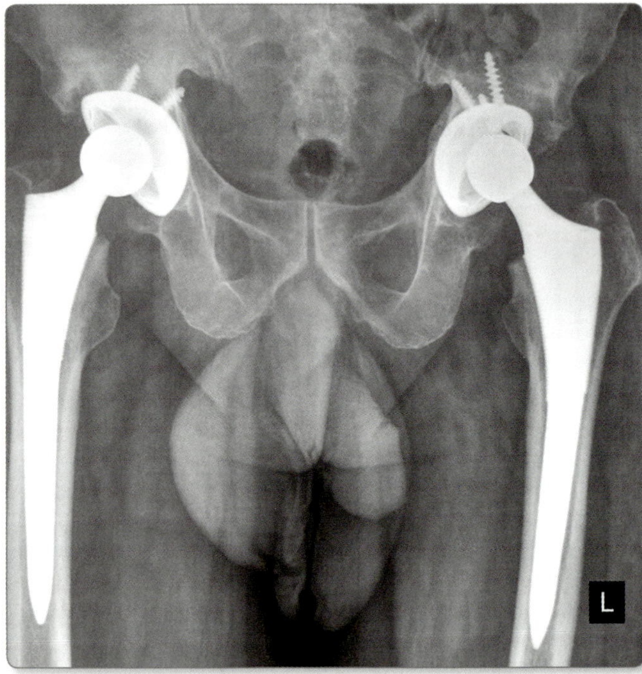

Fig. 8.18 Reconstruction of acetabular wall by bone graft taken from femoral head and application of uncemented cup and stem

2. Dysplastic hip:
   i. Acetabulum:
      - Shallow acetabulum
      - Proximal migration of acetabulum
      - Acetabular wall defect.
   ii. Femur:
      - Short or absent neck
      - Narrow neck and shaft of femur
      - Disproportionate neck and shaft of femur—narrow or broad neck in comparison to shaft.

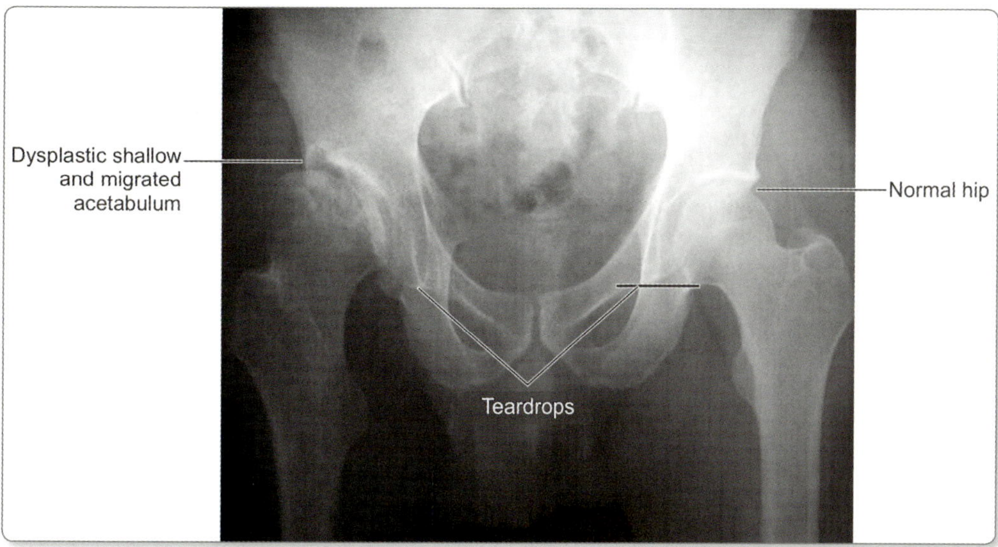

Fig. 8.19 Arthritis with dysplastic and migrated acetabulum in relation to teardrop

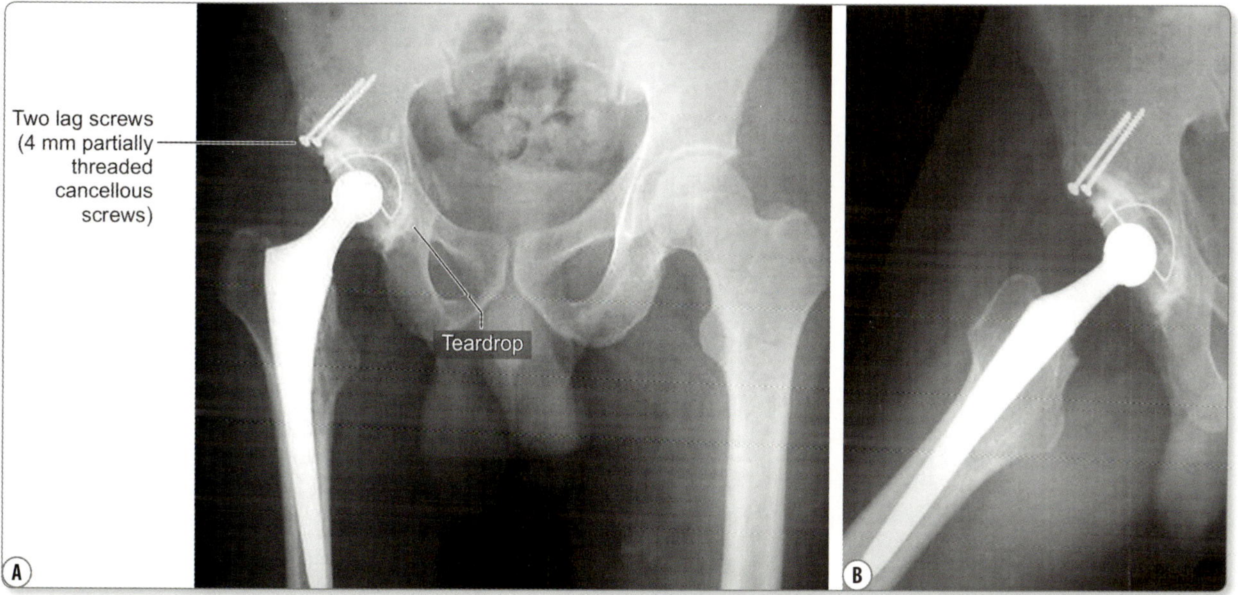

Figs 8.20A and B Reconstruction of acetabulum with bone graft taken from head of the femur and fixed with two lag screws, cup was implanted at the level of teardrop

In case of dysplastic hip with shallow acetabulum, reconstruction of acetabulum for medialization of cup is done by gradually increasing size acetabular reamer staring from size 36 mm reamer. Initially start reaming at 90° to some extent then tilt the reamer in 45° abduction and 20° anteversion till hemispherical dome is achieved. Decision for the size of acetabular cup is determined as described for insertion of acetabular cup. Dysplastic hips may be associated with acetabular wall defect especially posterosuperior which requires reconstruction by bone graft taken from femoral head **(Figs 8.19 and 8.20)**.

In case of short or absent neck, resection is made through the head keeping the saw blade one finger-breadth (10–15 mm) away from the lesser trochanter and reshapes it like femoral neck **(Figs 8.21 and 8.22)**. There may be narrow neck and shaft or disproportionate neck and shaft of femur and hence, usually requires smaller size stem **(Figs 8.23 to 8.28)**.

3. In case of ankylosis of hip, especially in ankylosing spondylitis, the dislocation of hip is not possible. Hence do femoral neck resection in situ after exposure of the hip joint. Make multiple drill holes by 2.5 mm drill bit in the neck near subcapital region perpendicular to

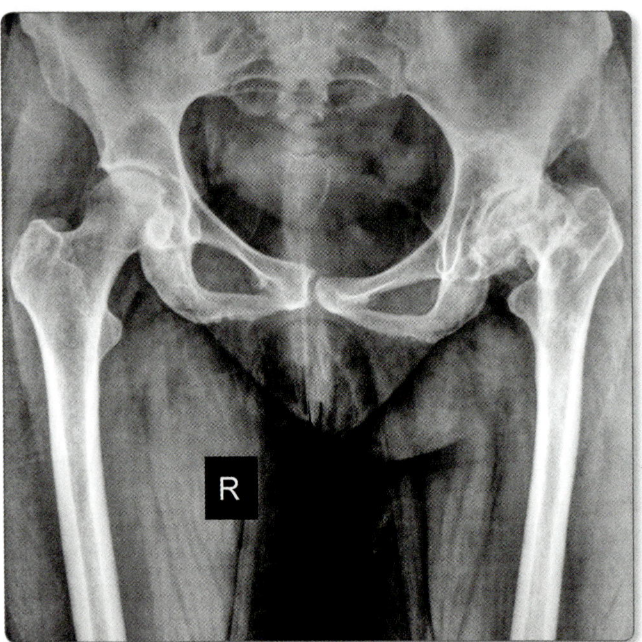

Fig. 8.21 Dysplastic left hip with shallow acetabulum and short neck

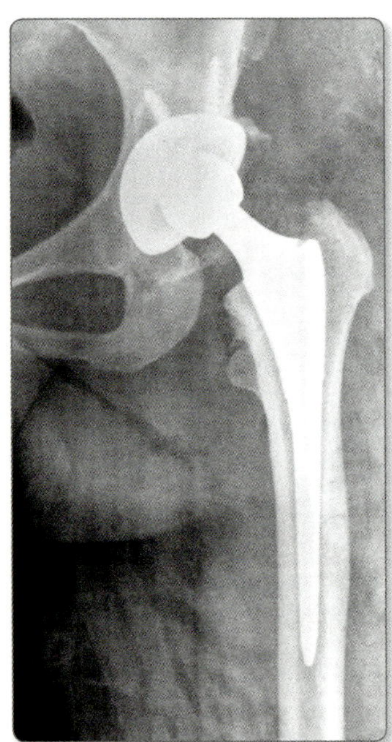

Fig. 8. 22 Reconstruction of acetabulum and medialization of cup (Duraloc shell)

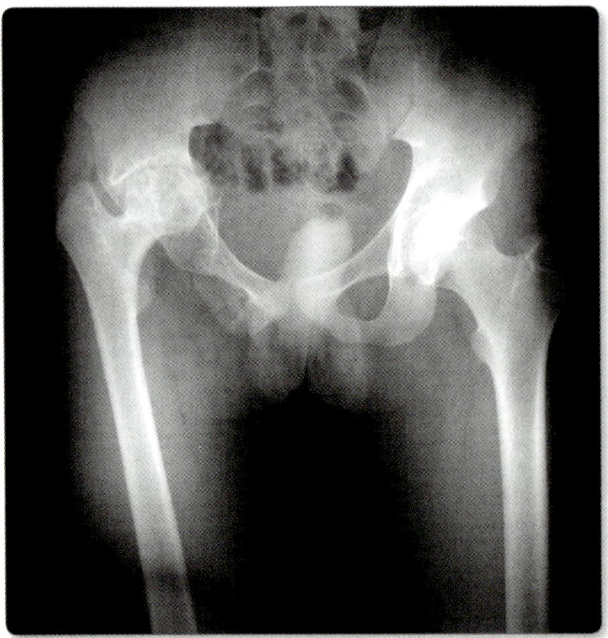

Fig. 8.23 Dysplastic right hip with narrow both neck and shaft

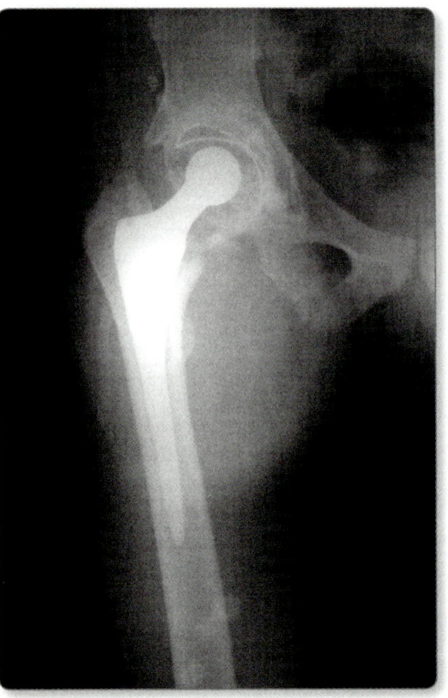

Fig. 8.24 Cemented cup with uncemented Summit stem

the surface of femoral neck and measure the depth of drill hole by depth gauge. This depth will tell the approximate length of oscillating saw blade which has to be introduced during cutting the neck of the femur. After cutting the neck by oscillating saw, complete the osteotomy by osteotome but avoid splintering of the neck. The assistant will support the proximal thigh on medial aspect while osteotomy to prevent the splintering of neck. Bring the limb in such a way that the sole of foot faces the ceiling and assistant will lift the thigh so that the femoral neck becomes parallel to the table. Revise the neck resection according to neck resection guide

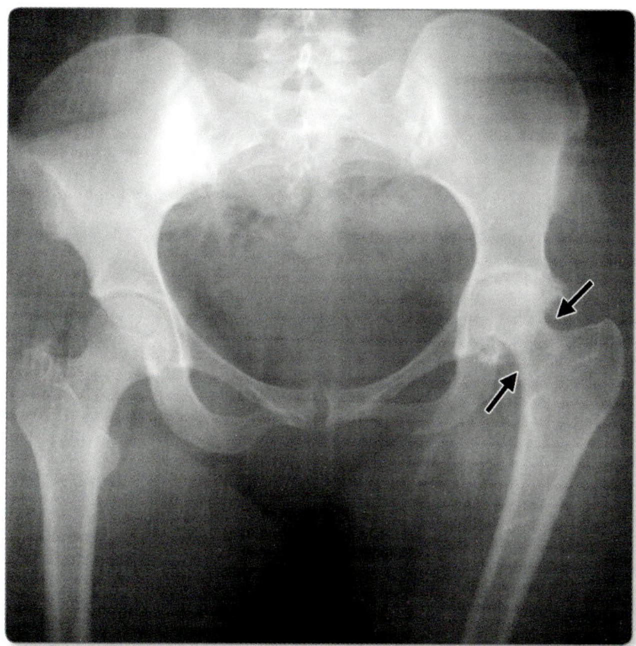

Fig. 8.25 Arthritis with narrow neck (Disproportionate neck and shaft), peroperatively, posterosuperior wall defect

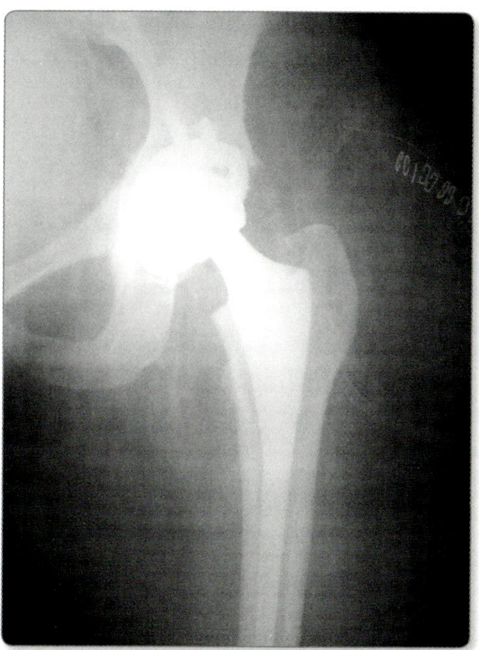

Fig. 8.26 Reconstruction of acetabulum by bone graft and implantation of uncemented Duraloc shell and Summit stem

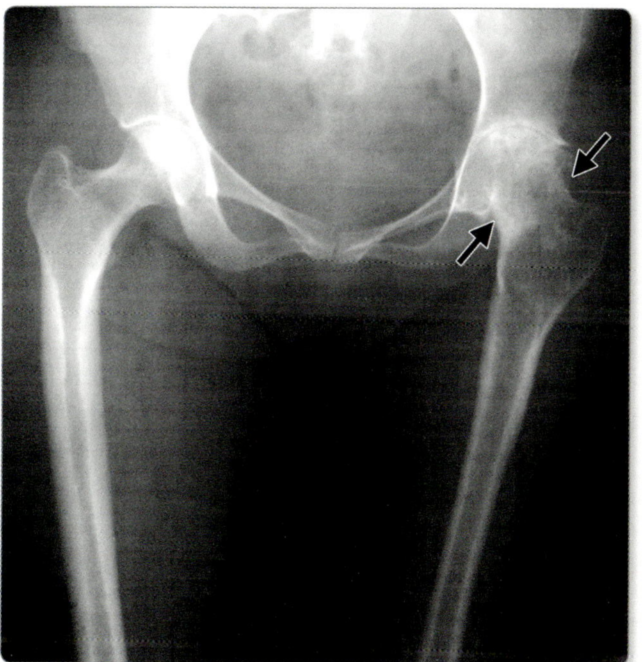

Fig. 8.27 Arthritis with broad neck (disproportionate neck and shaft) peroperatively, posterosuperior wall defect

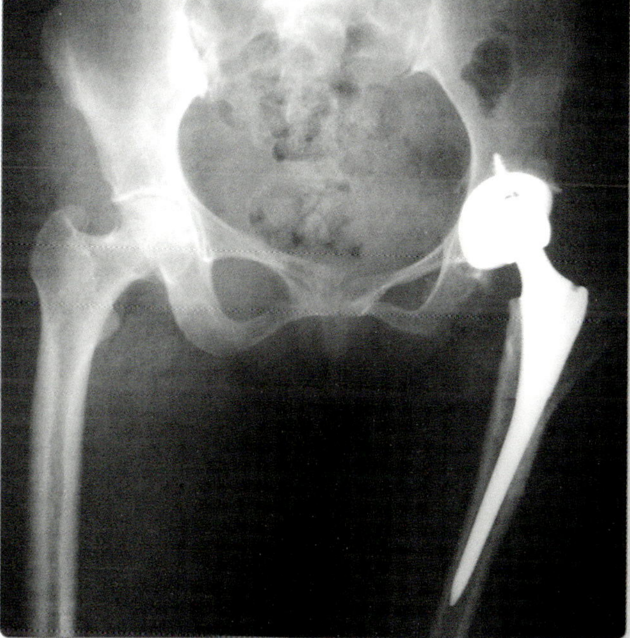

Fig. 8.28 Reconstruction of acetabulum by bone graft and implantation of uncemented Duraloc shell and Summit stem

keeping neck length 10–15 mm from lesser trochanter. Expose the acetabulum with remaining head up to 360° as described. Ream over the head in acetabulum by gradually increasing size reamer starting from size 36 mm reamer. Start reaming perpendicular to the hip to some extent and then tilt the reamer to 45° abduction and 20° anteversion. Remove the remaining head by ring curette. Ream acetabulum till the margin and floor of acetabulum is exposed and becomes hemispherical dome-shaped. Decision for the size of acetabular cup is determined as described for insertion of acetabular cup for uncemented THR (**Figs 8.29 and 8.30)** and for cemented THR **(Figs 8.31 and 8.32)**.

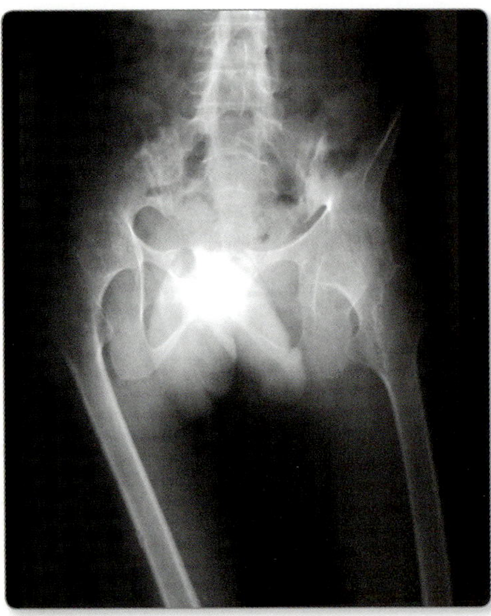

Fig. 8.29 Bony ankylosis of both hip joints in case of ankylosing spondylitis

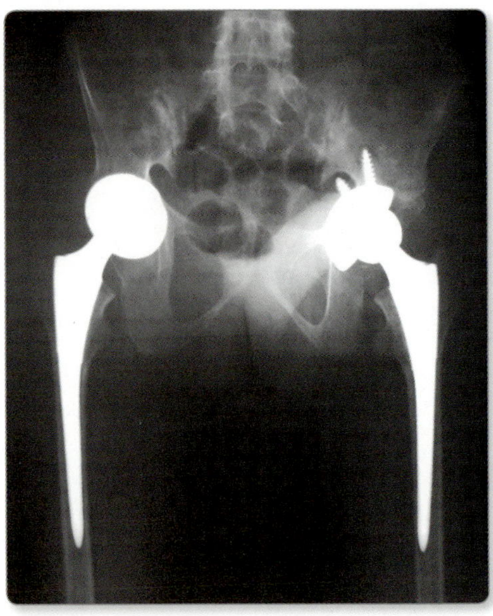

Fig. 8.30 Uncemented (Summit stem) bilateral total hip replacement after femoral neck resection in situ. 44 mm pinnacle cup on right side and Duraloc shell on left side

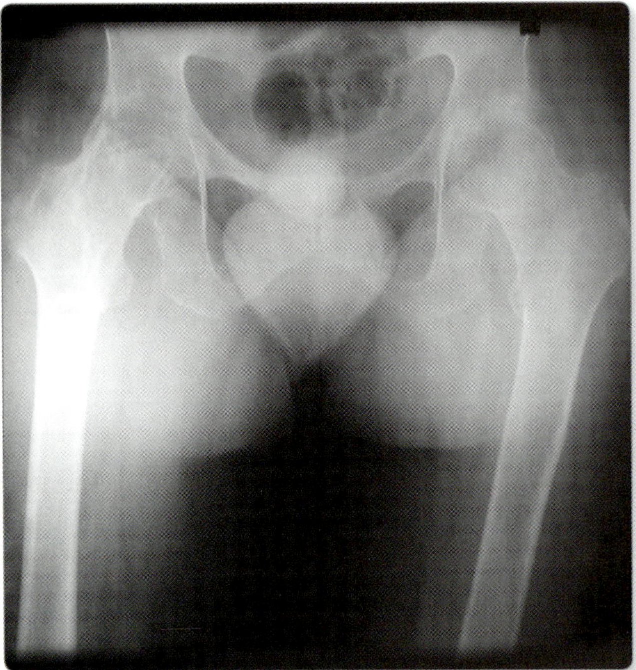

Fig. 8.31 Ankylosing spondylitis with bony ankylosis both hip Joints

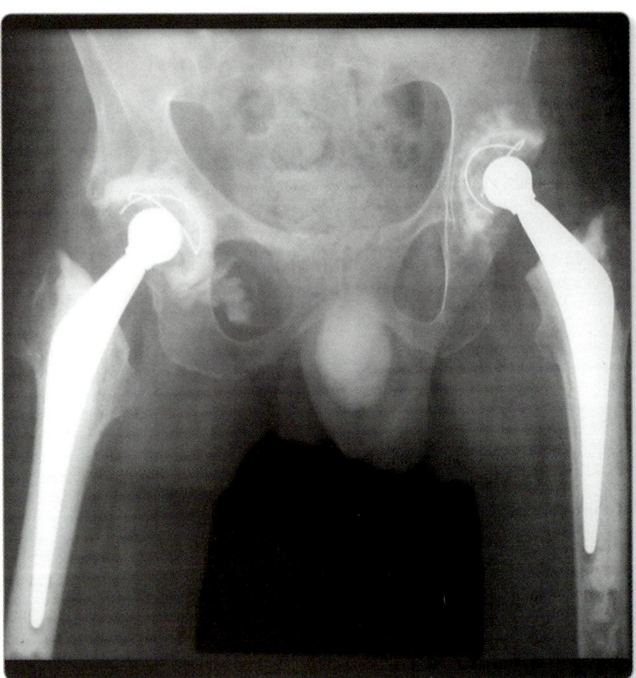

Fig. 8.32 C-Stem both hip joints after femoral neck resection in situ

4. Fixed external rotation deformity of hip is also one of the difficult situations where exposure and dislocation of hip is difficult and excessive force may result into fracture acetabulum or femur **(Figs 8.33 and 8.34)**. Gradual release including osteophytes removal should be done before dislocation of hip and sometimes may require osteotomy in situ.
5. In case of proximal migration of acetabulum **(Figs 8.35 to 8.39)** or acetabular wall defect due to fracture dislocation of the hip **(Figs 8.40 and 8.45)** where reconstruction is required (*See* classification of acetabular defect in revision THR), the bone graft is taken from the femoral head. Preoperative 3D-CT scan of hip is useful for assessing the amount of acetabular

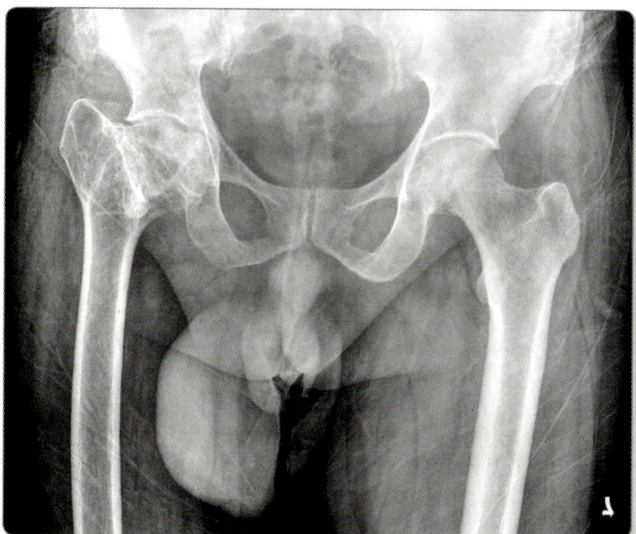
Fig. 8.33 Fixed external rotation deformity with absent neck following old trochanteric fracture

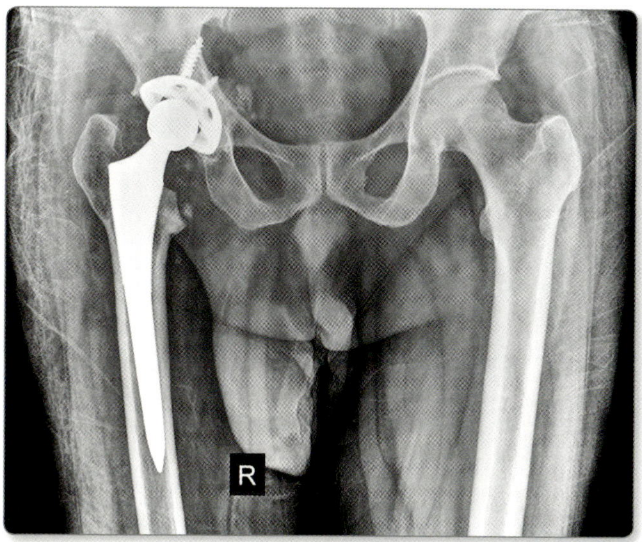

Fig. 8.34 Resection through head to preserve the neck and uncemented THR (Duraloc shell and Summit stem)

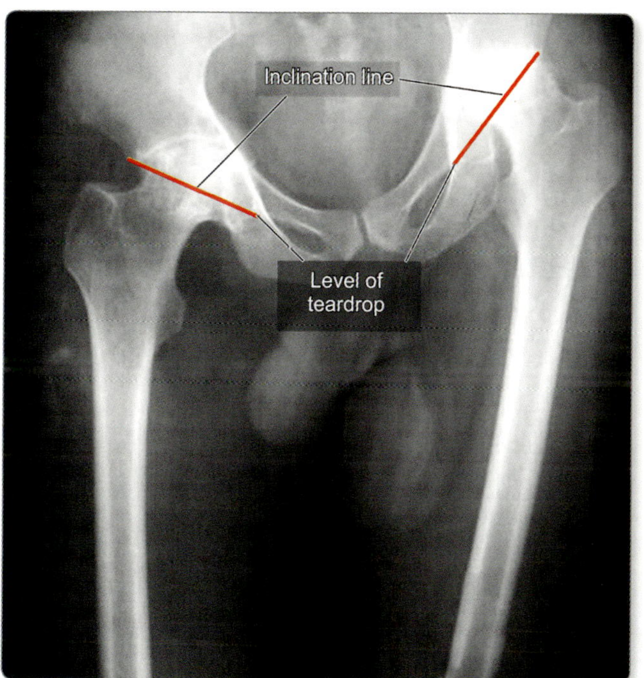

Fig. 8.35 AVN both hip with proximal migration of acetabulum

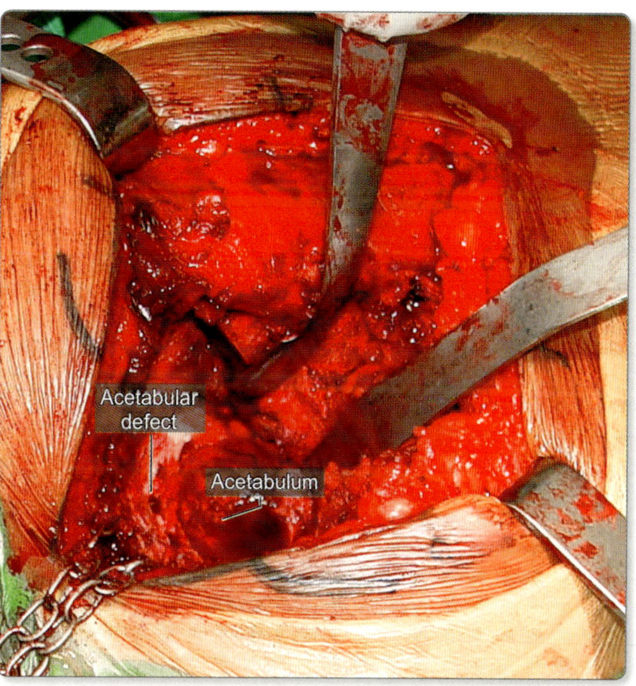

Fig. 8.36 Acetabulum after reaming with superior defect

wall defect. For taking the bone graft, the assistant will hold the femoral head by two towel clips and keep on the instrument trolley. The surgeon will divide the femoral head and neck by oscillating saw according to the size of the defect. Denude the cartilage from that part of head which will come in apposition with fractured surface of acetabulum. Make the shape of the graft according to defect with the help of saw blade, bone cutter and/or nibbler. Assess the congruity of graft by applying the acetabular trial. Temporarily fix the graft in the defect of acetabulum with one or two K-wires **(Fig. 8.51)**. Smoothen the graft surface by smaller size acetabular reamer-slowly and carefully to make it dome-shaped. Make one drill hole by 2.5 mm drill bit through graft to

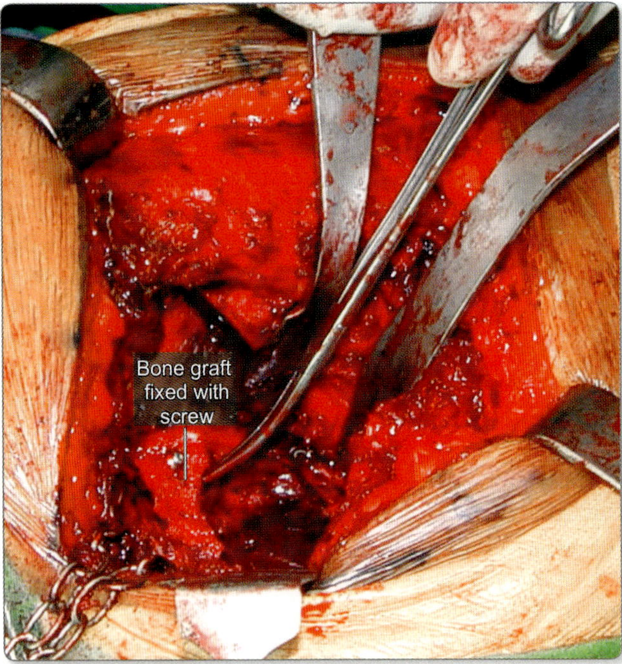

Fig.8.37 Reconstruction of acetabular defect by autograft from head of femur

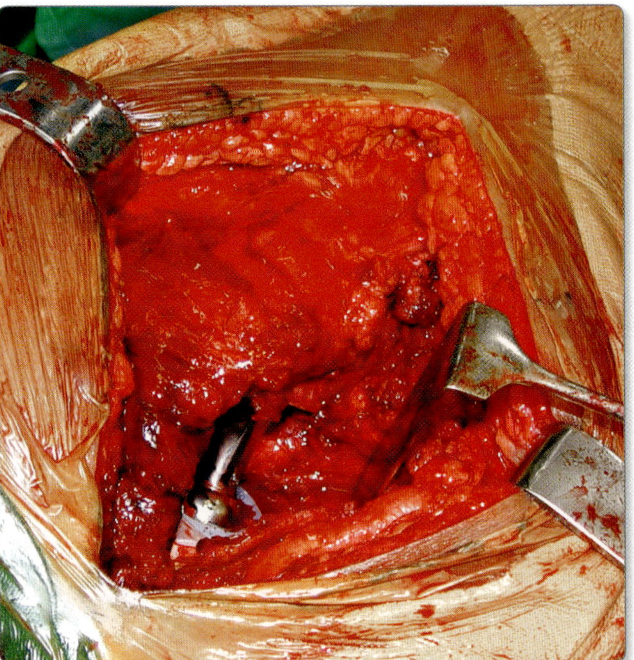

Fig. 8.38 Exposure of hip, bone graft at defect and cemented cup

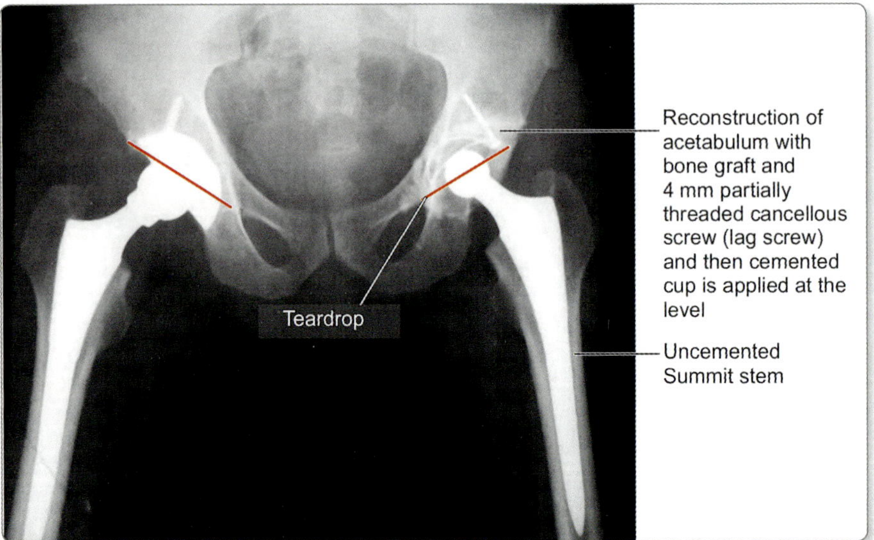

Fig. 8.39 Acetabular cup implanted at the level of tear drop after reconstruction in left hip

the acetabulum. Measure the length of screw by depth gauge. Tap with 3.5 mm tap. Countersink in graft or use washer and apply the appropriate length of 4 mm partially threaded cancellous screw (Lag screw). Remove the K-wires. Pass another screw in the similar way. After reconstruction of the acetabulum the cemented or uncemented (multihole cup) acetabular cup is placed at the level of teardrop **(Fig. 8.54)**. In case of uncemented cup (multihole cup), apply two or three 6.5 mm cancellous screws though the sound part of acetabular wall **(Fig. 8.52 and 8.56)**. Do not pass the cancellous screw through the holes of cup to the grafted bone. Finally apply the acetabular liner **(Fig. 8.53)**.

Associated Fractures

1. *Fracture acetabulum with AVN*: In old fracture acetabulum with AVN of femoral head, additional procedure of bone grafting **(Figs 8.40 to 8.42)** reinforcement ring **(Figs 8.46 to 49)** is required for lateralization and stable cup containment which is assessed during reaming and cup trial. Removal of reconstruction plate and screws depends on hinderance of cup placement by screws and/or plate **(Figs 8.43 to 8.48)**.
2. Fracture-dislocation of hip with posterosuperior wall defect with AVN **(Fig. 8.50)**: Posterosuperior acetabular wall defect is reconstructed by bone graft taken from resected femoral head **(Figs 8.51 to 8.56)** or freeze dried femoral head allograft.

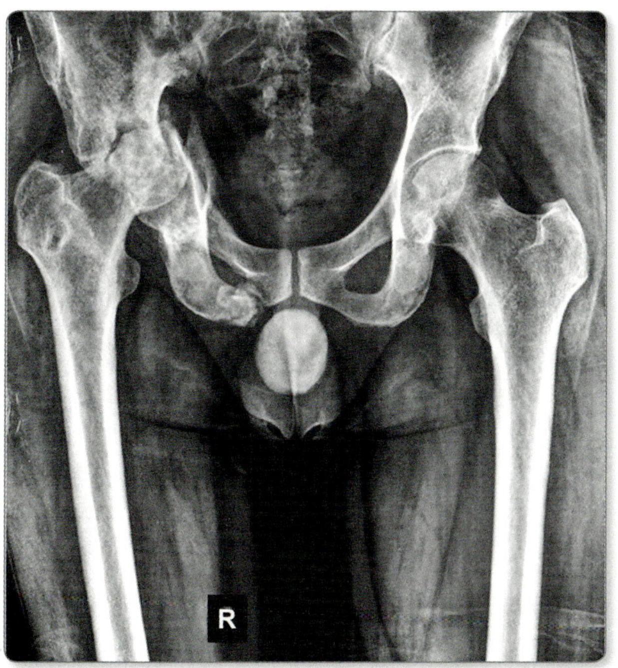

Fig. 8.40 X-ray showing central fracture-dislocation with AVN head

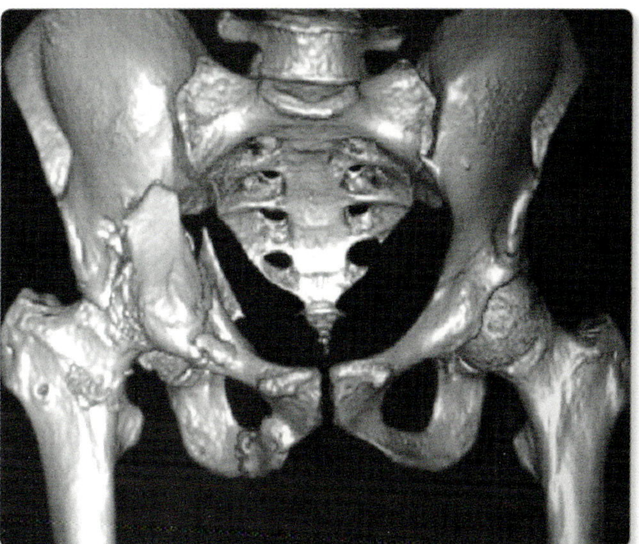

Fig. 8.41A 3D-CT scan anterior view

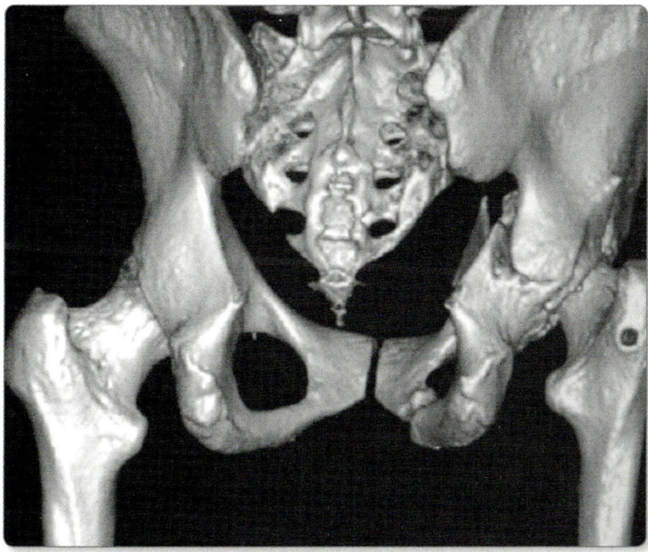

Fig. 8.41B 3D-CT scan posterior view

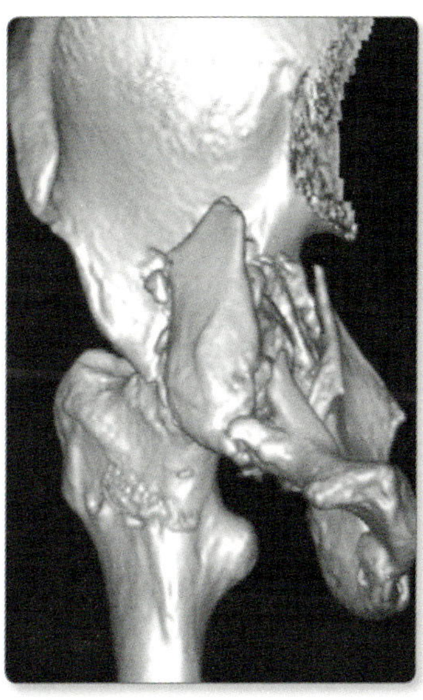

Fig. 8.41C 3D-CT scan lateral view

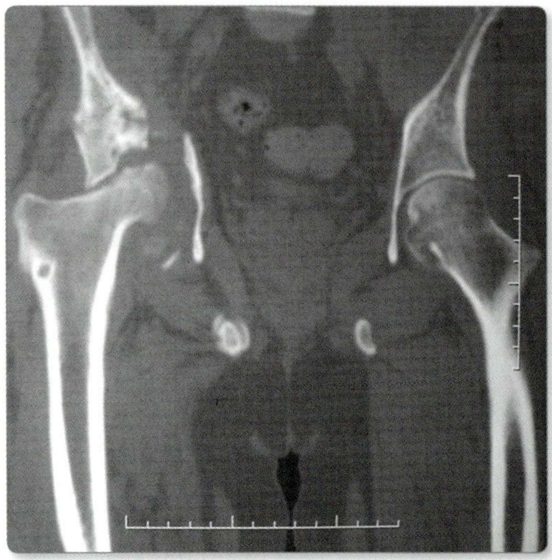

Fig. 8.41D CT scan sagittal view

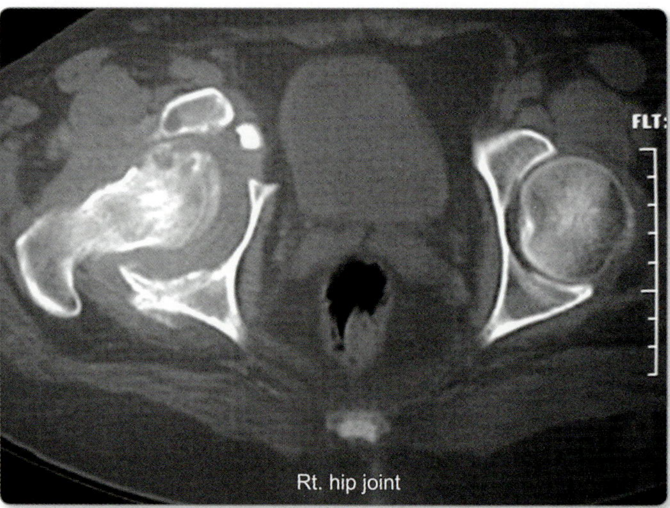

Fig. 8.41E CT scan transverse view showing medial wall defect

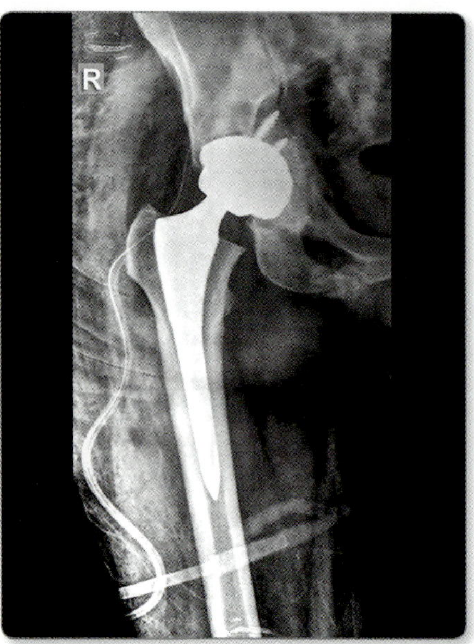

Fig. 8.42 THR after reconstruction of medial wall of acetabulum with autobone graft from femoral head

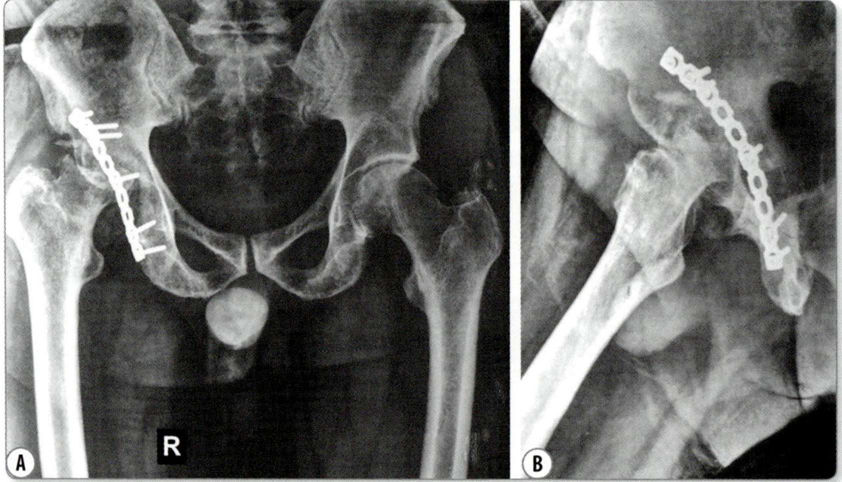

Figs 8.43A and B Old fixation of acetabulum with AVN and absorption of head

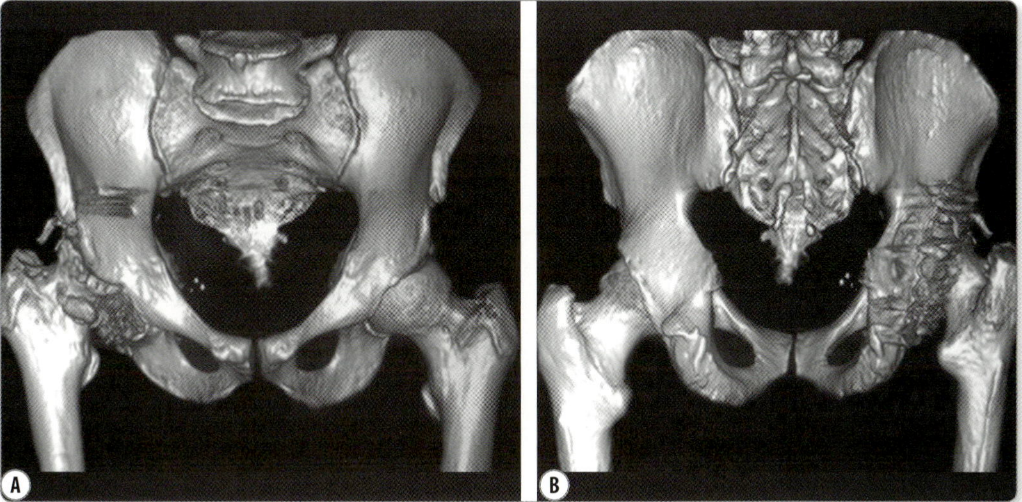

Figs 8.44A and B 3D-CT scan pelvis anterior and posterior view

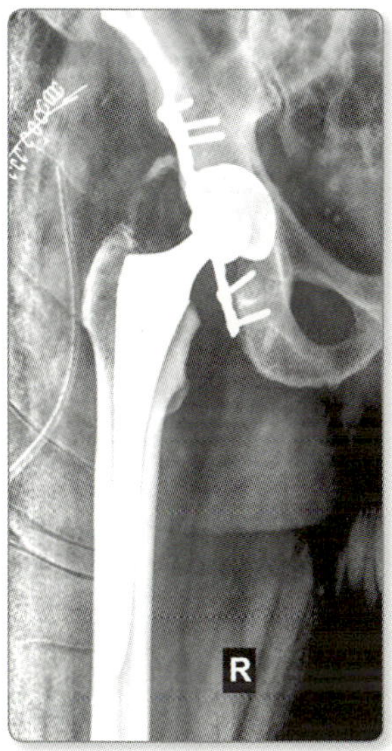

Fig. 8.45 Post-THR in old reconstructed acetabulum

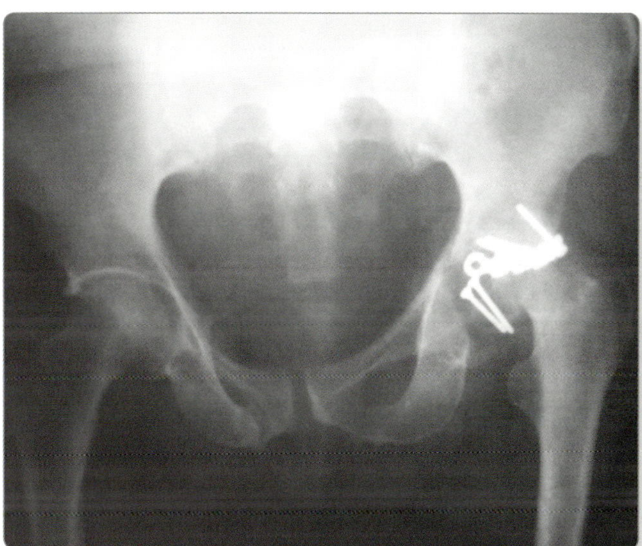

Fig. 8.46 Failed acetabular fixation for fracture acetabulum with AVN head and absorption of head

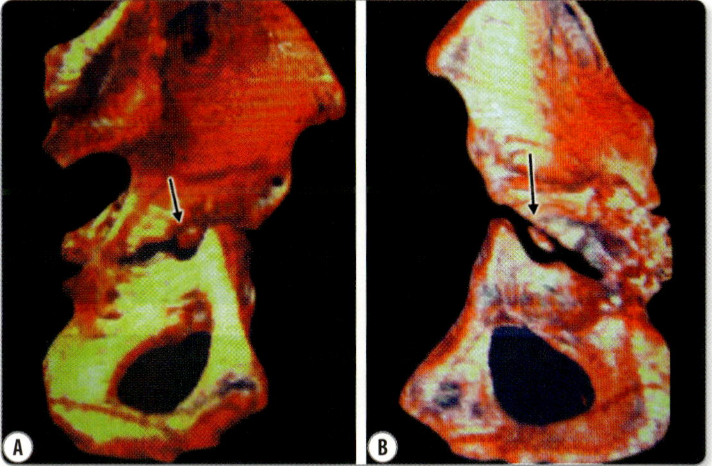

Figs 8.47A and B 3D-CT shows non-union fracture acetabulum

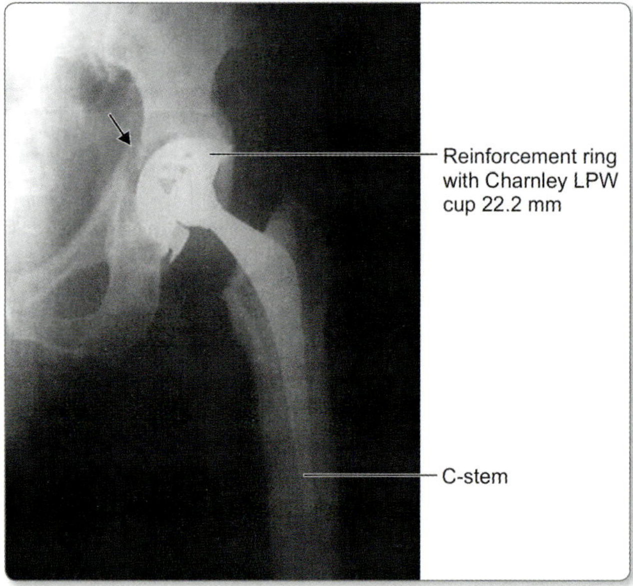

Fig. 8.48 C-stem and acetabular reinforcement ring with Charnley LPW cup

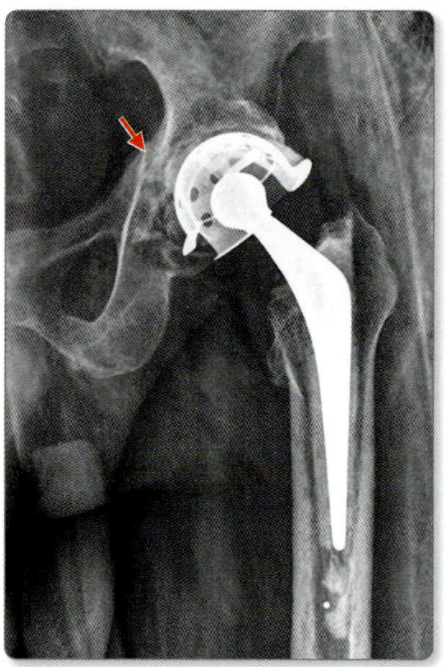

Fig. 8.49 Fracture acetabulum united (at 8 years follow-up)

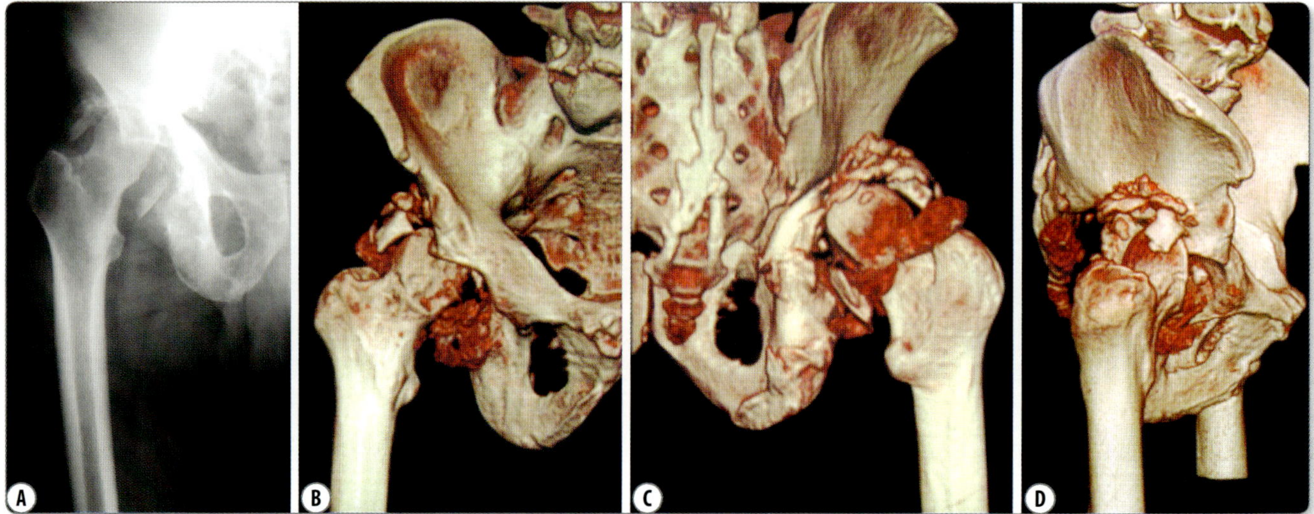

Figs 8.50A to D X-ray hip AP view and 3D-CT scan of hip anterior, posterior and lateral views showing fracture dislocation of the hip with posterosuperior acetabular wall defect

Important Points for THR in Fracture–Dislocation of Hip (Old Unreduced Hip or Failed Reconstruction of Acetabulum)

Finding the acetabulum is a difficult task due to filling of acetabular cavity by lot of fibrous tissues and disturbed outline of fractured acetabulum. In cases of failed acetabular reconstruction, remove all hardware. Six important points should be kept in mind while doing total hip replacement in cases of old unreduced fracture dislocation of hip or failed reconstruction of acetabulum.

1. *X-ray of both hip joints*: To assess the amount of migration of head as compared to the normal side hip joint and plan to compensate the limb length discrepancy **(Fig. 8.57)**.
2. *Preoperative 3D-CT scan of both hip joints*: To assess the level and amount of acetabular wall defect and position of femoral head in relation to acetabular cavity **(Figs 8.58A to D)**.

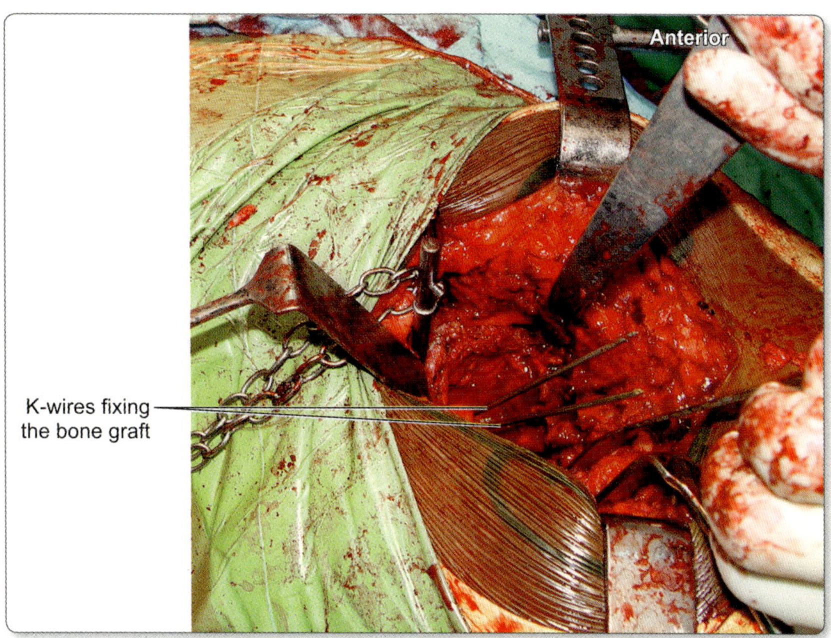

Fig. 8.51 Temporary fixation of graft by two K-wires

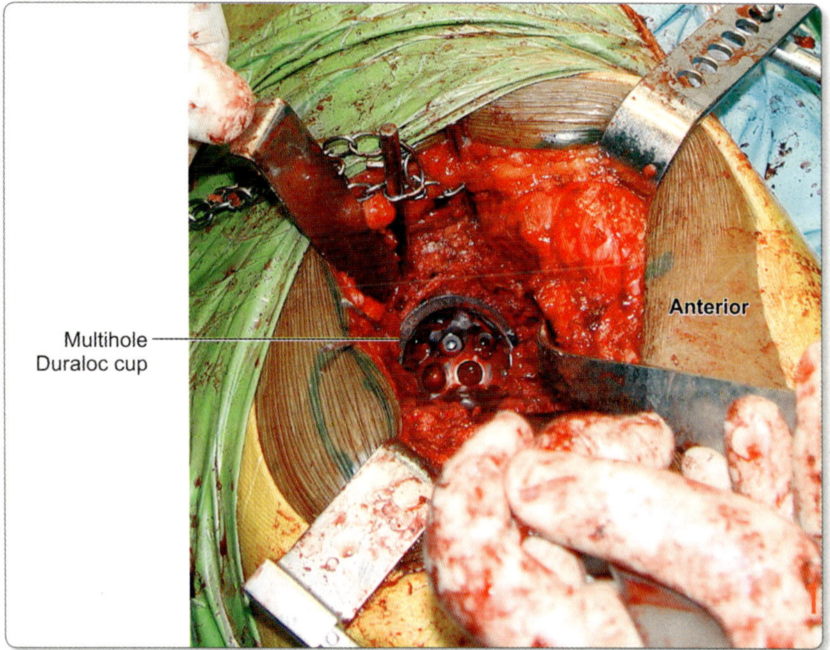

Fig. 8.52 Implantation of multihole Duraloc shell and fixation with cancellous screws

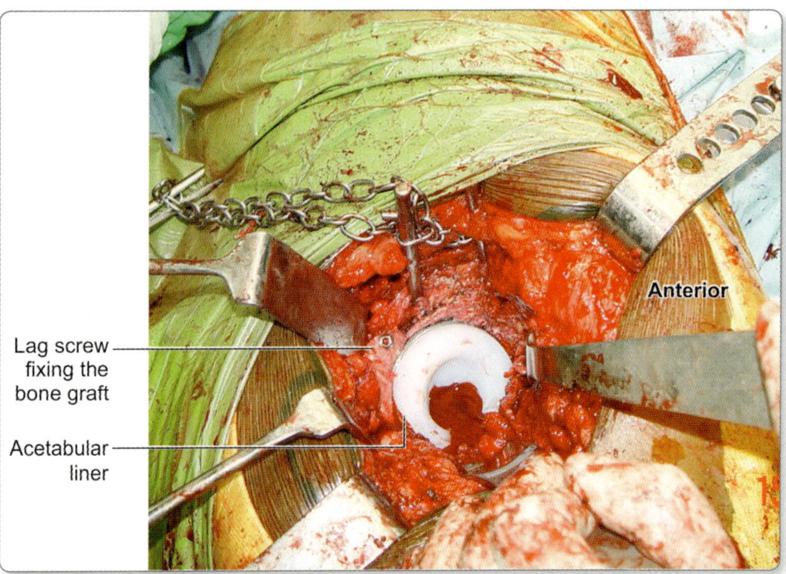

Fig. 8.53 Built-up defect by bone graft and 4 mm partially threaded cancellous screw (lag screw) and application of acetabular liner

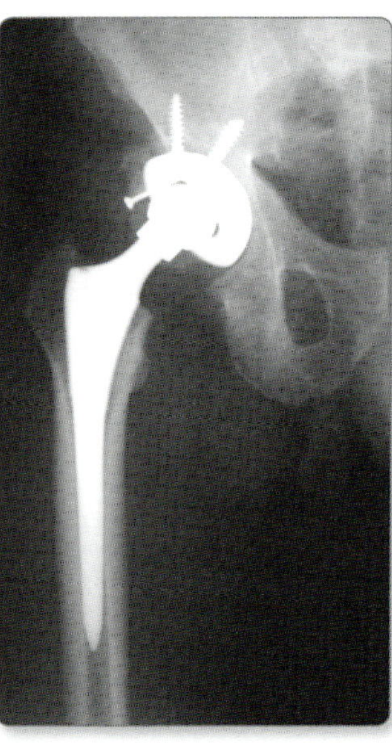

Fig. 8.54 X-ray AP view after final implantation of uncemented acetabular (multihole Duraloc shell) and femoral (Summit stem) components

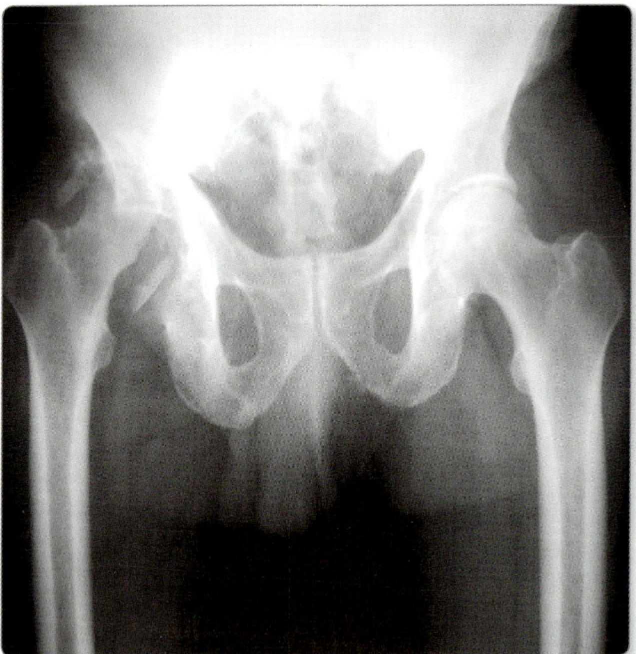

Fig. 8.55 Preoperative AP view of fracture dislocation of right hip with posterosuperior acetabular wall defect

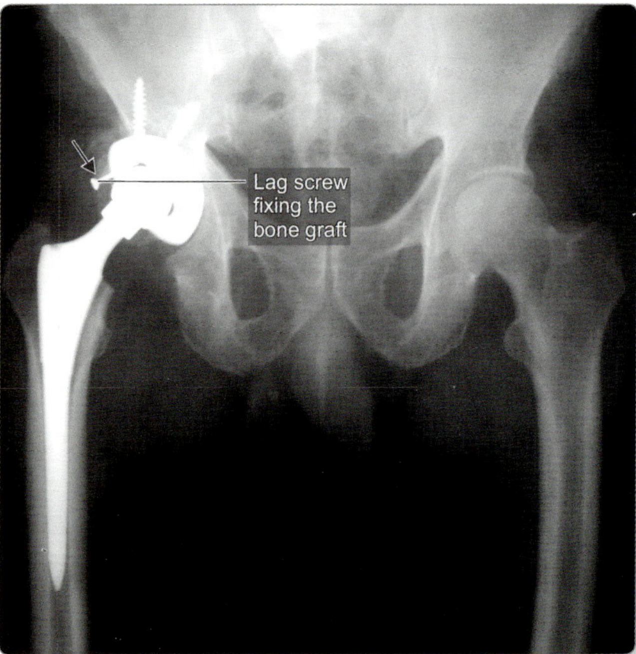

Fig. 8.56 Postoperative AP view with reconstruction of acetabulum and uncemented THR

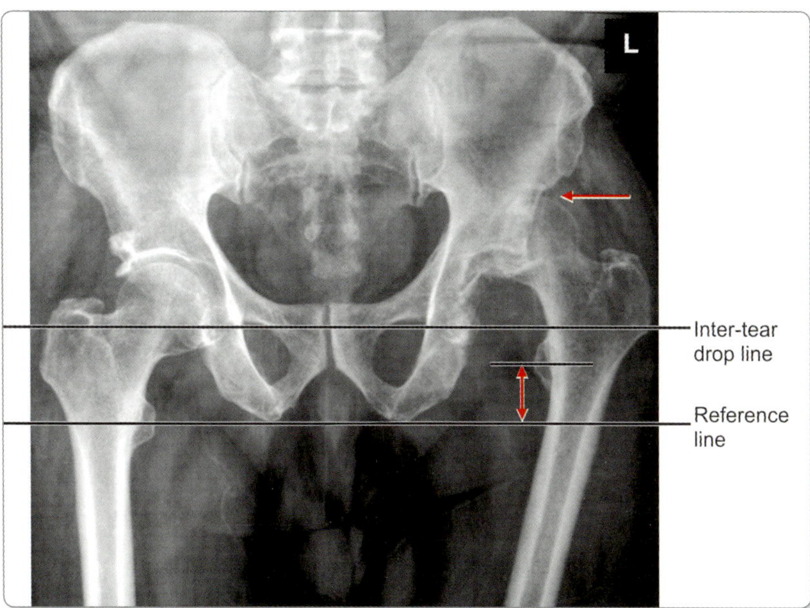

Fig. 8.57 Old unreduced fracture dislocation of left hip

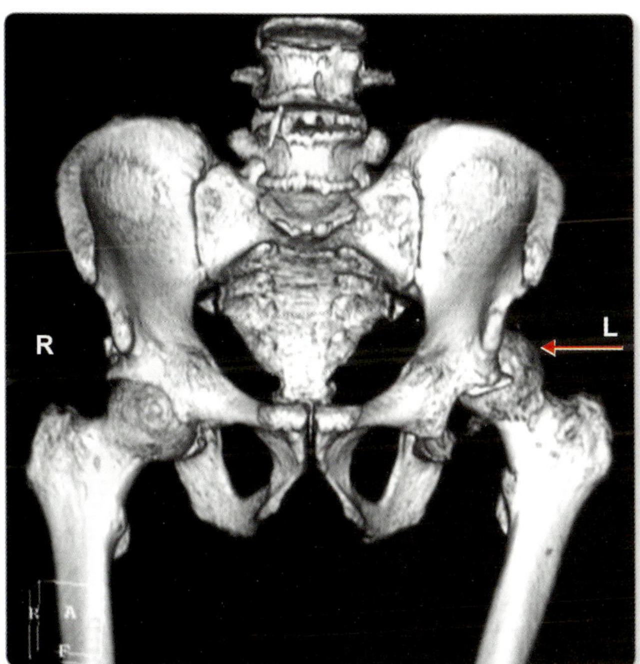

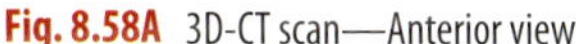
Fig. 8.58A 3D-CT scan—Anterior view

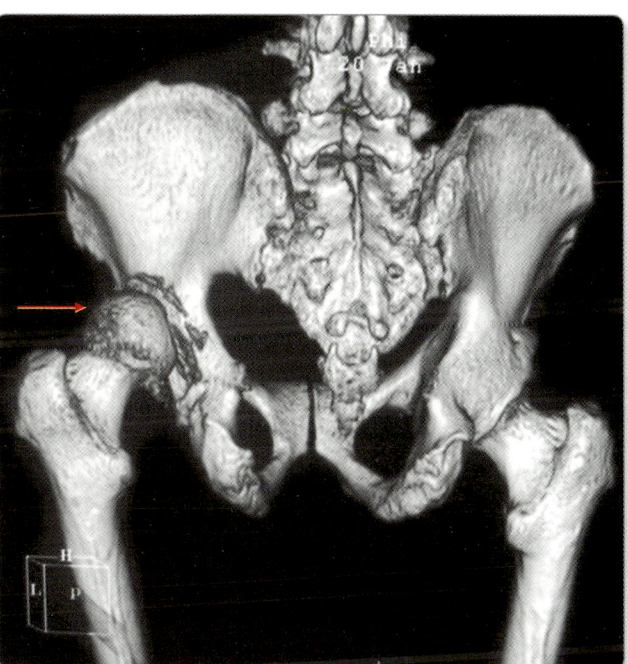

Fig. 8.58B 3D-CT—Posterior view

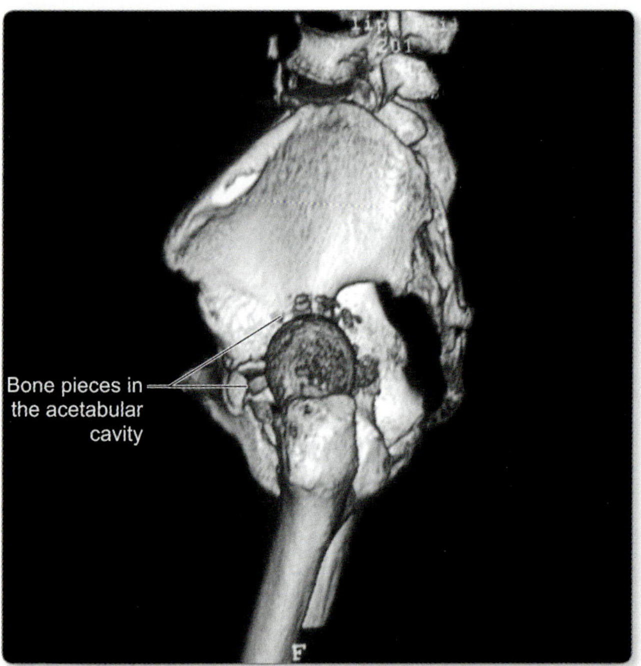

Fig. 8.58C 3D-CT lateral view of dislocated hip
(*Note:* 3D-CT scan showing dislocated hip with posterosuperior acetabular defect as compared from the normal hip. Figure 8.58C shows filling of acetabular cavity with bone pieces)

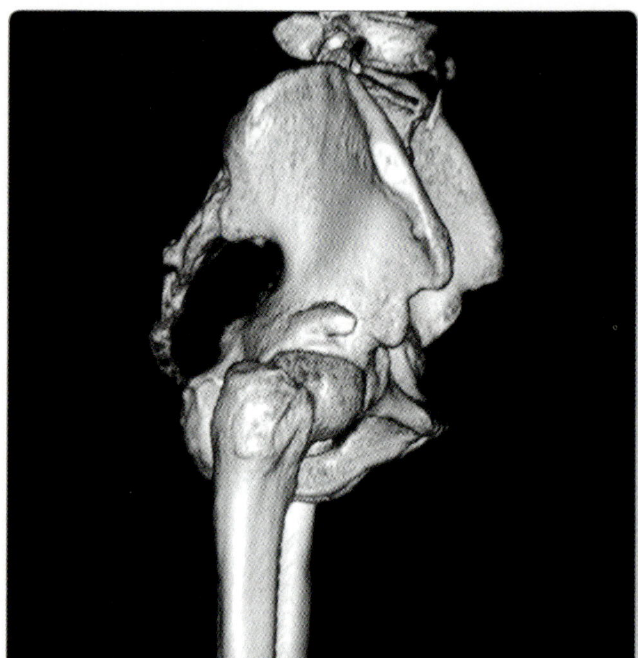

Fig. 8.58D Lateral view of normal hip (For comparison)

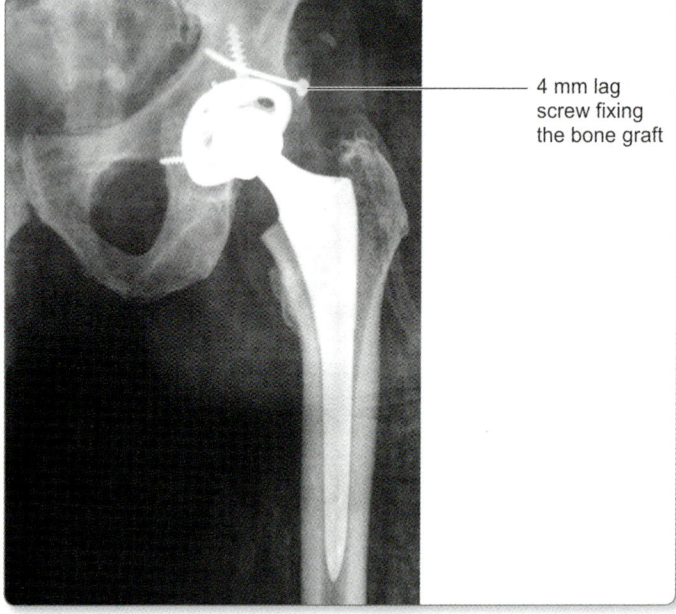

Fig. 8.59 X-ray showing reconstruction of posterosuperior wall by resected femoral head with 4 mm lag screw and implantation of uncemented multihole Duraloc shell securing with 6.5 mm three cancellous screws passing through sound parts of the acetabular wall

3. *Establish at least one of three landmarks of acetabulum*: Tear drop, ligamentum teres and fovea capitis, transverse ligament and acetabular notch after exposure of the hip joint. This is important to restore the center of rotation of hip to its anatomic location to establish normal joint mechanics.
4. *Reconstruction of acetabular wall*: Resected head alongwith neck autograft or freeze dried femoral head allograft is used to reconstruct the acetabular wall **(Fig. 8.59)**. Reconstruction of wall is done as described.
5. *Selection of multihole Duraloc/pinnacle cup*: To fix the cup with 2 or 3 cancellous screws (6.5 mm) in sound area of acetabular part. Do not pass the screw through the graft.
6. *Delayed ambulation*: Complete bed rest in supine position for 4 to 6 weeks. Physiotherapy like quadriceps exercise, ankle and toes movement, chest physiotherapy and continuation of low molecular weight heparin till the bedridden patient requires it essentially. After 4 to 6 week, patient is made ambulatory nonweight-bearing

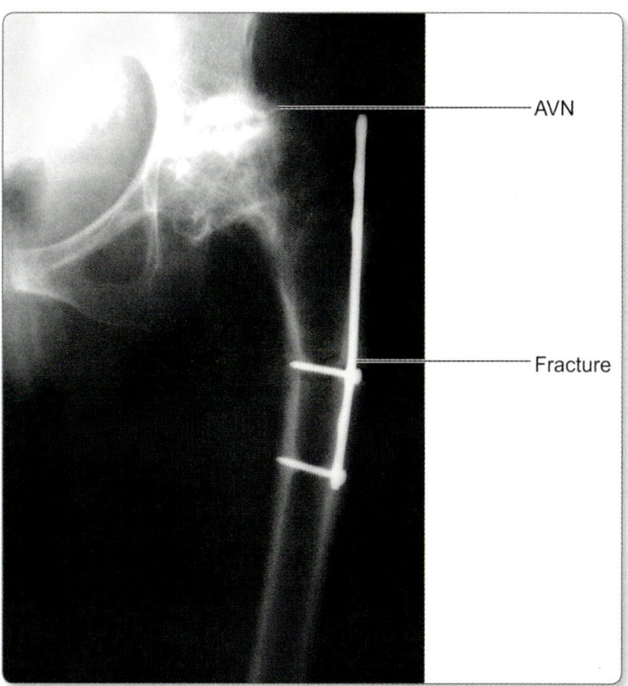

Fig. 8.60 AVN with subtrochanteric fracture femur

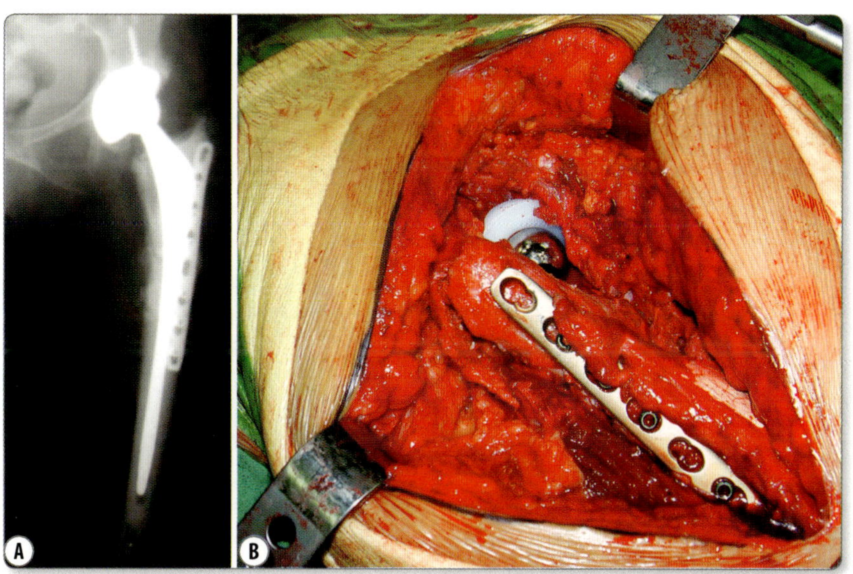

Figs 8.61A and B Fixation with LCP, uncemented cup and 200 mm long C-stem (Cemented)

walking with help of walker for further period of 6 weeks. After completion of 10 to 12 weeks, allow gradually from partial weight bearing to full weight-bearing walking.

i. AVN with subtrochanteric fracture femur **(Fig. 8.60)**—Expose the hip. Remove the loose implant if any. Implant the acetabular cup (cemented or uncemented). Expose the fracture site by extending the incision on posterolateral aspect of thigh. Reduce the fracture and fix with locking compression plate (LCP) and 12 mm locking screws (unicortical fixation) **(Fig. 8.61)** or LCDCP **(Fig. 11.78)**. One or two circlage wire may be applied for additional fixation. Prepare the femoral canal for distal fixation stem (cemented long C-stem 200 mm or 240 mm as per requirement or solution revision stem) **(Fig. 11.78)**. Do trial reduction. Implant the suitable size long C-stem after applying the Hardinge cement restrictor or solution revision stem. Reduce the hip. Take the bone graft from removed femoral head and apply over the fracture site. Close the wound in layers.

ii. In cases of comminuted fracture of neck and trochanter (cervico-trochanteric fracture) in elderly **(Figs. 8.62 and 8.64)** where chance of failure of internal fixation remains high or non-union trochateric fracture **(Fig. 8.66 and 8.68)** or failed fixation of trochanteric fracture **(Fig. 8.70)**, distal fixation uncemented (Solution revision stem) **(Figs 8.63, 8.67, 8.69 and 8.71)** or cemented stem (long C-stem) **(Fig. 8.65)** is good option. Remove the small loose pieces of bones.

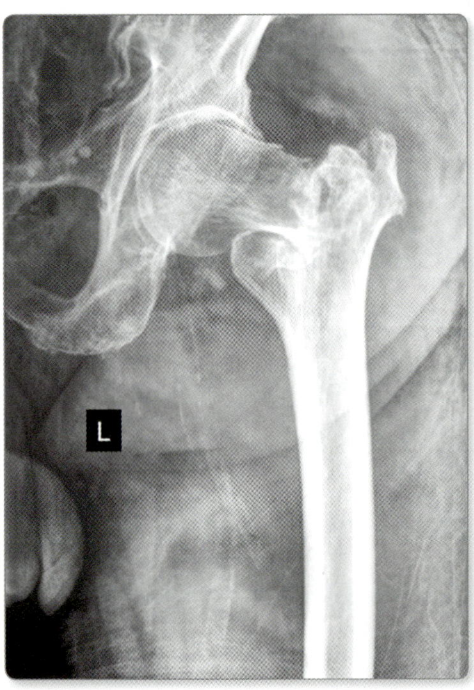

Fig. 8.62 Comminuted cervicotrochanteric fracture in elderly

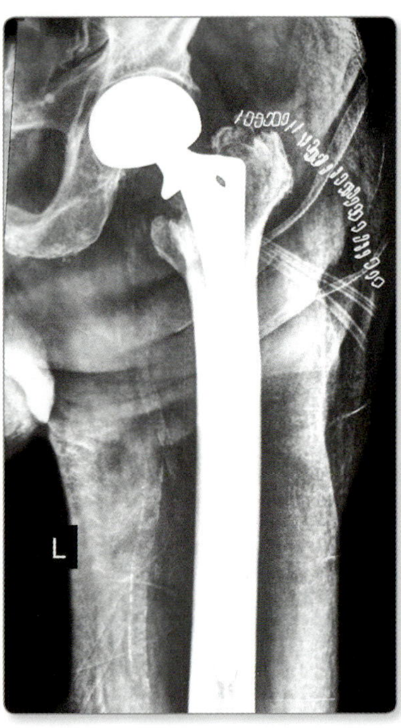

Fig. 8.63 Uncemented solution revision stem (200 mm), distal fixation with bipolar head

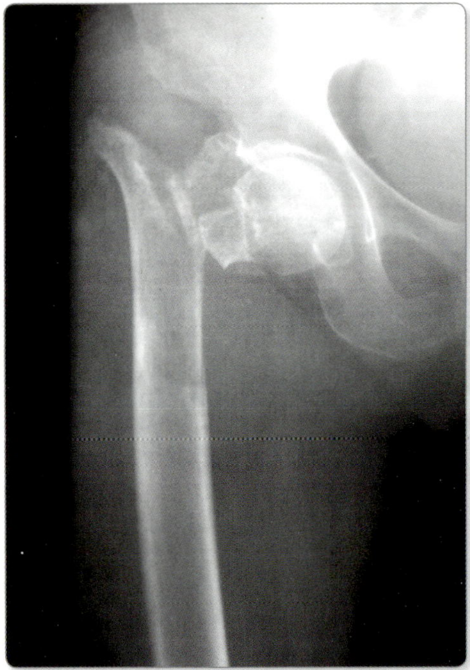

Fig. 8.64 Comminuted fracture neck and trochanter

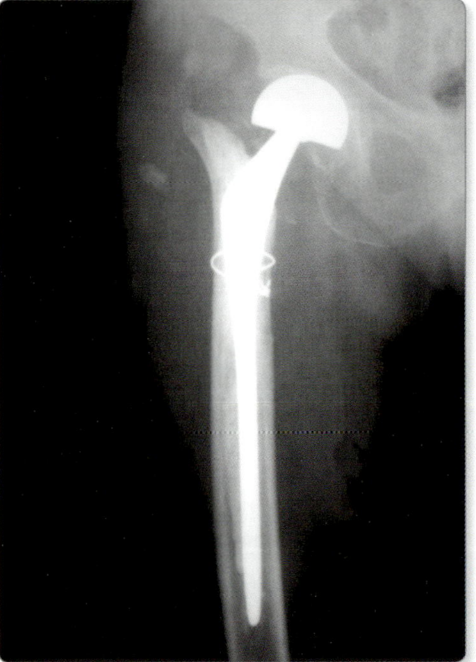

Fig. 8.65 Long C-stem with Bipolar head (split in femoral shaft was prevented by applying one cerclage wire

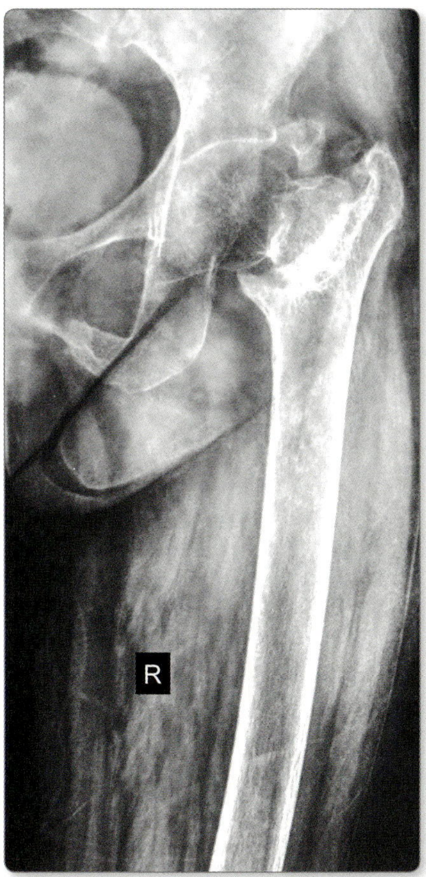

Fig. 8.66 Non-union trochanteric fracture left femur

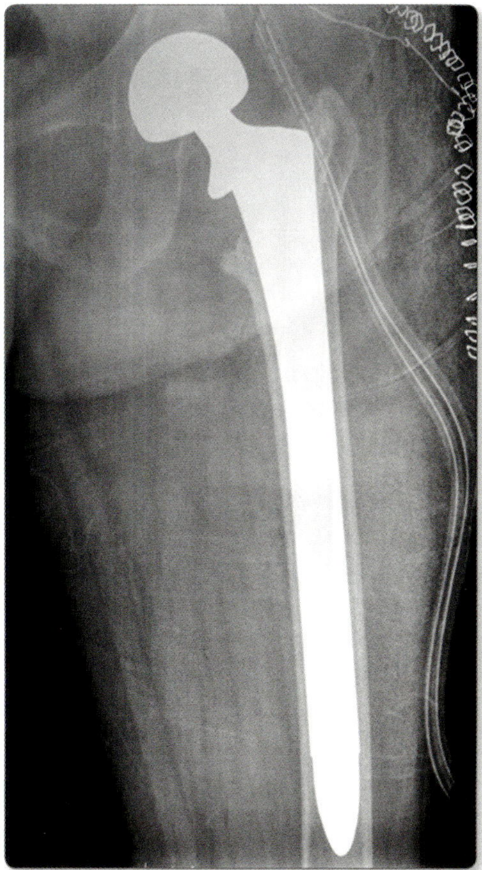

Fig. 8.67 Bipolar hip replacement with uncemented solution distal fixation stem

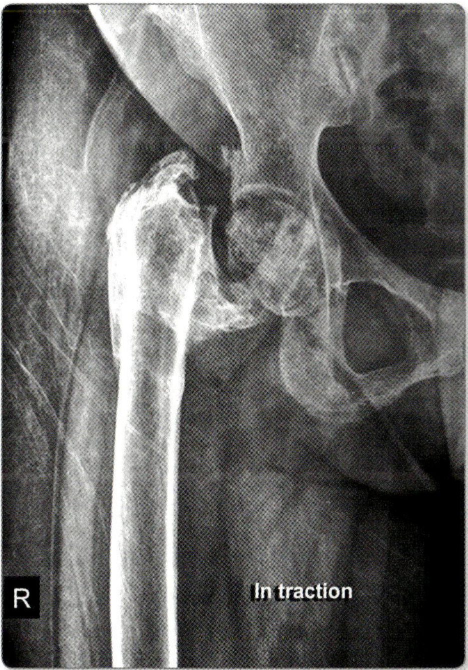

Fig. 8.68 Non-union trochanteric fracture right femur with AVN

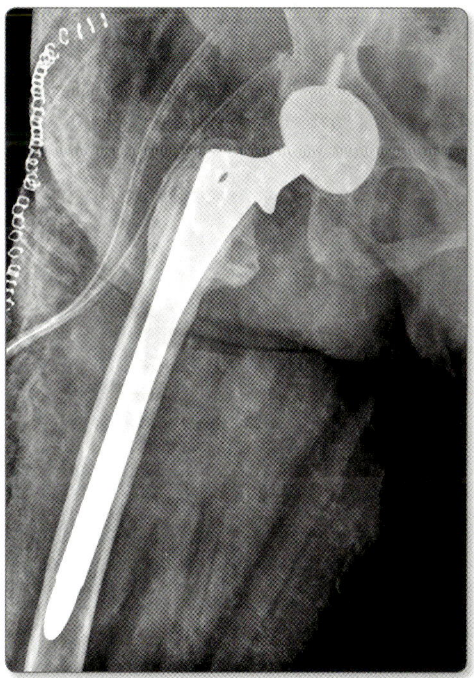

Fig. 8.69 Post-THR with distal fixation solution stem

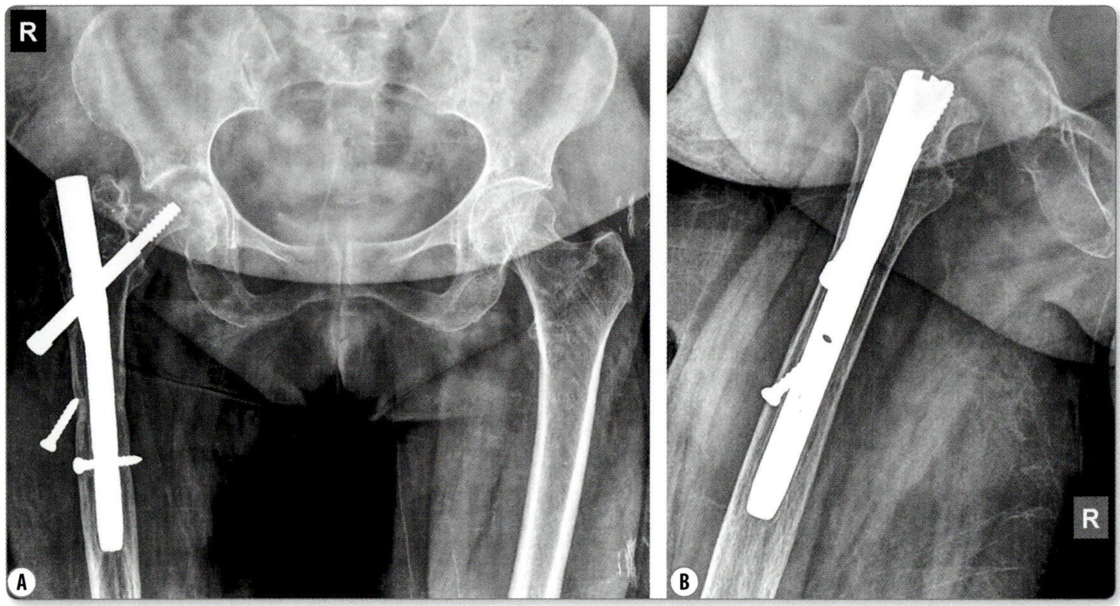

Figs 8.70A and B Failed fixation of trochanteric fracture right femur by PFN (proximal femoral nail) with AVN. (A) AP view; (B) Lateral view

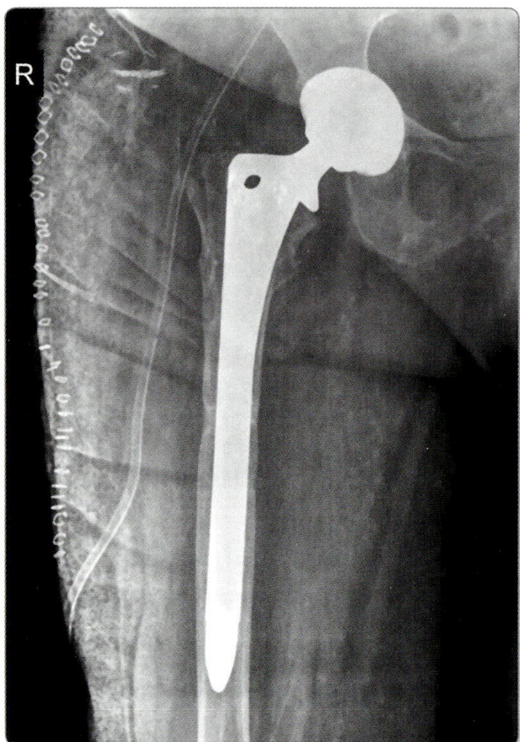

Fig. 8.71 Post-operative X-ray after removal of PFN and uncemented THR with solution stem

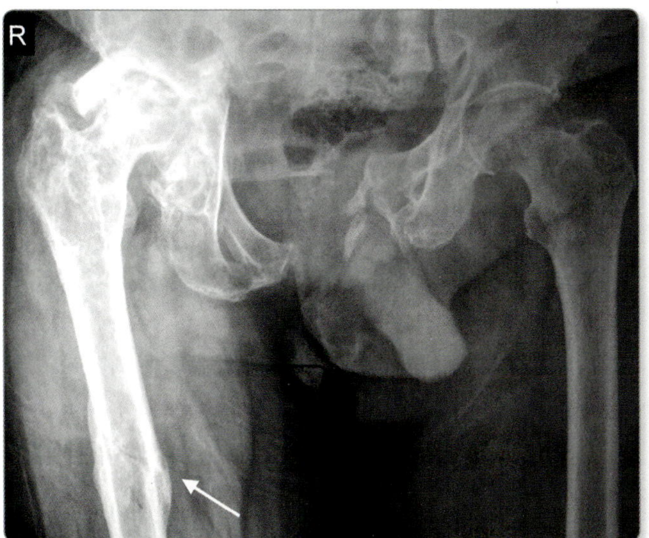

Fig. 8.72 Old fracture pelvis with acetabulum, AVN and united fracture shaft femur

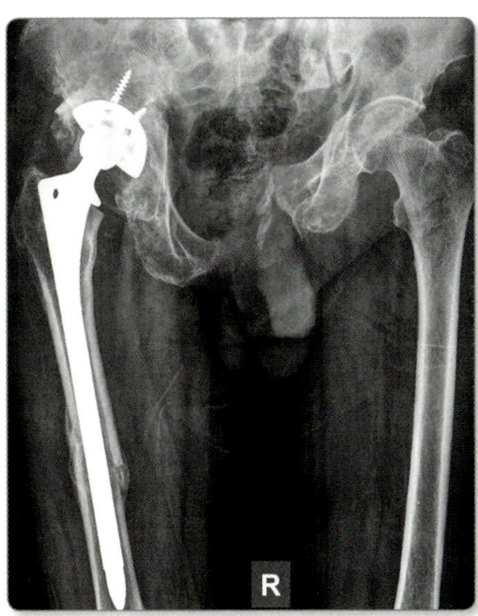

Fig. 8.73 Postoperative THR (distal fixation stem crossed the level of old united fracture femur

iii. In case of old fracture acetabulum with arthritis and fracture shaft femur **(Fig. 8.72)**, apply the multiholes acetabular cup with reconstruction if required and choose the distal fixation femoral stem to bypass the old fracture shaft of femur to avoid stress over fracture site **(Fig. 8.73)**.

Bone Cements

9

CHAPTER

CHAPTER OUTLINE

- Indications
- Contraindications
- Precautions
- Special Warnings
- Information for Use
- Undesirable Effects
- Package Quantities

Introduction

1. Used for positioning and securing metal or plastic prosthesis to living bone.
2. They have no adhesive properties but there is close mechanical interlock between the irregular bone surface and prosthesis, allowing even distribution of weight and other stresses between prosthesis and bone.
3. CMW1 Gentamicin bone cement: High viscosity cement for digital use. Used in fixation of knee components in TKR and acetabular cup in cemented THR.
4. CMW3 Gentamicin bone cement: Medium viscosity cement for syringe use. Used in fixation of femoral stem in cemented THR.
5. Composition:

Bone Cement Powder	CMW1 Gentamicin	CMW3 Gentamicin
Gentamicin sulfate (% w/w)	4.22*	4.22*
Polymethyl methacrylate (%w/w)	84.73	83.88
Benzoyl peroxide (% w/w)	1.95	1.90
Barium sulfate (%w/w)**	9.10	10.00
Bone Cement Liquid	**CMW1 Gentamicin**	**CMW3 Gentamicin**
Methyl methacrylate (%w/w)	99.18	97.50
N, N-dimethyl-p-toluidine (%w/w)	<0.82	<2.50
Hydroquinone (ppm)	25	25

* Equivalent to 1.0 g (1.0 MIU) Gentamicin base in 40 g unit, and 0.5 g (0.5 MIU) in 20 g unit

** Radiopaque agent.

Each bone cement is supplied as a two-component system, consisting of separate, sterile liquid and powder components, which are mixed together at the point of use to produce the cement.

Liquid Component

The liquid component is a colorless, flammable liquid with a distinctive odor. Its major component is the monomer methyl methacrylate. Hydroquinone is present in the liquid component as a stabilizer to prevent premature polymerization, which may occur when the liquid is exposed to heat or light. N, N-dimethyl-p-toluidine is added to promote cement polymerization following mixing of the liquid and powder components.

Powder Component

The powder component is a white, finely divided powder, composed of a polymethyl methacrylate-based polymer. Benzoyl peroxide is present in the powder component to initiate cement polymerization when the powder and liquid components are mixed. The powder component also contains the radiopaque agent barium sulfate.

Available in 40 g and 20 g unit packs.

Sterilization of the bone cement liquid is achieved via filtration. The sterile bone cement liquid is then aseptically filled into sterile ampoules. The blister pack is sterilized by ethylene oxide. The bone cement powder together with the peelable pouch is sterilized by gamma irradiation.

Indications

For the fixation of prostheses to living bone in arthroplasty. It should be used with appropriate prosthesis.

Contraindications

Myasthenia gravis, hypersensitivity to gentamicin.

Precautions

1. The use of bone cement requires collaboration and consultation between surgeon and anethetist. The anesthetist should be told during the operation when the bone cement is inserted.
2. The preparation of the bone marrow cavity results in marrow contents entering the blood stream. Prior to the application of bone cement to the bone, the cavity should be thoroughly cleaned by brushing and washing (lavage) to remove fat, marrow and other debris. The cavity should be kept as dry as possible to prevent blood and debris becoming mixed with the cement. Thorough cleaning of bone reduces the risk of marrow content being forced into the vascular system during the insertion of bone cement and subsequent pressurization. The expulsion of bone marrow has been associated with the occurrence of pulmonary embolism and this risk has been found to be increased in patients with highly osteoporotic bone and patients diagnosed with femoral neck fracture. Reaming of the marrow cavity can have similar effects on mean arterial pressure as the introduction of bone cement.
3. The premature insertion of cement may lead to a drop in blood pressure, which has been linked to the availability of methyl methacrylate at the surface of the product, although this has not been proven. This drop in blood pressure, on top of hypotension induced either accidentally or intentionally, can lead to cardiac arrhythmias or to an ischemic myocardium. To reduce the risk, the surgeon should avoid the early insertion of the cement. As a general guide, prior to insertion, the cement surface should appear dull and should not adhere excessively to the surgeon's gloves. The hypotensive effects of methacrylate are potentiated if the patient is suffering from hypovolemia.
4. Upon application of the cement, it is important to maintain the positioning of the prosthetic component until the completion of polymerization process. This must be done in order to achieve proper fixation.

Special Warnings

1. Special training is required for the safe and effective use of bone cements and bewares of their handling characteristics, their limitation of use and their proper application.
2. The powder and liquid components of CMW gentamicin bone cements are premetered to give optimum results. It is essential to add the entire liquid component when mixing the cements. Ensure that the powder and liquid to be mixed together have the same lot number, since the monomer and polymer components are individually formulated for each batch. To prevent any possible contamination of the cement with glass fragments, do not break the ampoule over the mixing device.
3. Properly cemented-in prostheses are stable and durable. However, loosening and fracture of either the cement or the prosthesis, or both, because of disease, trauma, inadequate cementing technique, mechanical failure of the material or latent infection may occur. Therefore, long-term follow-up is advised for all patients on a regular basis.
4. The liquid component is volatile and flammable. The operation theater must be properly ventilated and the liquid component and its vapor must not be exposed to a naked eye.
5. Continuous inhalation of the liquid vapors may have a soporific effect. Excessive exposure to the concentrated vapors may cause irritation to the respiratory tract and eyes, so should be avoided. If the liquid component comes into contact with the eyes, wash with copious amounts of water.
6. Contact of monomer with the skin or mucous membranes should be avoided. The liquid component is a powerful lipid solvent which might cause contact dermatitis in susceptible individuals. The wearing of a second pair of surgical gloves and strict adherence to the mixing instruction will diminish the possibility of hypersensitivity reactions.
7. The liquid component should not be allowed to come into contact with rubber.
8. Concentrated vapor of the liquid component may have an adverse reaction with contact lenses. Personnel wearing contact lenses should be informed and limit their exposure.

Information for Use

1. Bone cements are heat sensitive. Any increase or decrease in temperature (either ambient, and/or of the cement components and mixing equipment) from the recommended temperature of 23°C will affect the handling characteristics and setting time of the cement. Manual handling and body temperature will reduce the final setting time.
2. Variations in humidity will affect the handling characteristics and setting time.
3. The handling characteristics and setting time may vary if the cement components or mixing equipment have not been fully equilibrated to 23°C before use.
4. Store the bone cement below 25°C and protect from light to minimize the variation in setting time.

5. The setting time of the cement can be reduced if a vacuum mixing system is used.

Cement Preparation

The protective pouch, the peelable pouch and blister pack are opened by circulating nurse. The sterile powder bag and sterile ampoule of the same batch are aseptically transferred into the sterile operating area.

The powder bag is opened with sterile scissors and the entire contents emptied into a suitable clean, dry, sterile mixing vessel made from an inert material (stainless steel bowl). The ampoule of bone cement liquid is opened and the entire components are emptied evenly onto the powder in the mixing vessel and mixed with a stainless steel spoon.

A dose is prepared by mixing the entire components of the ampoule with the entire components of the bone cement powder bag. The amount of mixed material required is determined by the clinical judgment of the surgeon in each individual case.

Mixing and Digital Application: (CMW1 Gentamicin)

The cement is mixed thoroughly to minimize the entrapment of air. When a dough is formed the surgeon should wait until the cement no longer adheres to the glove. The cement can then be taken into gloved hands and kneaded thoroughly. It is vital that premature insertion of cement is avoided as this may lead to a drop in the patient's blood pressure. To avoid this, the appearance of the cement should be observed to ensure the surface has become dull as opposed to shiny. Also cement should not adhere excessively to the surgeon's gloves.

In general, implant insertion should be delayed until the cement has developed a sufficient degree of viscosity to resist excessive displacement by the implant. However, implant insertion should not be delayed such that there is a risk that the procedure cannot be completed due to cement hardening.

Following introduction, the implant must be firmly held in position to avoid movement and pressurization must be maintained until the cement finally hardens. Excess bone cement must be removed before the cement has completely hardened.

Syringe Application: (CMW3 Gentamicin)

The bone cement is prepared and mixed, as described previously by adding all the liquid component to all the powder component. The cement is then transferred into a suitable cement gun cartridge. The surgeon should use their experience to judge when the cement has reached an appropriate viscosity to be extruded. This will not occur until after the cement has formed a dough. A small amount of cement should be extruded from the syringe and visually assessed to ensure that the surface of the cement appears dull and excessive flow under gravity has ceased.

Prior to extrusion, a cement restrictor should be introduced into the femur at the required depth. Introduction of cement should be carried out in a retrograde fashion. Once the cavity is filled, it is strongly advised that adequate pressurization is applied and maintained up to the point of hardening. In general, implant insertion should be delayed until the cement has developed a sufficient degree of viscosity to resist excessive displacement by the implant. However, implant insertion should not be delayed such that there is a risk that the procedure cannot be completed due to cement hardening.

Undesirable Effects

Serious

1. Myocardial infarction.
2. Cerebrovascular accident.
3. Cardiac arrest.
4. Sudden death.
5. Pulmonary embolism.
6. Anaphylaxis.

Most Frequent

1. Transitory fall in blood pressure
2. Thrombophlebitis
3. Hemorrhage and hematoma
4. Loosening or displacement of the prosthesis
5. Superficial or deep wound infection
6. Trochanteric bursitis
7. Short-term cardiac conduction irregularities.

Reported

1. Heterotopic new bone.
2. Trochanteric separation.

Storage

1. Store below 25°C and protect from light.
2. Store at a recommended mixing temperature of 23°C for a minimum of 24 hours before use.

Package Quantities

Pack size (g)	CMW 1 Gentamicin		CMW 3 Gentamicin	
	Powder (g)	Liquid (g)	Powder (g)	Liquid (g)
40	40	18.37	40	17.90
20	20	9.19	20	8.95

Ultrasonic System for Cemented and Uncemented Revision Surgeries

10

CHAPTER

CHAPTER OUTLINE

- Goal
- Principle
- Ultrasonic System
- Technique
- Factors that Affect Risk of Thermal Energy
- Precautions during Surgical Procedures

Introduction

Efficient and safe cement removal is critical in revision arthroplasty. Conventional manual cement removal by hand or power-driven instruments can be time-consuming, require osteotomy, and be associated with complications such as cortical perforation, fracture, or bone loss. Ultrasonic devices offer an alternative method of cement removal by converting mechanical vibrations into thermal energy, liquefying the cement. This facilitates selective cement removal, preserves bone, decreases cortical perforation risk, and eliminates the need for osteotomy.

Goal

The goal in revision surgeries is to remove the unwanted implants and cement and preserve the integrity of the normal host tissue.

Principle

The ultrasonic device consists of a console to generate ultrasound power, an ultrasonic handpiece, and a variety of tool tips and extenders that are controlled by a foot switch during surgery. With the use of a piezoelectric transducer, the console converts electrical energy into mechanical energy. The mechanical energy passes through the tool tip as high frequency energy acoustic waves (20,000 to 100,000 cycles/sec or hertz). The energy from the acoustic waves is transferred from the tool tip to the cement, causing intermolecular friction. This friction produces heat, which is preferentially absorbed by the polymethylmethacrylate (PMMA) due to its high capacity for energy absorption and a low thermal conductivity. As the PMMA absorbs this energy, its temperature rises causing it to soften, allowing its rapid removal from the bone.

Ultrasonic System (Figs 10.1 and 10.2)

The system has generator with:

1. Five modules.
2. LED (Liquid Crystal Display) indicators.
3. Handsets.
4. Cables.
5. Probes and.
6. Osteotomes.

Five modules

The first three modules are powering the handset. The fourth smaller module is the supply conditioning input module. The fifth module contains the endoscopic light source and the connection to the camera. The three modules running the handset are microprocessor controlled and are designated to produce ultrasonic energy at the resonant frequency of the attached handset within a range of 27.9 to 28.6 kilohertz. Careful control of the generator output ensures that the energy delivered to the cement removal

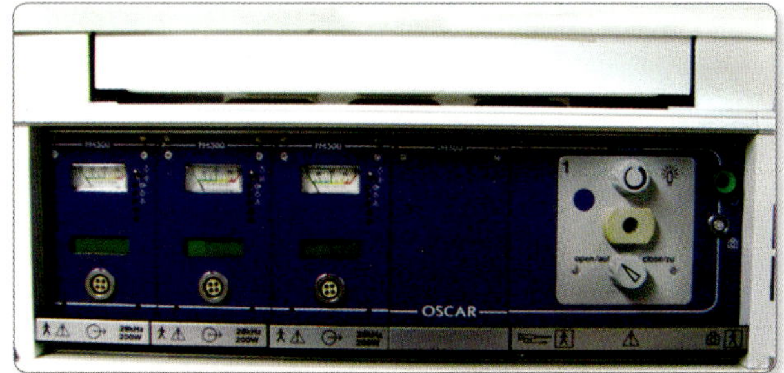

Fig. 10.1 Generator of ultrasonic system

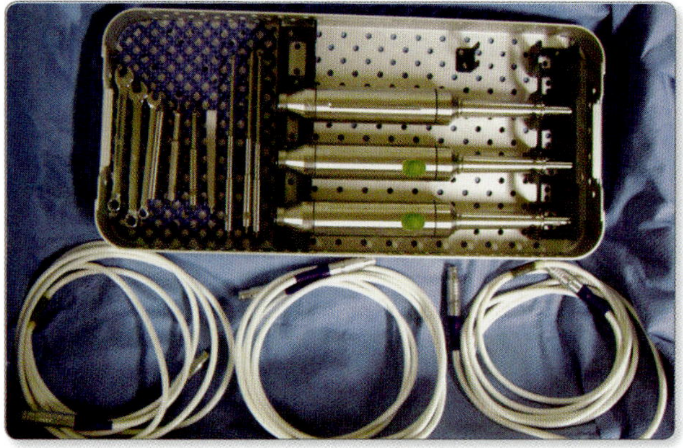

Fig.10.2 Handsets, probes, spanners and cables

probes increases automatically in response to the increased load. In effect, as the probe is pushed into the bone cement, more energy is supplied to the handset, ranging from a few watts to a 150-watt output. In practice the peak loads do not exceed 130-watts when piercing solid cement.

LED indicators

This indicates the current status of the handset by displaying a series of messages and system readings. Red indicator shows power status of module. Yellow indicator illuminates when handset is activated. Red indicator illuminates when the module is heavily loaded or when the module has shutdown due to much pressure exerted on the handset, module could not find a handset resonance in the correct frequency range, power device within the module became too hot or the countdown timer has timed out. The maximum time the handset can be run continuously is 25 seconds.

Handsets

Each handset contains a piezo-ceramic sandwich transducer—the ultrasonic "motor" and a mechanical focusing device—the "horn". These are enclosed in water and pressure tight stainless steel casing which incorporates a small hand operated switch. This switch when depressed once and held will operate the handset; a click will be felt. The electrical connection is at the rear end of the handset. The shroud and end cap are removed from the handset prior to autoclaving. A variety of probes may be fitted to the output end of the horn via a screwed coupling. Each probe consists of a waveguide, which is an integral number of half wavelengths long, its shape and overall length being chosen to suit a particular case. The signal from the generator induces the crystals within the handset to vibrate, producing ultrasonic energy. This energy is focused along the waveguide to the tip of the probe, which will vibrate at approximately 28.3 KHz. The rapid oscillatory movement produces heat when the tip of the probe is in contact with bone cement, causing the cement to liquefy for a fraction of second. There is separate handset (osteotome handset) to cut both cortical and cancellous bone for porous coated prosthesis extraction. In this handset, the transducer generates axial vibration so that its output impedance is compatible with bone tissue. This results in reduced displacement amplitude and the ability to sustain a higher distal load. The bone cutting handsets are identified by their blue or gold colored anodised case and larger size connecting thread at the output end).

Cables

Silicon rubber cables screened conduction wires are supplied with the equipment to connect the handset to the generator.

Probes

The ultrasonic device comes with a variety of tool tips to aid in the different aspects of cement removal. The tool tips are manufactured from titanium alloy. These are separate for cement removal and prosthesis extraction. The tool tips are groover, scraper (6 mm, 8 mm and 10 mm), piercer (6 mm, 8 mm, 10 mm, 11.5 mm, 13 mm), acetabular probe.

Osteotomes

Following osteotomes are available for the use of removing the prostheses during cemented and uncemented revisions.

1. 6 mm flat serrated osteotome
2. 6 mm flat nonserrated osteotome
3. 6 mm curved serrated osteotome.

These flat narrow osteotomes are coupled with the blue bone cutting handset for accurate cutting of the cancellous bone interface surrounding the implant component that makes prosthesis extraction easier. These are used for:

1. Removal of well-integrated uncemented acetabular cups.
2. Loosening and extraction of proximally coated press fit stem.
3. Loosening and removal of tibial and femoral components in TKR.

Technique

Correct cement removal is initiated by creating troughs 1 to 2 cm deep approximately 120° apart. These troughs facilitate cement removal by acting as access channels for the ultrasonic device and serve as tracks on which the softened cement can be removed. In order to create the troughs, the device is turned on and the tip is inserted into the cement. Within a few seconds of applied energy, the cement will begin to soften. The ultrasound tip then is withdrawn, dragging the softened cement with it **(Fig. 10.3)**.

The cement should be removed from the medullary canal superficial to deep, progressing 1 to 2 cm at a time, with frequent cold, irrigation, and suction between probe tip passes. Care should be taken to avoid plunging the ultrasound tip deep into the medullary canal and trying to pull softened cement past a column of intact hard cement. The bursts of ultrasound usage and cement heating should be intermittent and last several (3–5) seconds. The ultrasound device should not be used continuously for prolonged times, as this can lead to tissue injury.

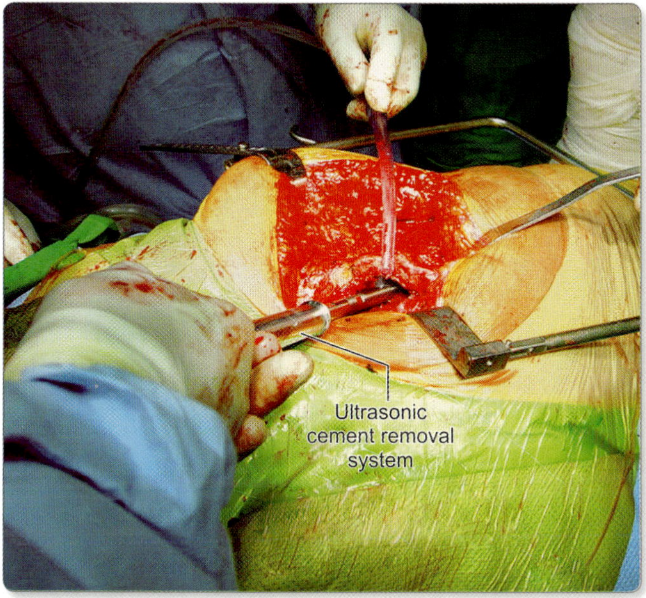

Fig.10.3 Removal of bone cement by ultrasonic system

In contrast to manual cement extraction with hand tools or burs under power, ultrasound devices also provide the surgeon with both tactile and auditory feedback. When the ultrasound device contacts bone, a high-pitched screech occurs. Furthermore, when the tip contacts hard cortical bone, it can recoil, providing tactile feedback. Smoke is produced when the ultrasound device is within cement. However, when it contacts bone, no smoke is produced. The factors, unique to ultrasound, facilitate selective removal of cement and preservation of host bone.

Studies have demonstrated that when the tip of the probe is in contact with the endosteal bone surface for a period of 10 seconds, cell death to a depth of only 50 micron occurs. This contrast with cell death to a depth of 500 microns, which occurs when conventional PMMA is applied to the endosteal surface during pressurized cementing of the prosthesis.

For well-fixed femoral components **(Figs 10.4 and 10.5)**, it is recommended that the flexible osteotome be used between the stem and cement. The implant can then be removed with a slap hammer. The remaining cement mantle usually consists of a cement tube proximally and a cement plug or mantle distally. To remove the proximal cement, the ultrasonic flat osteotome is used to develop three or four slices or troughs down the sides of the cement tube. It is important to maintain a side-to-side oscillating motion when using the device to widen the slice or trough.

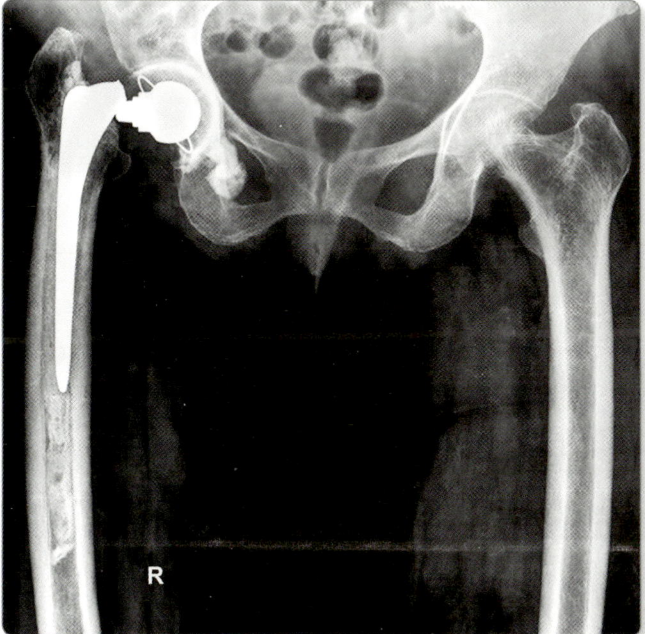

Fig.10.4 Broken neck of stem

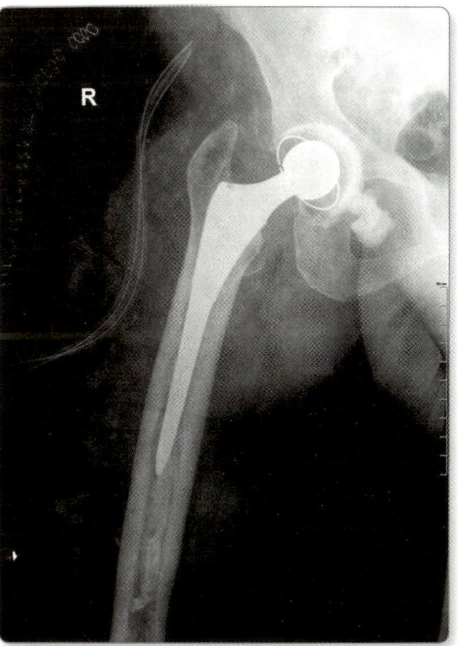

Fig. 10.5 After removal of broken stem by ultrasonic cement removal system and application of uncemented summit stem

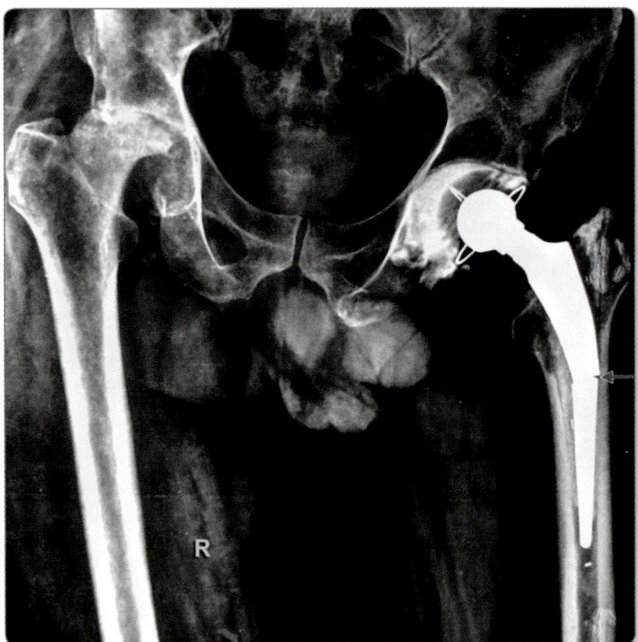

Fig. 10.6 AVN right hip and broken stem of prosthesis of left hip

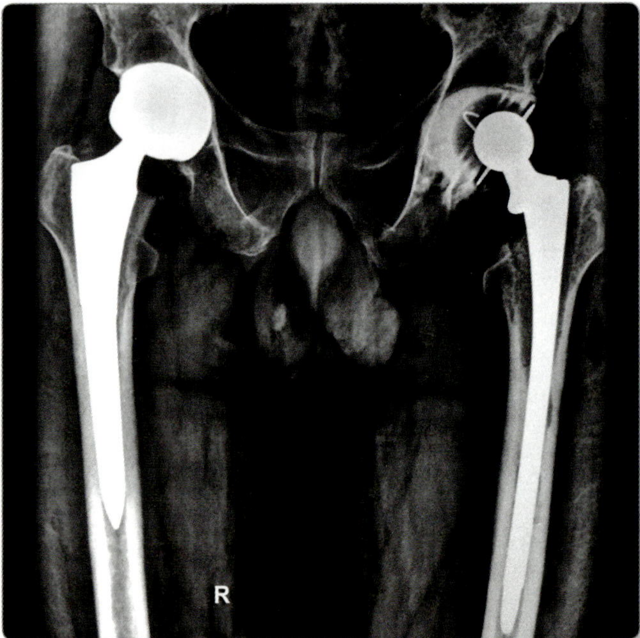

Fig. 10.7 uncemented THR on right side with summit stem and delta motion cup and revision solution stem left side after removal of cement by ultrasonic cement removal system and removal of broken implant by push up technique (chapter 11)

An ultrasonic tip is then used to section the cement perpendicular to the longitudinal slices. The short ultrasonic osteotome can then be used to develop a plane between the cement and host bone. A manual hand osteotome is then used to remove these large segments of proximal cement.

Removal of distal cement plug or mantle: The distal cement plug or mantle has been classified into three types: A, B, and C **(Figs 10.6 and 10.7)**. Type A distal cement plug/mantle is one that is located proximal to the isthmus of the femur and is therefore more narrow distally. This is easily removed using the ultrasonic plug puller tool with the extender. The distal tip is driven straight into the center of the distal cement and the power turned off. The tool is then immediately rotated 90 degrees and held in place until the cement hardens. Once hard, the slap hammer is applied to the device and the cement plug/mantle can often be removed in its entirety. Type B distal cement plug/mantle is at the isthmus. The short osteotome must be used first to free the cement from the host bone, and the plug puller can then be used as described above. Type C distal cement plug/mantle is distal to the isthmus; and as a result, the distal cement is larger than the more proximal cement. In this case, the ultrasonic disc drill should be used to convert the solid cement into a cylinder of cement. Once a cylinder is formed, the cement can then be removed in a similar fashion as the proximal cement mantle. Removal of acetabular cement is performed using the ultrasonic acetabular gouge to disrupt the cement-acetabular component interface. Once the acetabular component is removed, the ultrasonic short osteotome can be used to section the remaining cement into thirds to aid in removal.

Factors that Affect Risk of Thermal Energy

Following factors affect risk of thermal energy when using ultrasound for cement removal:

1. Intrinsic factors:
   i. Thermal conductivity of material: Cancellous bone > Cortical bone > Cement.
   ii. Bone thickness
   iii. Bone density (i.e. osteopenia).
2. Device parameters:
   i. Amplitude of ultrasonic waves on variable setting devices
   ii. Size of device tip (surface area)
   iii. Shape of device tip.
3. Operative technique:
   i. Length of continuous energy application
   ii. Magnitude of pressure of device tip within cement
   iii. Lack of device tip movement in cement
   iv. Use of irrigation including frequency, volume and type
   v. Adequacy of irrigant removal
   vi. Use of tourniquet.

Heat production is influenced by the inherent thermal conductivity of each material that the ultrasound device contacts. Thus, PMMA, bone, muscle, and nerve all have different thermal conductivities and will become heated to different degrees with the same ultrasound parameters. For example, heat conduction is greatest in cancellous bone followed by cortical bone followed by cement.

Operative technique also can influence heat production. Longer, continuous bursts of energy lead to higher temperatures than shorter, intermittent bursts. Increased heat occurs when the device tip is maintained in one position instead of steady movement within the cement mantle. Furthermore, firm, constant pressure can increase friction at the interface, leading to higher heat production. Thus, slow, gentle advancement of the instrument tip is important to allow the ultrasonic waves to penetrate and soften the cement in a manner that generates less heat. Although use of a tourniquet does not contribute to heat production, it may limit heat dissipation and contribute to thermal injury.

In addition, changing the ultrasound device parameters can alter heat production. The higher power settings increase the amplitude of the sound waves and produce greater heat. Higher power settings also produce more aerosolization of irrigation fluid and blood, decreasing the volume of liquid at the bone-cement surface and the dissipation of heat. The ultrasonic tip design influences heat production based on the magnitude of tip surface area contacting the cement interface. Device tips are manufactured in assorted sizes and shapes to optimize function during various phases of cement removal and for use in different bones. Probes with higher surface area result in increased frictional heat generation.

Precautions during Surgical Procedures

1. The instrument tip should not touch any metal component whilst the handset is engaged. Even a brief contact with a screw, retractor or part of the prosthesis can result in serious damage and impair the performance of the instrument. Spark may sometimes be seen if the probe tip comes into contact with metal. The back scraper will lose its sharp cutting edge if it is in contact with hard cortical bone. Cracks in the piercer head will reduce its cutting efficiency, although it will still function.
2. While liquefying bone cement, small amount of smoke will be present. Smoke should be extracted by suction to create a safe environment for the operating room staff.
3. If a probe becomes damaged during a procedure, it is possible to replace it by unscrewing it from the distal part of the horn using a spanner. While replacing a probe in this way, it is most important not to get talcum powder, blood or any form of contamination on the mating surfaces as this will cause them to become eroded and materially affect the ultrasonic conduction of the wave guide, making it less efficient.
4. Cables should not be compressed during cement removal as this can cause fracture of the component of the cable.
5. Any damage to the probes or cables should be repaired or replaced at the earliest.
6. Irrigation during cement removal should be used intermittently following use of the scrapers or groover probes and the frequency of irrigation should be more frequent when using the piercer probes. Do not irrigate during ultrasonic energy application, this will compromise the speed of removal and efficiency of transmission. The irrigation of bone canal following a period of cement removal clears the canal of cement debris and maintains safe operating temperatures.

In irrigation during uncemented revision, it is important to maintain a steady flow of saline around the prosthetic stem during insertion of the prosthesis extraction osteotome probe, particularly when cutting cortical bone. This ensures that the metal on metal interface is kept cool and lubricated whilst the active edges of the osteotome are cutting bone.

Complications and Revision THR

11
CHAPTER

Complications

1. Early complications:
   i. Nerve palsy: Sciatic, femoral, obturator and peroneal.
   ii. Hemarthrosis.
   iii. Thromboembolism.
2. Late complications:
   i. Loosening.
   ii. Stem failure (deformation or fracture).
   iii. Osteolysis.
3. Complications at any time:
   i. Infection.
   ii. Dislocation.
   iii. Periprosthetic fracture.

Revision THR

Problem—Deficient proximal bone of femur and acetabular defect.

Goal—To provide axial and rotational stability of the components and restoration of limb length.

Following implants and techniques have been used to overcome the problems and to achieve the goals for revision THR:

1. Femoral stems—
   i. Cemented—C-stem
   ii. Uncemented—Solution revision stem or REEF (Distal fixation stem).
2. Acetabular cup—Cemented or uncemented.
3. Wire mesh (with stem or acetabular cup to reinforce the defect).
4. Re-enforcement ring.
5. Cemented—Protrusio large acetabular reconstruction cup.
6. Uncemented:
   i. Multihole Duraloc shell, multihole pinnacle cup, cancellous bone screws 6.5 mm, hooded acetabular liner.
   ii. Octopus ring, octopus cementless cup, reorientation polyethylene insert.
7. Cerclage wires.
8. Impaction bone grafting.
9. Frozen femoral head allograft for acetabular reconstruction.

Whenever there is defect in the shaft of femur, long stem is selected to bridge the defect at least 4–6 cm below the level of defect (stem must bypass two times outer diameter of the diaphysis). In addition, impaction bone grafting (IBG) by freeze dried allograft is done to fill the bone defect.

Acetabular Defects

These are resulting from osteolysis caused by loosening or infection, excessive bone reaming at the time of previous surgery, preexisting bone deficit like acetabular dysplasia and inadvertent destruction of bone during removal of previous component or cement.

Objectives of Acetabular Reconstruction

1. To restore the center of rotation of hip to its anatomic location to establish normal joint mechanics.
2. To reestablish the structural integrity of the acetabulum and to obtain initial rigid fixation of bone graft.
3. Adequate containment of the new prosthesis and rigid fixation of the revision prosthesis to host bone.

Paprosky Classification of Acetabular Defects

The classification of acetabular defects is it based on the integrity of:

1. *Kohler's line (ilioischial line)*: It is the line connecting most lateral aspect of pelvic brim and most lateral aspect of obturator foramen on AP view of pelvis **(Fig. 11.1)**. Medial migration of the component relative to the Kohler's line represents a deficiency of the anterior column.
   i. *Grade 1*: Medial aspect of the implant is lateral to the Kohler's line.
   ii. *Grade 2*: There is migration to Kohler's line or slight remodeling of iliopubic and ilioischial lines without a break in continuity.
   iii. *Grade 3*: Migration medial to the line.
2. *Osteolysis of teardrop*: It indicates bone loss from inferior and medial aspect of acetabulum, and inferior aspect of anterior column, lateral aspect of pubis, and medial wall.
3. *Osteolysis of ischium*: It is quantified by measuring distance from most inferior extent of lytic area to superior obturator line. It indicates bone loss from the inferior aspect of the posterior column including the posterior wall.
4. *Acetabular component migration* (superior migration of the hip center): It is measured as the distance in millimeters (adjusted for magnification) relative to the superior obturator line. Superior migration of the hip center represents bone loss in the acetabular dome involving the anterior and posterior columns. Superior and medial migration indicates a greater involvement of the anterior column. Superior and lateral migration indicates a greater involvement of the posterior column.

Classification

1. Type I: Rim is intact without significant distortion of the rim. Acetabulum is hemispherical but there may be small focal areas of contained bone loss **(Fig. 11.2A)**. Anterior and posterior columns are intact. Hemispherical cementless implant is almost completely supported by native bone and has full inherent stability. There is no migration of the component and no evidence of osteolysis in the ischium or teardrop. Kohler line has not been violated (medial most aspect of the component is lateral to the Kohler line).
2. Type II: Distorted but intact rim with adequate remaining bone to support a hemispherical cementless implant.
   i. *Type IIa*: Anterior and posterior columns are supportive and the rim is intact. Bone loss is superior and medial **(Fig.11.2B)**. There is superior migration of the hip center less than 3 cm above the obturator line. Failed component migrates into a cavitary defect medial to the thinned remaining superior rim. Most defects are treated with particulate allograft because the defect is contained.
   ii. *Type IIb*: Anterior and posterior columns will support an implant but there is a small superior rim defect which is not contained **(Fig. 11.2C)**. Remaining anterior and posterior rims and columns are supportive for an implant. Superior rim is deficient for less than one-third of the rim circumference. Migration is less than 3 cm above the obturator line directly superior or in combination with lateral migration. Femoral head allograft may be appropriate but majority of segmental defects are

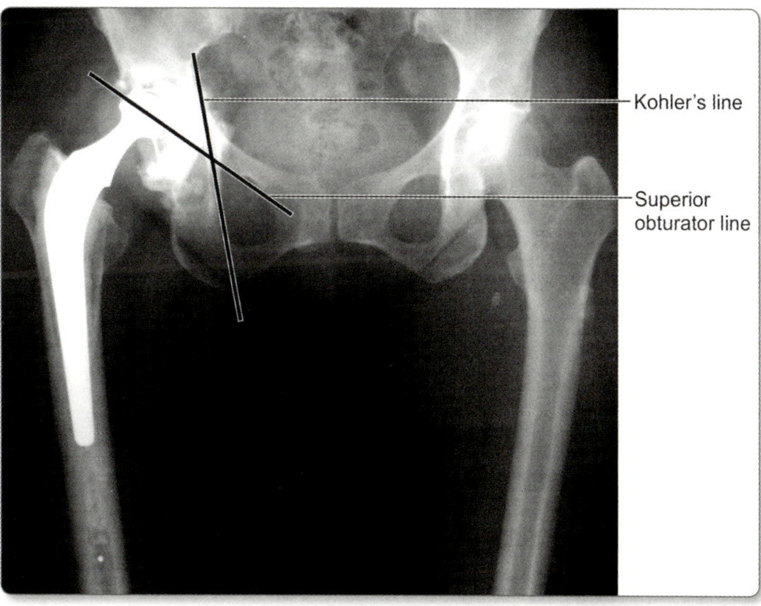

Fig. 11.1 Type I acetabular defect

not grafted. Particulate graft is not an option with the Type IIB defects because there is no buttress to contain the graft.

iii. *Type IIc*: There is medial wall defects and migration of the component medial to Kohler's line **(Fig. 11.2D)**. Rim of the acetabulum is intact and will support the component. Reconstructions involve particulate graft placed medially. If the medial membrane is not a sufficient buttress for the particulate graft, then insert a wafer of femoral head into the defect. Graft is then placed over the wafer buttress.

3. *Type III*: Acetabular rim is not adequate for initial stability of the component. Allograft is necessary to help restore deficient host bone in order to restore stability of the implant. Posterior column may require reconstruction.

i. *Type IIIa*: It is characterized by greater than 3 cm of superior migration of the femoral component cephalad to the superior obturator line **(Fig. 11.2E)**. There is moderate teardrop and ischial lysis, and an intact Kohler line. Host bone is adequate for ingrowth but the acetabular rim is not entirely supportive. Defects are associated with a nonsupportive superior dome. Anterior and posterior columns remain intact but hemispherical shell will have less than 50 percent host bone contact. Migration of implant is superior and lateral. Surgical options include figure 7 shape distal femoral allograft, use of a bilobed implant or a trabecular metal acetabular component with a superiorly placed trabecular metal augment, or cup placement in the high hip center.

ii. *Type IIIb*: There is less than 40% of host bone available for ingrowth. Rim defect is greater than 1/2 circumference **(Fig. 11.2F)**. Failed component has migrated superior and medial. High risk of occult pelvic discontinuity (posterior column reconstruction necessary). Massive allografting and reconstruction cages are typically needed.

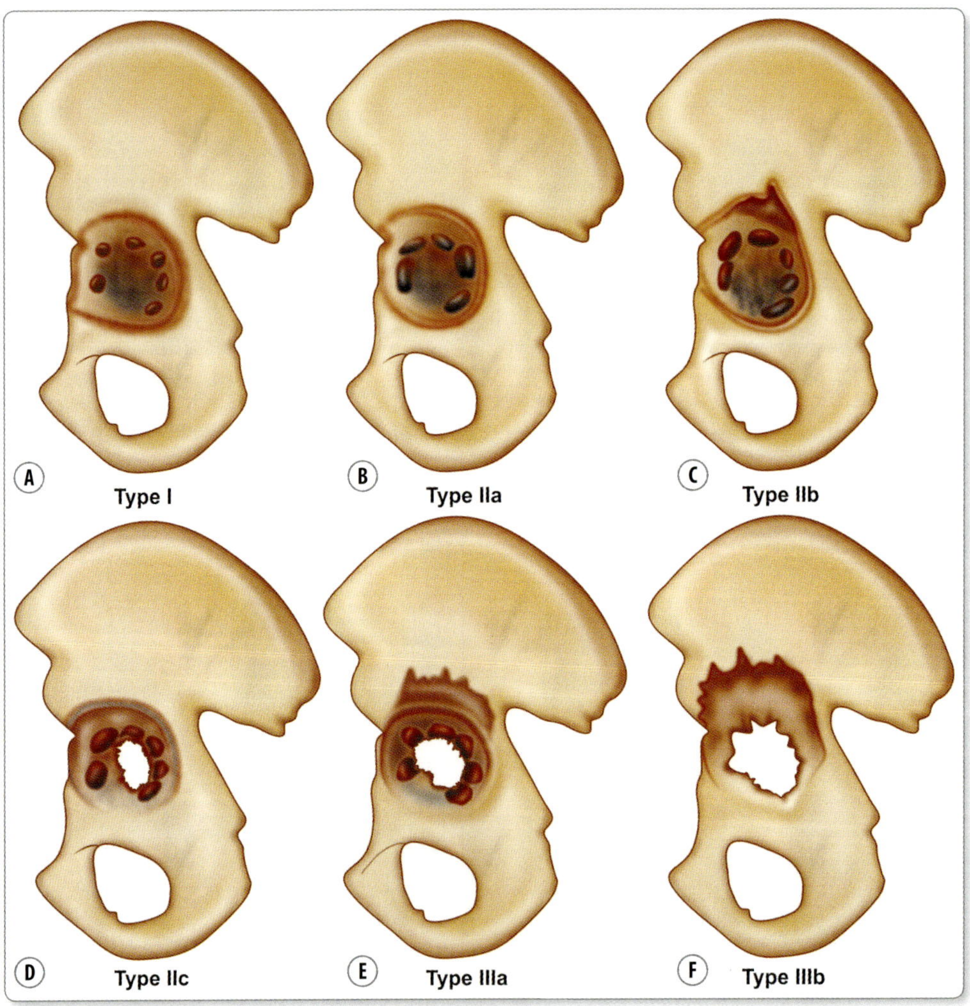

Figs 11.2A to F Types of acetabular defects

Type	Relationship of component to the Kohler line	Vertical migration	Ischial lysis	Tear drop
I	Lateral	Minimal	Minimal	Intact
IIa	Lateral	Minimal	Minimal	Intact
IIb	Lateral	Approaching 3 cm	Minimal	Intact
IIc	Medial	Minimal	Minimal	Violated
IIIa	Lateral	>3 cm	Mild/moderate	Intact
IIIb	Line violated	>3 cm	Severe	Violated

Preoperative Planning

Take X-rays of both affected and unaffected hips with femur AP and true lateral views to determine the amount of bone loss proximally and distally, to assess the curvature of femur to avoid perforation of anterior femoral cortex and to assess limb length discrepancy to determine whether extra long neck segments will be required to restore the limb length. Template on AP and lateral views of X-rays to assess the size of components.

Loosening

Patient complains of groin pain or thigh pain. Increased limp and shortening are signs of subsidence. Prosthesis is sunken and/or tilted. X-ray shows periprosthetic osteolysis. It may be aseptic or septic loosening. It is sometimes difficult to differentiate aseptic from septic loosening. Septic loosening requires two-stage revision THR. Remove the infected implants. Do thorough debridement and apply either antibiotic spacer or put the patient on skeletal traction till infection is controlled by systemic antibiotics.

Technique

Expose the hip as described. Dislocate the hip by bone hook passing around the neck of the implant and pulling it out from the acetabulum in place of pump handle technique to avoid undue force over stem which may lead to femoral shaft fracture. Remove the loose prosthesis with the help of bone hook, stem remover and/or radius-ulna punch and mallet. Remove the cement by cement splitter, cement removal forceps and/or ultrasonic cement remover. High speed drill and microdrive plus are useful for removal of implant, cement and sclerosed area of bone. Loose acetabular cup is removed by acetabular cup remover **(Fig. 11.3)**. Cemented or uncemented cup is implanted as per requirement **(Fig. 11.4)**.

Acetabular defect **(Figs 11.5 to 11.7)**, if any, is built by the bone graft **(Figs 11.8 to 11.10)**, wire mesh, re-enforcement ring, protrusio large acetabular reconstruction cup, octopus ring depending on the type of the defect.

Femoral Defects

These are encountered in revision surgery situations resulting from osteolysis, periprosthetic fractures, deep sepsis, and iatrogenically induced during the stem or cement removal. They may be also present during primary complex hip arthroplasty due to previous fracture, post infection, in local tumors and tumor-like conditions, as well as due to dysplastic and developmental causes.

Paprosky Classification of Femoral Defects

1. Type I: Supportive calcar region, minor cancellous bone loss anteriorly/posteriorly, intact metaphysis and diaphysis **(Fig. 11.11A)**.

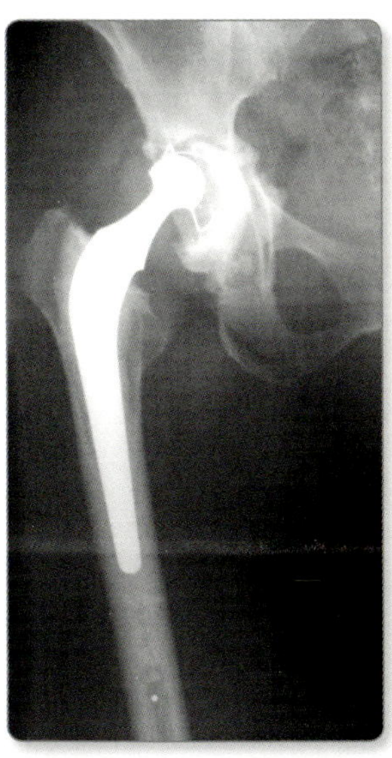

Fig. 11.3 Type I acetabular defect with loose cemented acetabular cup

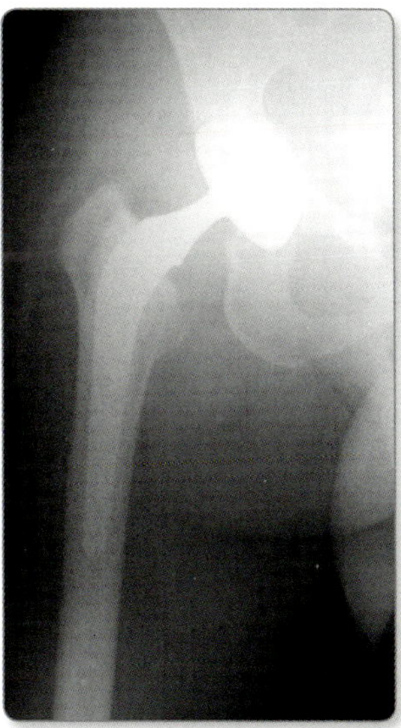

Fig. 11.4 Revision of cup by uncemented Duraloc shell with 22.2 mm plastic liner

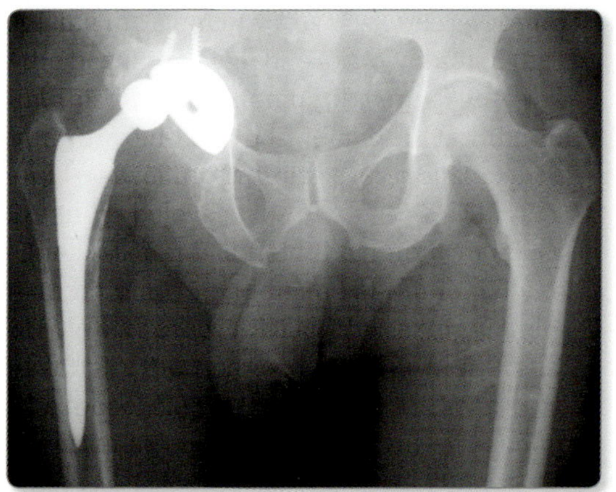

Fig.11.5 X-ray shows dislocation of head and migration of cup

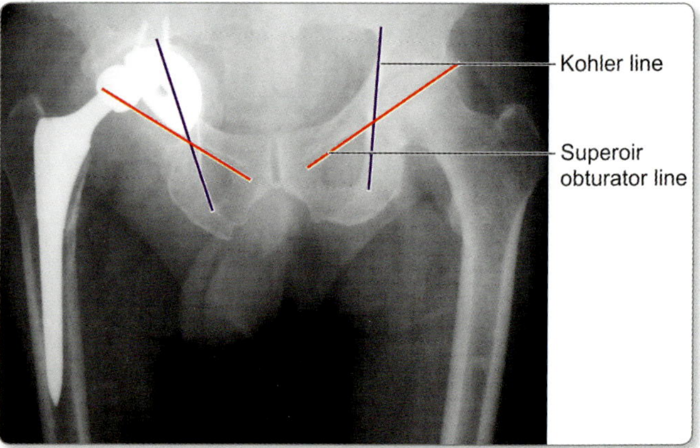

Fig. 11.6 Kohler's lines and superior obturator lines indicate the amount of migration of cup (Compare from normal side)

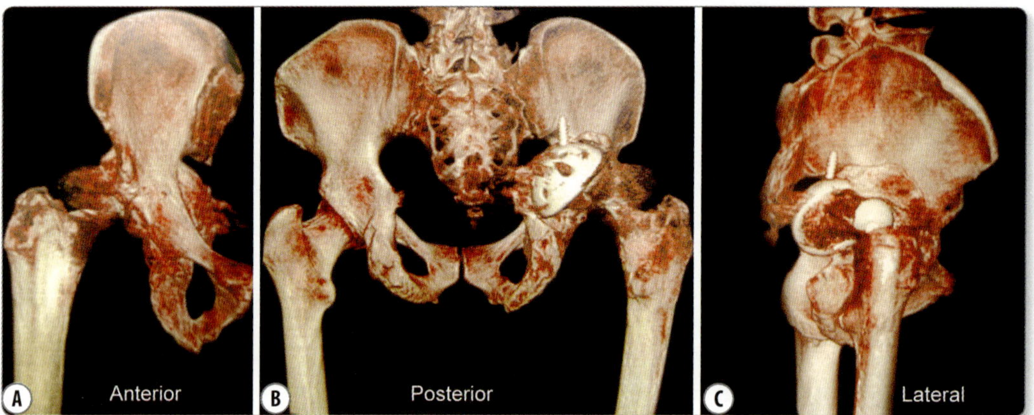

Figs 11.7A to C Type IIIb acetabular defect, 3D-CT scan shows posterior and medial wall defect with superior and medial migration of cup

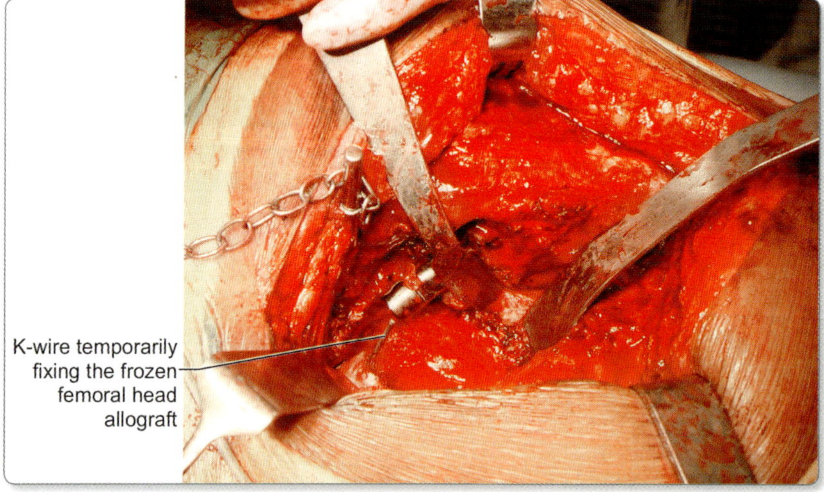

Fig. 11.8 Temporary fixation of allograft by K-wire

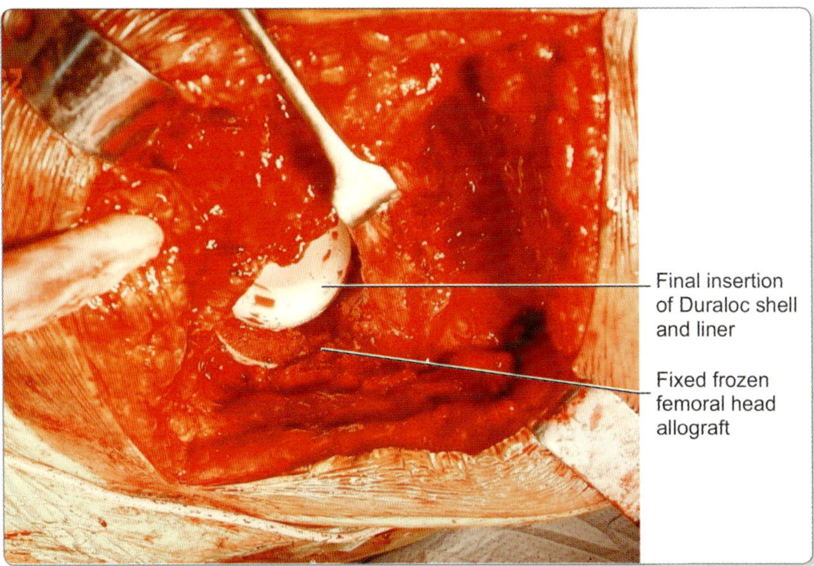

Fig. 11.9 Final implantation of duraloc shell and liner over fixed frozen femoral head allograft

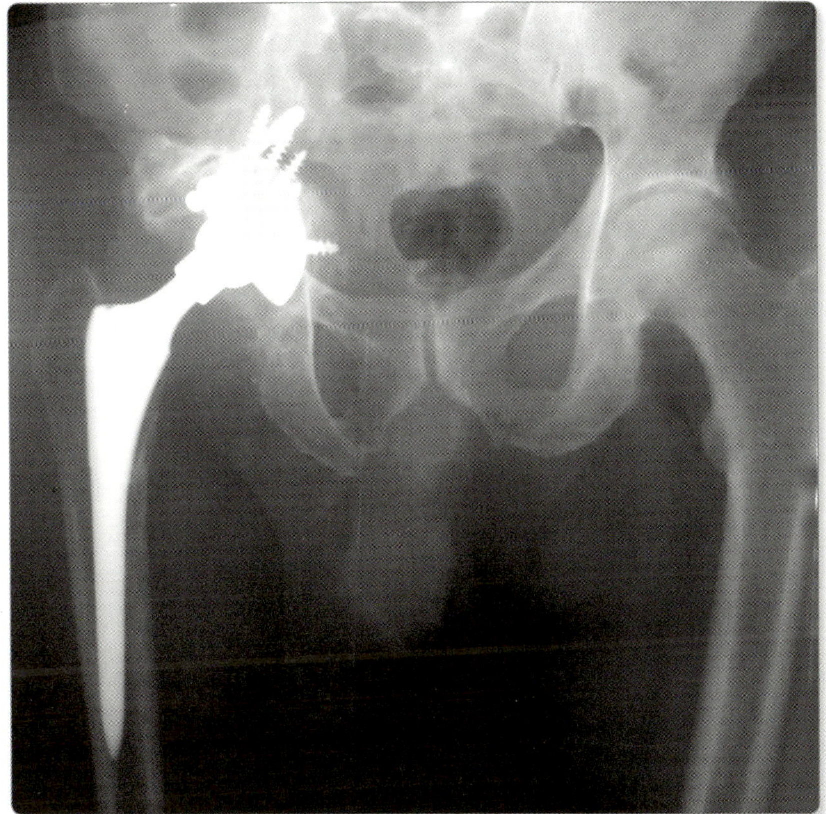

Fig. 11.10 Posterior column reconstruction by frozen femoral head allograft fixed by 6.5 mm cancellous 16 mm threaded lag screw and insertion of uncemented multihole Duraloc shell and exchange of head of higher offset

2. Type II: Nonsupportive calcar region, absent cancellous/cortical structural bone, metaphysis not intact, minimal diaphyseal damage **(Fig. 11.11B)**.
3. Type III:
   i. IIIA—Nonsupportive metaphysis and diaphysis due to bone loss, distal fixation over 4 cm can be achieved near the isthmus **(Fig. 11.11C)**.
   ii. IIIB—Nonsupportive metaphysis, diaphysis not intact due to severe bone loss, distal fixation over 4 cm can be achieved at the isthmus **(Fig. 11.11D)**.
4. Type IV—Extensive metadiaphyseal damage, erosion of the cortical isthmus **(Fig. 11.11E)**.

Recommendations for management of various defect types according to Paprosky classification are:

1. Type I—As primary, young uncemented, old cemented.
2. Type II—As primary, young uncemented, old cemented or distal fixation stem.
3. Type IIIA—Distal fixation, straight or bowed stem.
4. Type IIIB—Distal fixation, longer bowed stem, IBG (Impaction bone grafting).
5. Type IV—Proximal massive femoral allografting, or IBG— C-stem.

For implantation of stem, follow the four steps—reaming, broaching, trial stems and implantation. Reaming should be done till good endosteal cortical contact is obtained. Implant is selected as per type of defect.

Type I and Type II defects are managed by cemented standard C-stem **(Fig. 11.12 to 11.15)**. If all cement cannot be removed and there is no femoral defect, then standard C-stem can be applied. Cement should be removed till trial reduction could be done by trial prosthesis. Apply the hardinge cement restrictor at appropriate level. Cementing may be done on remaining cement by good pressurization. Type II defect is also managed by uncemented distal fixation stem (Solution hip stem) **(Figs 11.16 and 11.17)**.

Type III A and B femoral defects are managed by distal fixation stem. Cemented long C-stem or uncemented solution hip stem or REEF is applied. The femoral defect with uncemented stem is filled up by freeze dried morselized bone graft (IBG by allograft).

Cement removal or removal of failed implant from femoral canal may require opening of window (open technique). Presently, open technique is replaced by ultrasonic cement removal system for removal of bone cement and implant. For open technique, pass 3 to 4 cerclage wires by wire passer around the shaft of femur. Make a series of drill holes by 2.5 mm drill bit on lateral aspect of femur longitudinally along the linea aspera till the end of the cement/failed implant **(Fig. 11.18)**. Use of osteoclasis drilling template is helpful for drilling a series of holes. It is held in place with two drill sleeves. Make drill holes transversely for horizontal osteotomy at end of the longitudinal drill hole on the anterolateral location on the femur. Make few drill holes parallel to the longitudinal drill holes. Connect the multiple drill holes by saw along the linea aspera and transverse drill holes **(Fig. 11.19)**. By the help of 10 mm curved osteotome, gradually open the window keeping the periosteal hinge on the anterolateral location of the femur **(Fig. 11.20)**. Care should be taken to avoid further damage of existing lesions and the soft tissue attachments and the muscles are handled very gently in order to preserve

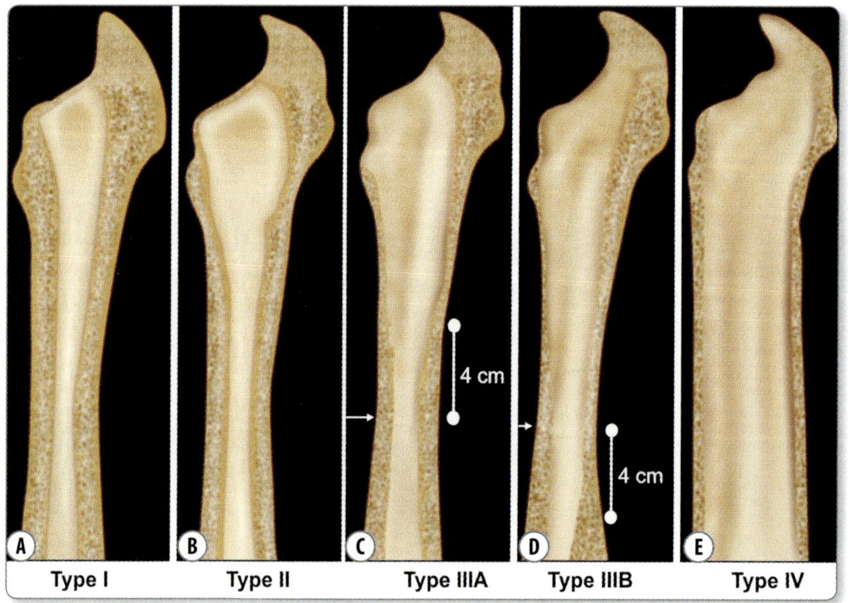

Figs 11.11A to E Types of femoral defects

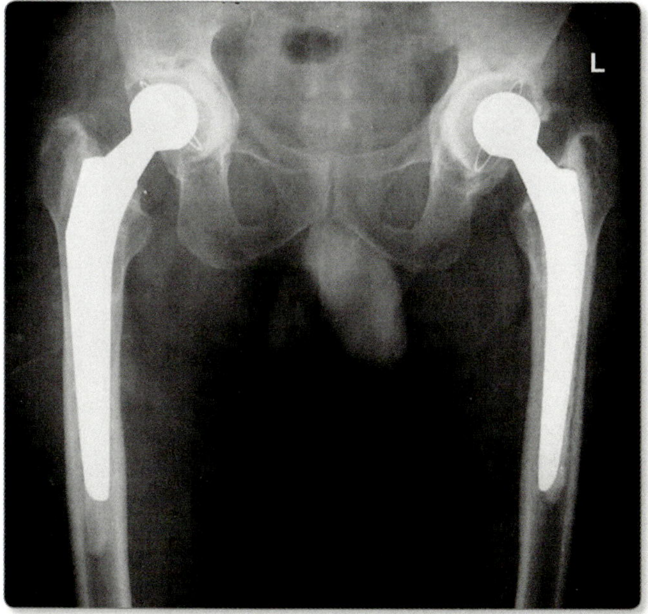

Fig. 11.12 Type I defect bilateral loose prosthesis (both cups and stems)

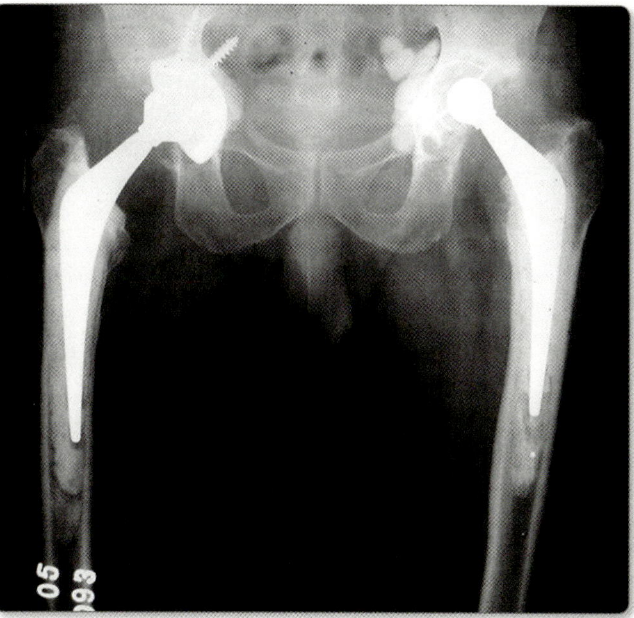

Fig. 11.13 Bilateral revision by standard C-stem

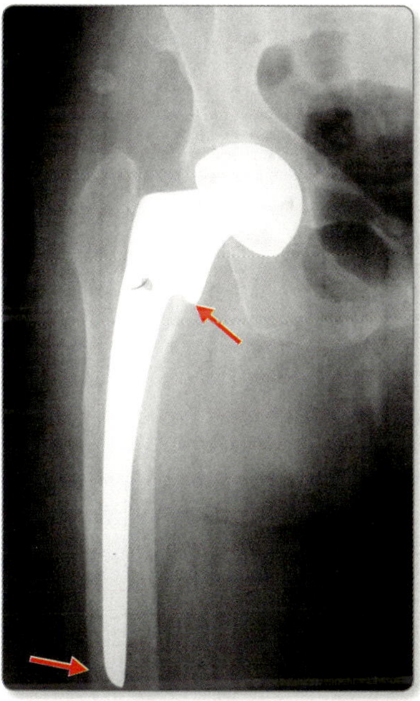

Fig.11.4 Type II defect sunken and tilted prosthesis

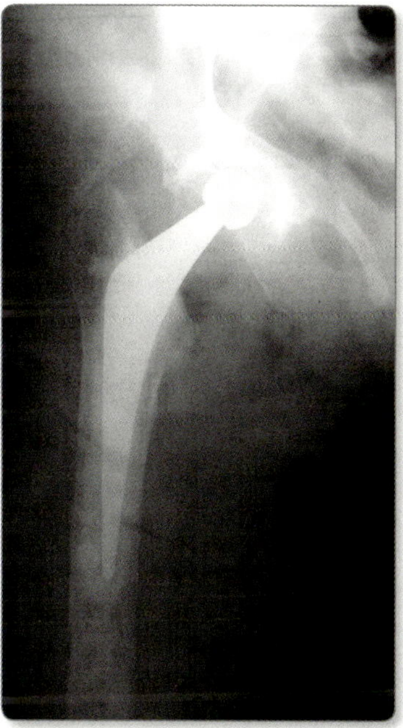

Fig. 11.15 Revision THR by standard C-stem

the bone's blood supply. Remove the bone cement/failed implant carefully **(Fig. 11.21)**. Select the long femoral stem either cemented (Long C-stem) or uncemented which will bridge the defect (minimum of 4–6 cm below the level of defect). The long uncemented stem options are solution revision stem (extensively porous-coated femoral implant) or REEF (distally interlocked modular femoral reconstruction prosthesis with fully hydroxyapatite coated and the position of most proximal screw hole should be at least 5 cm below the most distal defect).

For solution revision stem, use rigid reamer for straight stem and flexible reamer (thin-shaft) for bowed stem. If the rigid reamers are used, under-ream the femoral canal by 0.5 mm. If the flexible reamers are used, ream the femoral

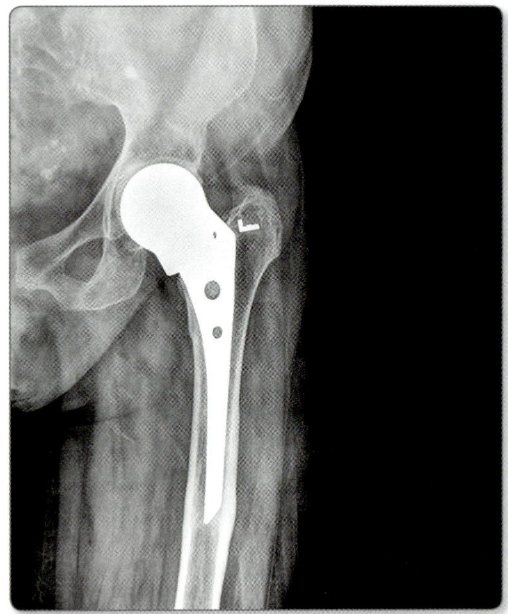

Fig.11.16 Type II defect with loose prosthesis

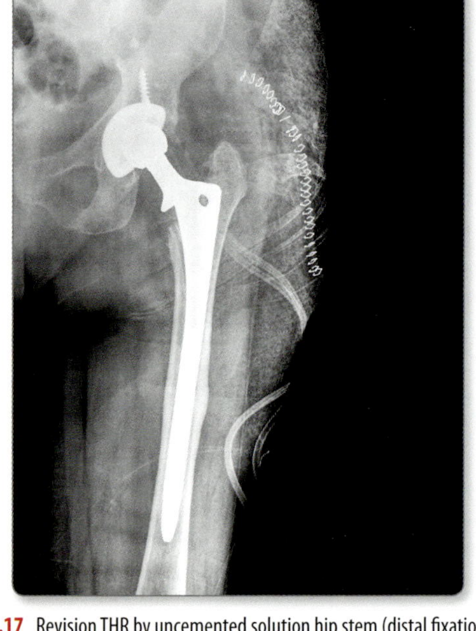

Fig. 11.17 Revision THR by uncemented solution hip stem (distal fixation stem)

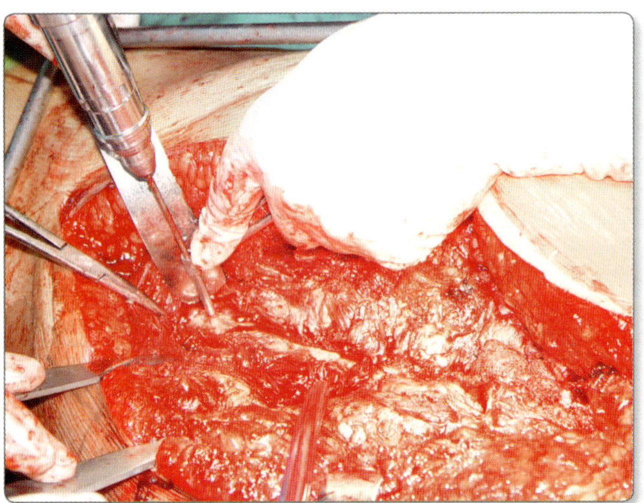

Fig. 11.18 Drilling on lateral aspect of femur for making window

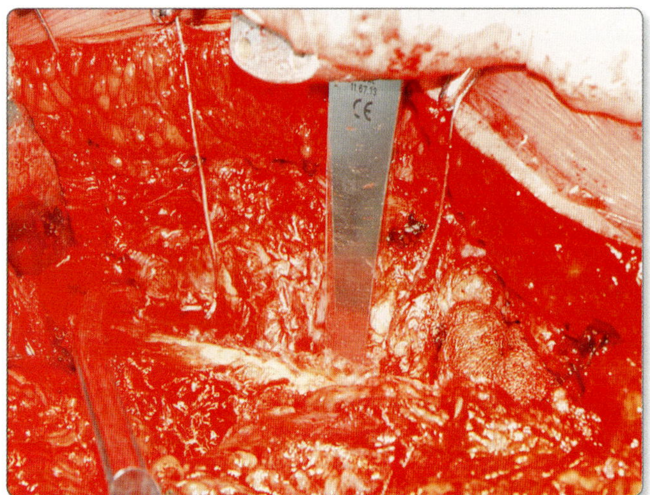

Fig. 11.19 cutting by saw

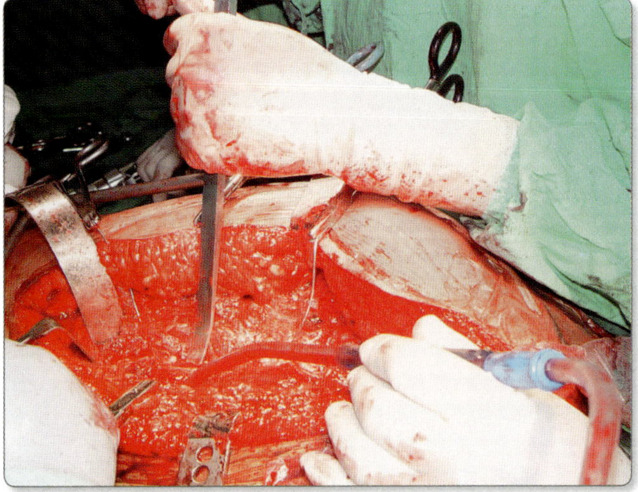

Fig. 11.20 Cutting by osteotome

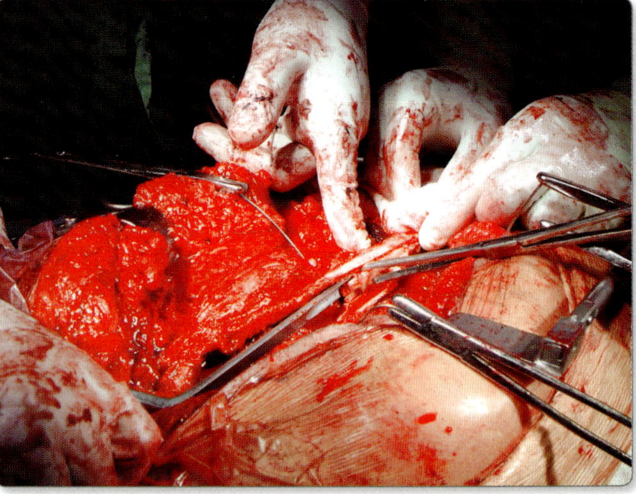

Fig. 11.21 Removal of cement from medullary canal

canal line-to-line or 0.5 mm over the stem diameter. Select the stem length in such a way that a minimum of 4–6 cm of "scratch-fit" can be achieved below the level of the defect.

REEF implant is having four components—Distal stem with proximal flared and anteroposterior face metaphyseal part having degressive horizontal macrostructures to avoid subsidence, 100 mm length and 26 mm proximal diameter and distal cylindrical and bowed diaphyseal part having vertical macrostructures to avoid rotation with holes for interlocking screws, trochanteric component with or without collar having horizontal step macrostructures to avoid subsidence and medial cerclage cable holes with neck-shaft angle of 135°, locking screw to tighten the trochanteric component with distal stem and lateral wing to fill the major defect in the region of greater trochanter. Proximal reaming upto 5" to 6" (i.e. 125 mm to 135 mm) of the femoral canal is done at least 23 mm diameter. Distal Reaming of the femoral canal is done line-to-line of the stem diameter for proper fitting. Trial stem is applied by the help of stem inserter in the femoral canal. The anterior surface is marked "ANT" to facilitate the orientation with respect to the femoral curvature. The marker groove on the trial stem denotes the junction of metaphyseal and diaphyseal part of the definitive stem. Trial trochanteric component is tightened with distal stem in proper version (+10° or –10° as per marked) by locking screw. Trial head is applied on the taper and trial reduction is done. After selection of final components, the targeting device is attached with definitive stem to ensure that locking screw holes are correctly aligned. The selected stem is attached with stem inserter and impacted to the level measured during trial reduction. The appropriate targeting device (right or left) is attached with stem. Drill for proximal screw first by 3.5 mm drill bit through stab incision and drill guide. Measure the depth by screw length gauge and apply the appropriate size 5 mm diameter interlocking screw by screw driver. Similarly, apply the distal interlocking screw. Trial trochanteric component is applied and trial reduction is done to check the limb length, stability and anteversion. Then the selected trochanteric component is impacted. Lateral wing may be applied in case of major defect of greater trochanter. Re-attach the flap by cerclage wires. Impaction bone grafting with morselized bone graft may be done to fill the defect.

If there is marked osteolysis, use of wire-mesh with long C-stem is helpful for re-enforcement of the femoral shaft **(Figs 11.22 and 11.23)**. Apply the trial femoral stem and tighten the cerclage wires by the help of wire tensioner **(Fig. 11.22 and Figs 11.24 to 11.26)**. Remove the trial femoral component and fix the femoral cemented **(Fig.11.23)** or uncemented stem **(Figs 11.27 to 11.29)**. In uncemented stem, fill the defect with freeze dried morselized bone graft.

Type IV femoral defect is managed by long stem (Cemented C-stem or uncemented REEF or solution revision stem) with proximal massive allograft **(Fig. 11.30 and 1.31)**.

Stem Fracture

Proximal, middle or distal stem.

Push-up or push-down—for distal part of broken stem.

a. Push-up: If the broken distal part of prosthesis is larger **(Figs 11.32A and B)**. Remove the proximal part of broken prosthesis **(Fig. 11.33)**. Make a window in the femoral shaft distal to the tip of broken prosthesis in the anterolateral location on the femur in line with the neutral bending axis and it should be <30% of the bone diameter. The approximate level of the site of window is decided preoperative on X-ray and peropertaively by measuring with scale. Expose the lateral aspect of femoral shaft at approximate level of the site of window by splitting the vastus lateralis muscle through separate

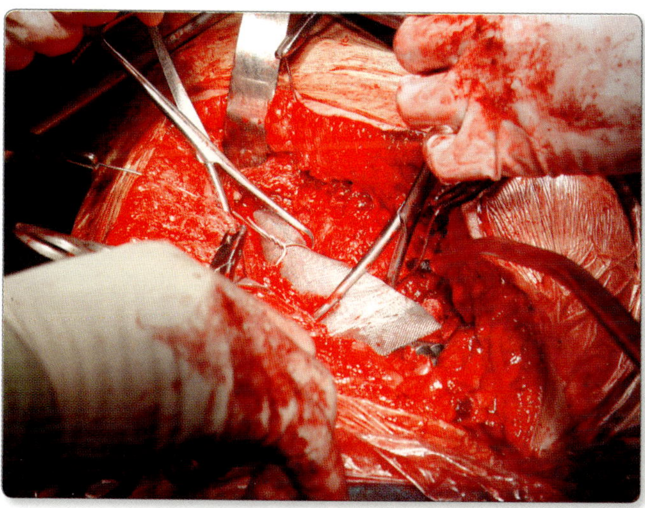

Fig. 11.22 Reinforcement by wire mesh with trial stem

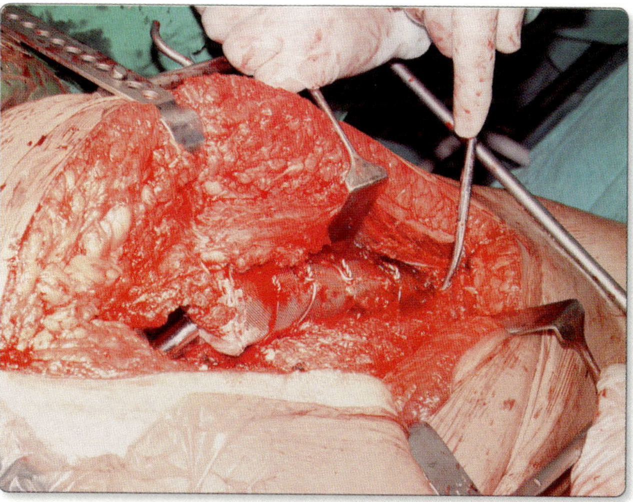

Fig. 11.23 After application of long C-stem and reduction

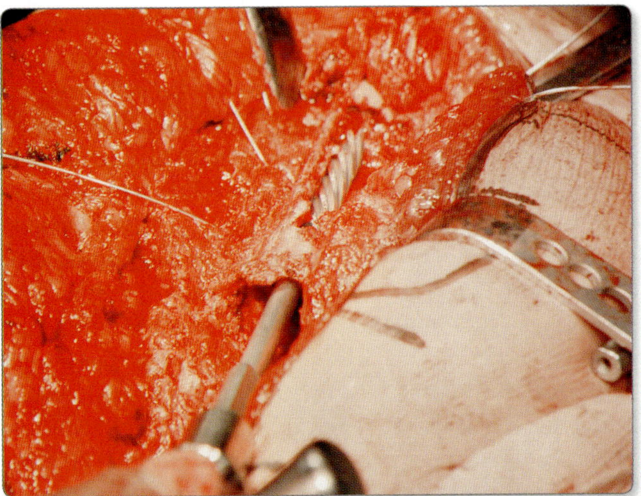

Fig. 11.24 Reaming for solution stem (Uncemented)

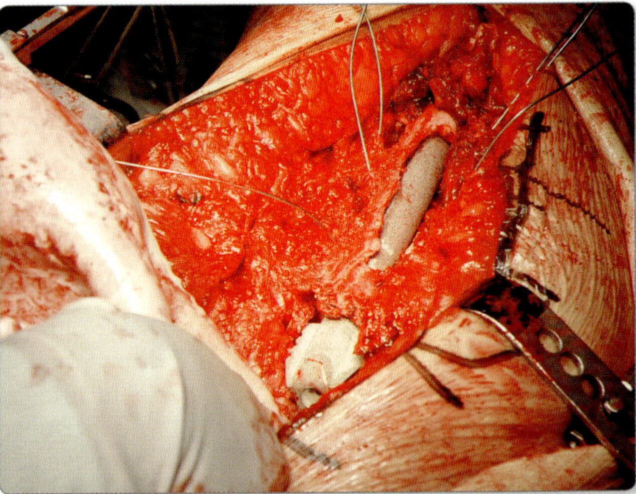

Fig. 11.25 Implantation of solution revision stem

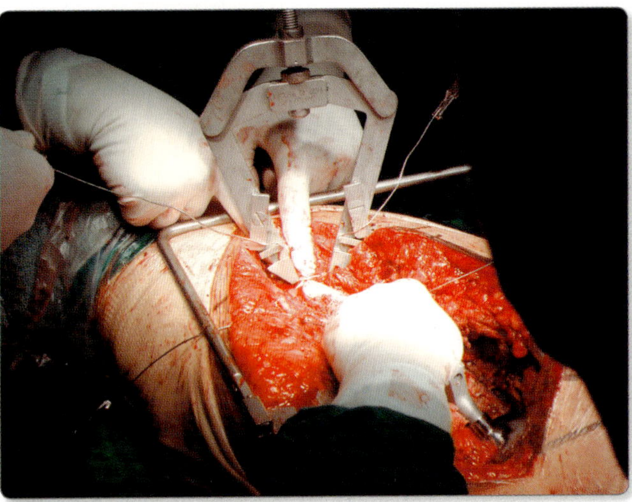

Fig. 11.26 Tightening of wires around the femur by wire-tensioner

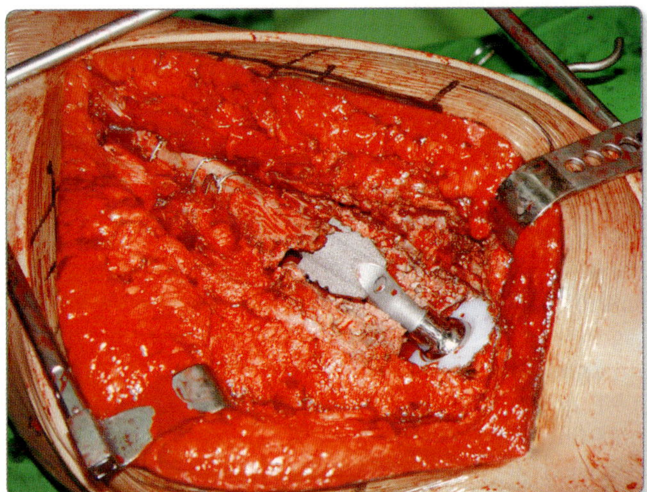

Fig. 11.27 After final reduction

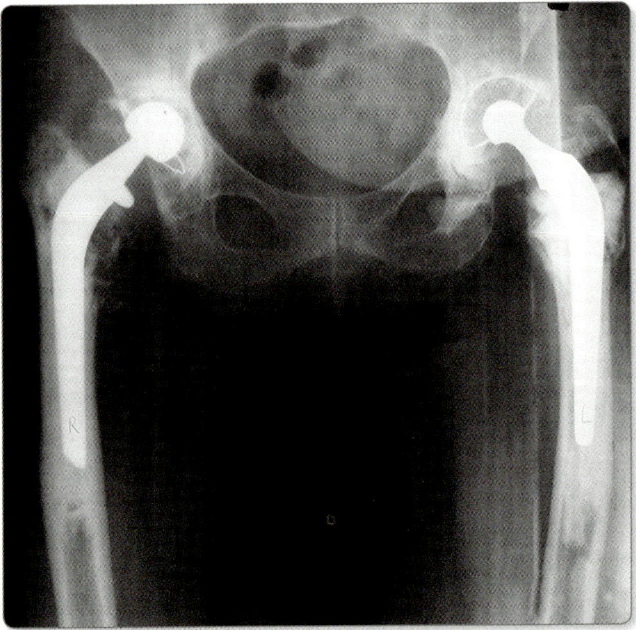

Fig. 11.28 Type III A and B femoral defects

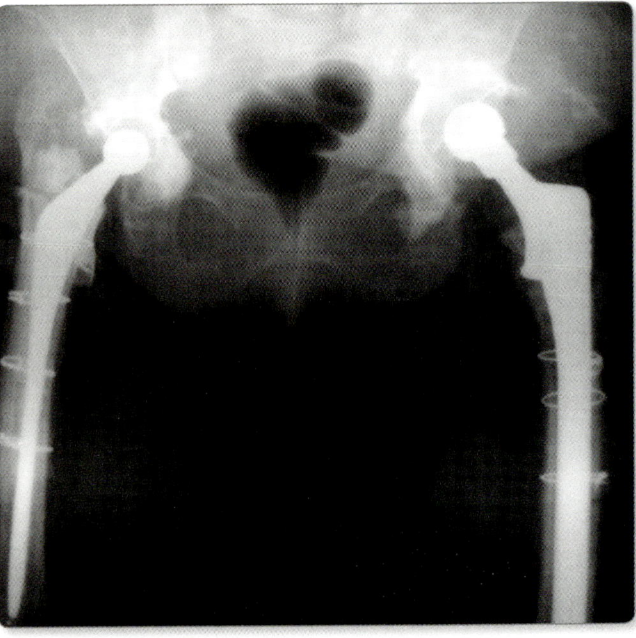

Fig. 11.29 Long C-stem with wire mesh and cerclage wires in right hip and solution revision stem with cerclage wires in left hip

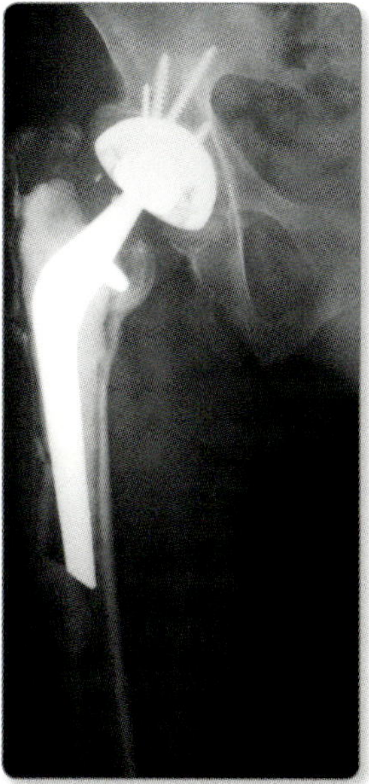

Fig. 11.30 Type IV femoral defect

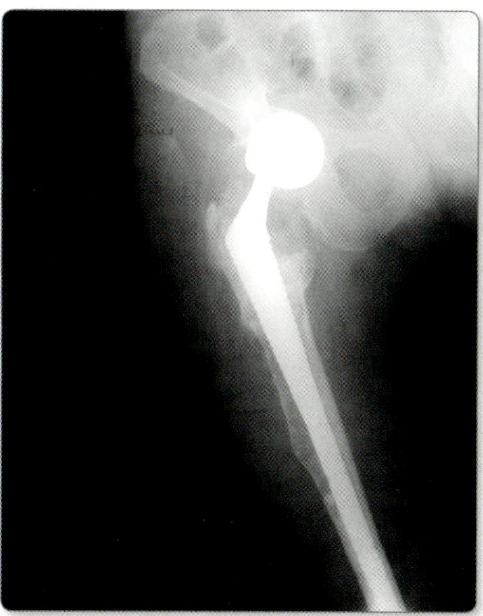

Fig. 11.31 Uncemented THR (REEF stem), proximal bone defect is filled up by freeze dried morselized bone graft

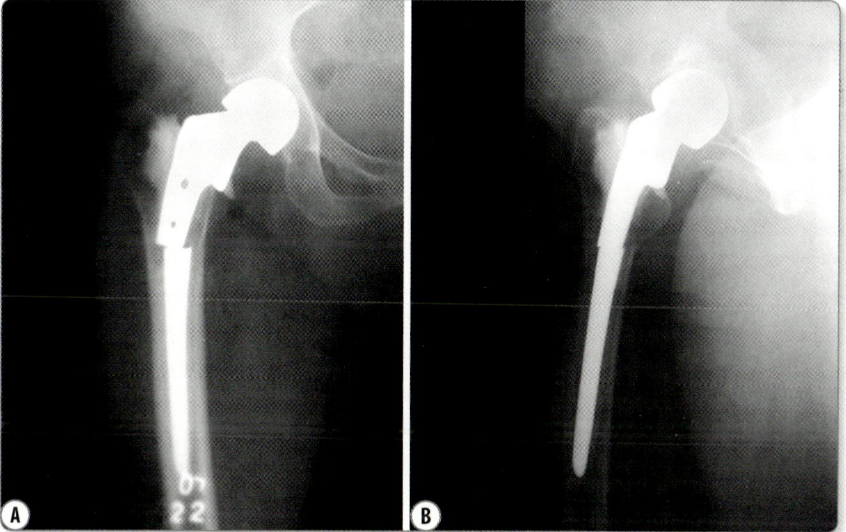

Fig. 11.32 A and B Broken prosthesis with larger distal part

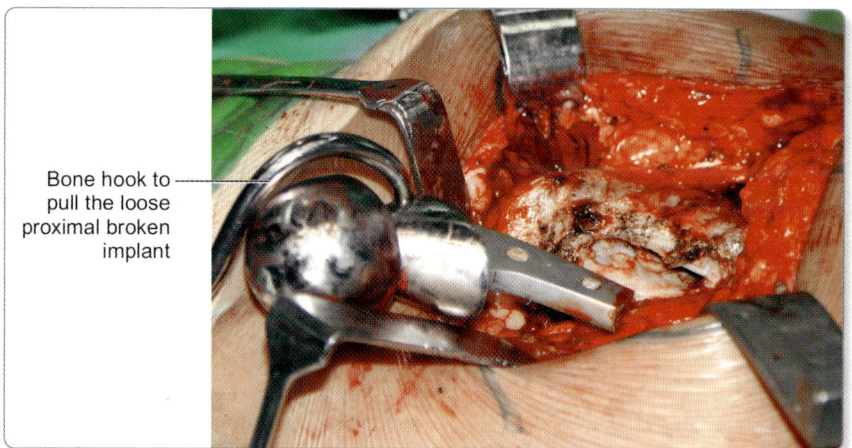

Fig. 11.33 Removal of loose broken implant

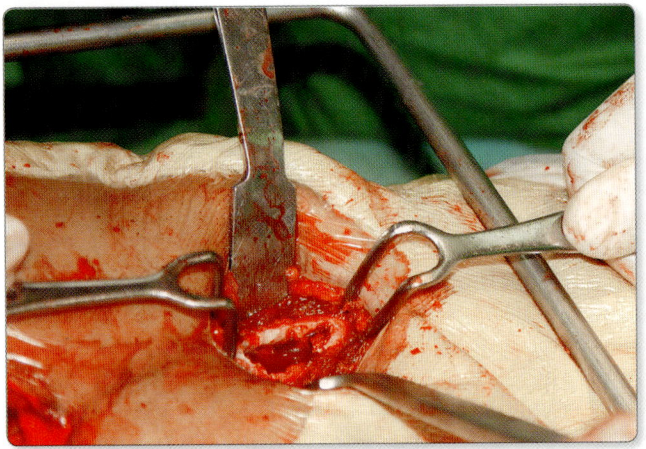

Fig. 11.34 Window on the anterolateral cortex to push up the distal piece of broken implant by curved punch

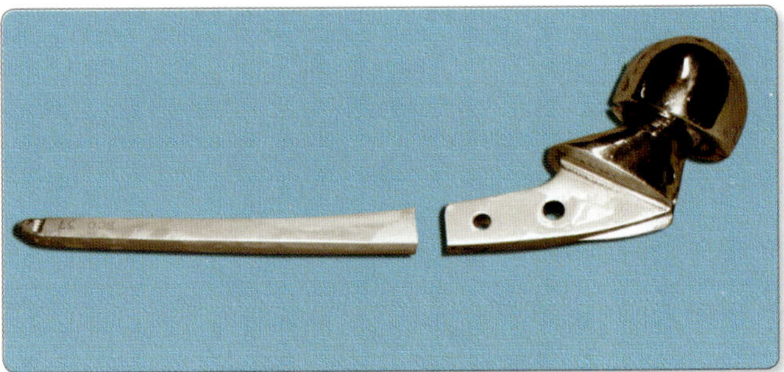

Fig. 11.35 Removed broken implant

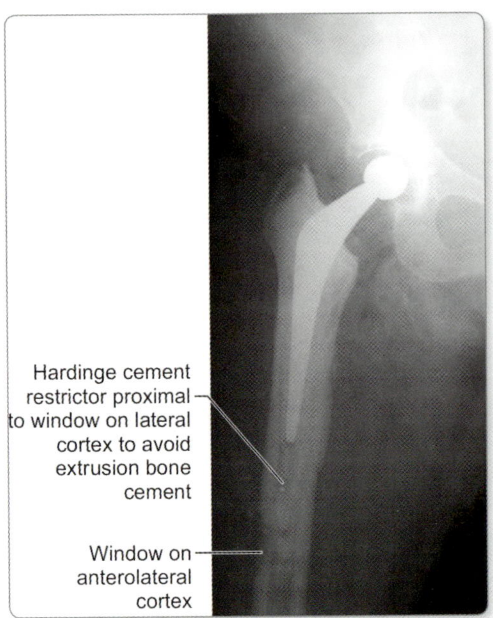

Fig. 11.36 Revision THR with C-stem

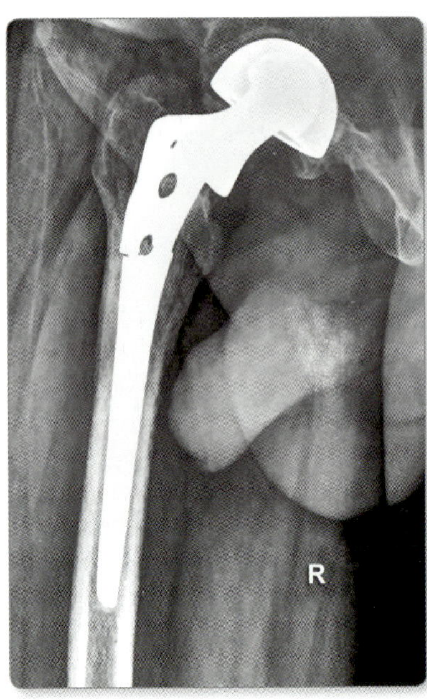

Fig. 11.37 Broken stem

incision. Make two or three drill holes in one line by 4.5 mm drill bit in the lateral cortex and to find out the tip of broken prosthesis. At the level of tip, widen the window by 2.5 mm drill bit and 10 mm osteotome **(Fig. 11.34)**. Pass curved punch and gently hammer to deliver the broken stem out **(Fig. 11.35)**. Care should be taken to avoid fracture of femur. If the broken part is not coming out then use the open technique as described. Hardinge cement restrictor should be applied just proximal to the level of window to avoid extrusion of cement **(Fig. 11.36)**. Window is closed by the pieces of bones which were removed during opening of window.

In case of open technique, long stem implant is selected to bridge the level of horizontal osteotomy.

Alternatively uncemented Summit stem can be used **(Figs 11.37 and 11.38)**. In case of calcar deficit, implant distal fixation stem (solution revision stem) **(Chapter 10, Fig. 10.7)**.

b. Push-down: If the broken distal part of prosthesis is smaller and loose **(Figs11.39 and 11.41)**, push it by Charnley's punch almost 2 ½ inches beyond the tip of the expected size of stem (usually beyond 18 cm) from the level of the opening of the femoral canal. Implant the cemented stem **(Figs 11.40A and B)** or uncemented Summit stem **(Fig. 11.42)**.

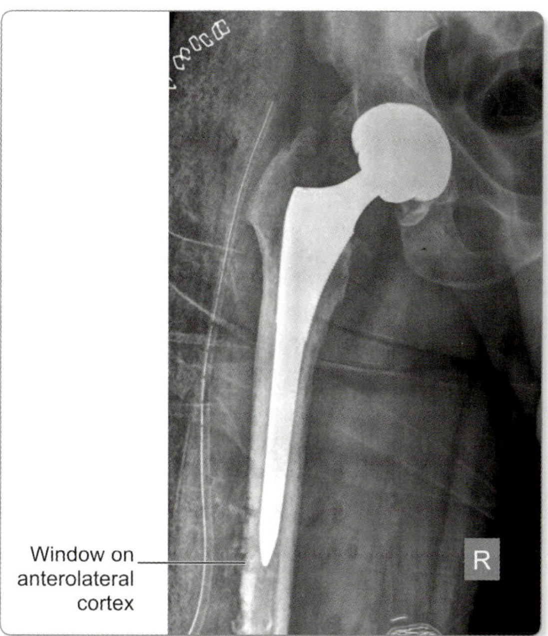

Fig.11.38 Revision THR with uncemented Summit stem after removal of broken stem by technique as described above

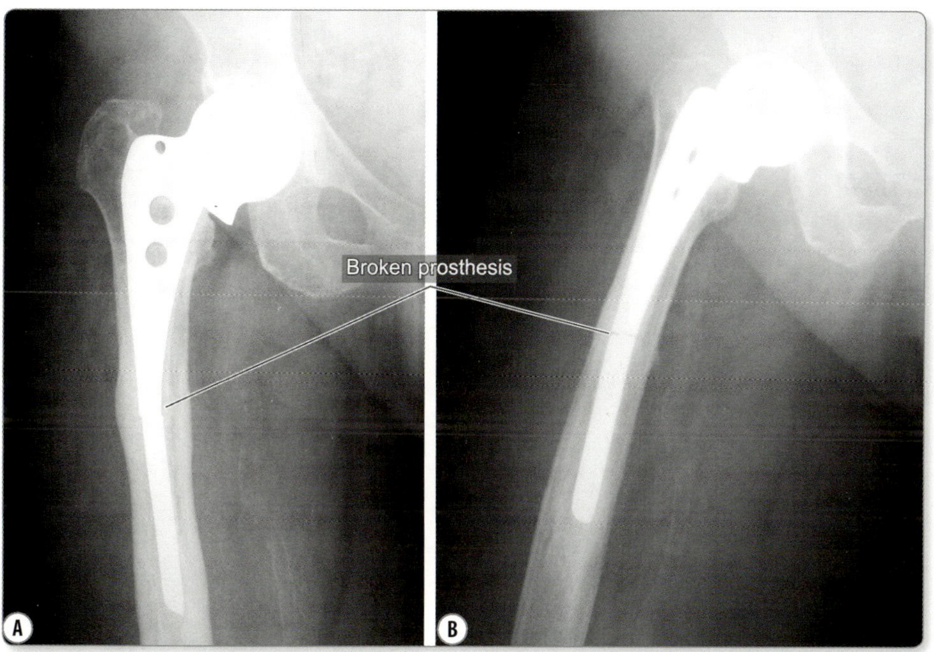

Figs 11.39A and B Broken prosthesis. (A) AP; (B) Lateral views

Periprosthetic Fracture

Fracture of the femoral shaft around a hip prosthesis presents the simultaneous problems of prosthetic stability and femoral-fracture management. Treatment options include nonoperative stabilization (traction) and operative stabilization by means of intramedullary fixation, extramedullary fixation, or proximal femoral prosthetic replacement.

Classification

Vancouver Classification

Type A : Fracture in the trochanteric region
- AG: Greater trochanteric region
- AL : Lesser trochanteric region.

Type B : Fracture around or just distal to the stem
- B1 : Stable prosthesis
- B2 : Unstable prosthesis

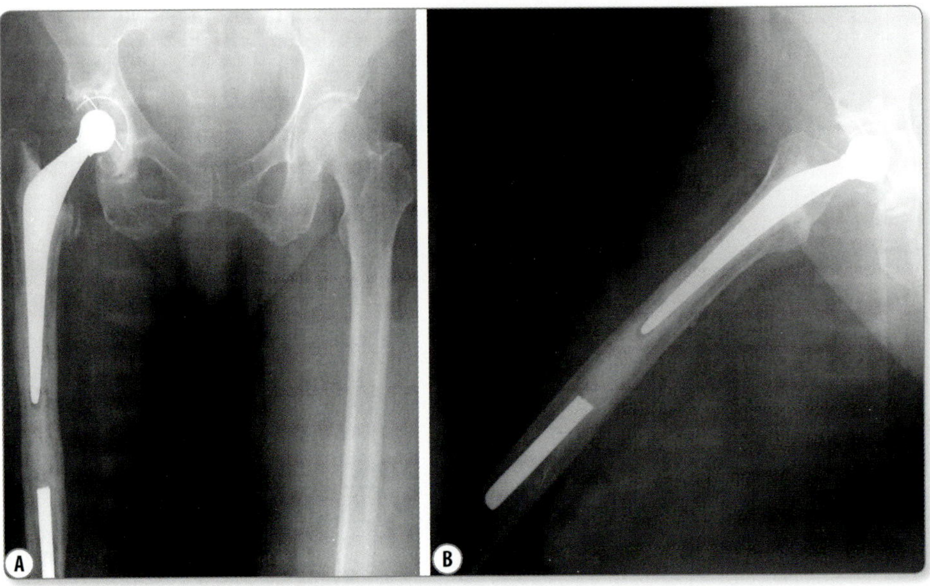

Figs 11.40A and B Small distal broken part of prosthesis pushed down and implantation of C-stem (AP and lateral views)—Cemented THR

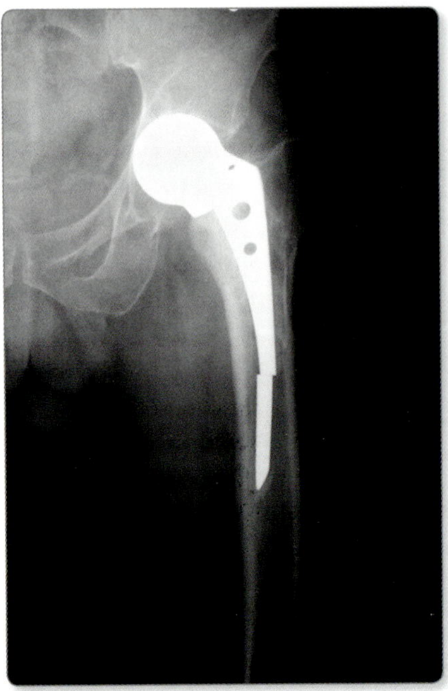

Fig. 11.41 Boken prosthesis with acetabular erosion

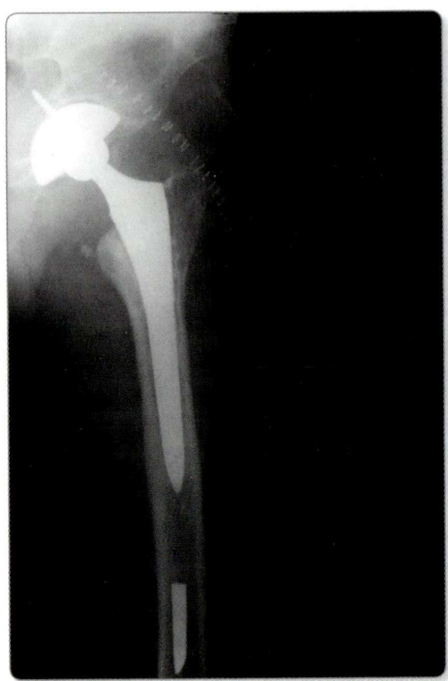

Fig. 11.42 Small distal broken part of prosthesis pushed down and implantation of Summit stem (AP views)—Uncemented THR

B3 : Unstable prosthesis with inadequate bone stock.
Type C : Fracture well below the stem.

Treatment Principles

1. Treatment depends on:
   i. Location of the fracture.
   ii. Stability of the prosthesis—loose stem requires revision.
   iii. Bone stock.
   iv. Age and medical condition of the patient.
   v. Accurate reduction and secure fixation.
2. Options include:
   i. Conservative treatment: Limited weight bearing, brace, cast, or traction.
   ii. Open reduction and internal fixation (with plate and screws or cable and/or strut allograft).
   iii. Revision plus open reduction and internal fixation

Type A Fractures

1. These are usually stable and minimally displaced.
2. Open reduction and internal fixation (ORIF) is used to maintain abductor function with wide displacement.
3. Revision of acetabular component is indicated with severe polythene wear.

Type B1 Fractures

1. These are usually treated with internal fixation.
2. Options for fixation include:
   i. Wires or cables.
   ii. Plate and screws and/or cables/wires with wire mount.
   iii. Cortical onlay allograft.
   iv. Combination.
3. Long-term results depend on:
   i. Implant alignment.
   ii. Preservation of the periosteal blood supply.
   iii. Adequacy of stress riser augmentation.
4. Routine bone graft is used with open reduction and internal fixation (ORIF).

Type B2 Fracture

1. Revision arthroplasty and ORIF is used.
2. Choice of implant includes:
   i. Uncemented prosthesis :
      - Extensive coated long-stem curved prosthesis.
      - Fluted long stem prosthesis.
   ii. Cemented prosthesis.

Type B3 Fractures

1. No sufficient bone stock supports the revision prosthesis.
2. Options include:
   i. Proximal femoral reconstruction—composite allograft.
   ii. Proximal femoral replacement.
3. Treatment depends on:
   i. The age of the patient.
   ii. The severity of the bone defect.
   iii. The functional class of the patient.

Type C Fractures

1. Treat independently of the arthroplasty.
2. Use a plate and screws and/or cables with or without a strut allograft.
3. Do not make any new stress risers.

Acetabular Fractures

1. Undisplaced fractures should be observed and treated with crutches and limited weight bearing. There is a high incidence of late loosening of the acetabular component requiring revision.
2. Displaced fractures should be treated by ORIF, and the component should be revised.

Sometimes, due to severe osteoporosis, fracture shaft of femur may occur peroperatively during dislocation or trial reduction which requires fixation by LCP in transverse or short oblique fractures and cerclage wiring in long oblique or spiral fractures. Use the long stem femoral implant (Long C-stem for cemented or Solution stem for uncemneted) to bridge the defect **(Figs 11.43 to 11.46)**.

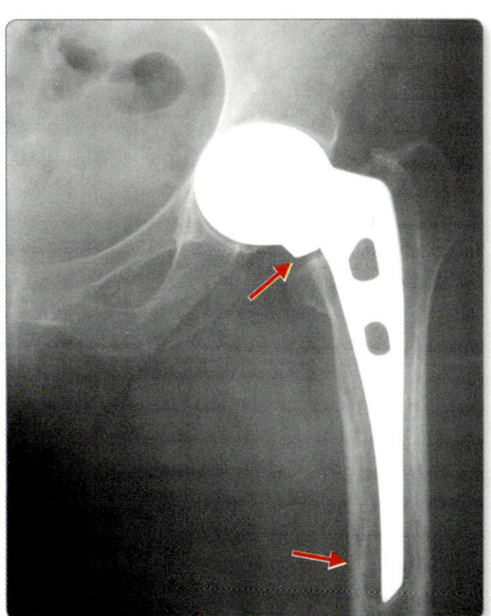

Fig. 11.43 Loose prosthesis with severe osteoporosis

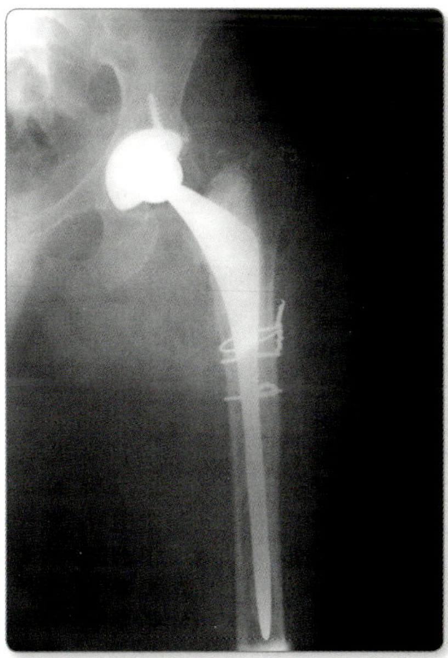

Fig. 11.44 Uncemented cup and long C-stem. Cerclage wires were applied for spiral fracture shaft of femur which occurred peroperatively

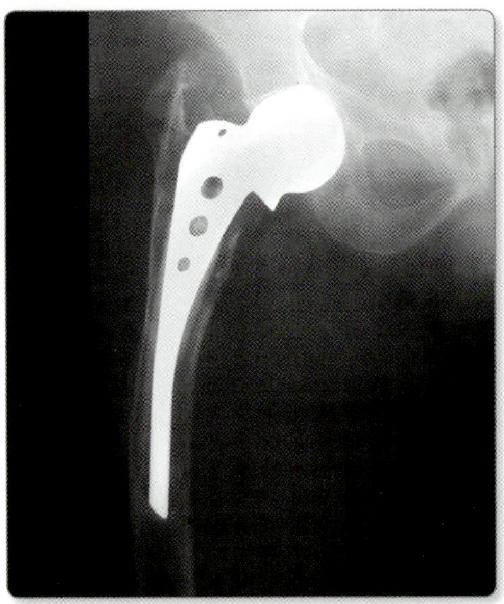

Fig. 11.45 Loose prosthesis with severe osteoporosis

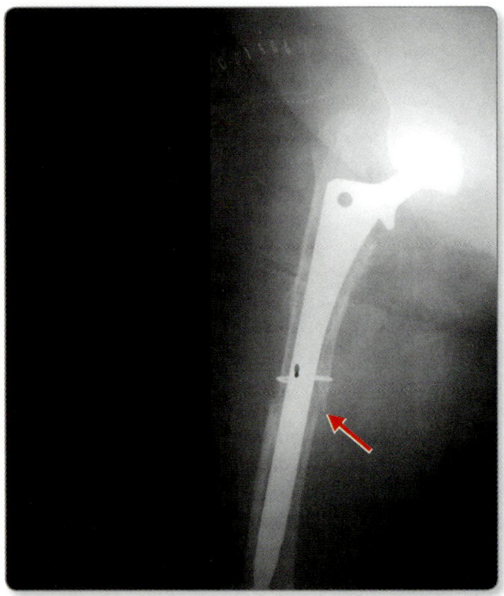

Fig. 11.46 Uncemented long solution stem with bipolar hastings head and 22.2 mm cobalt chrome articul/eze. Fracture occurred peroperatively. Cerclage wire was applied for split in proximal fragment

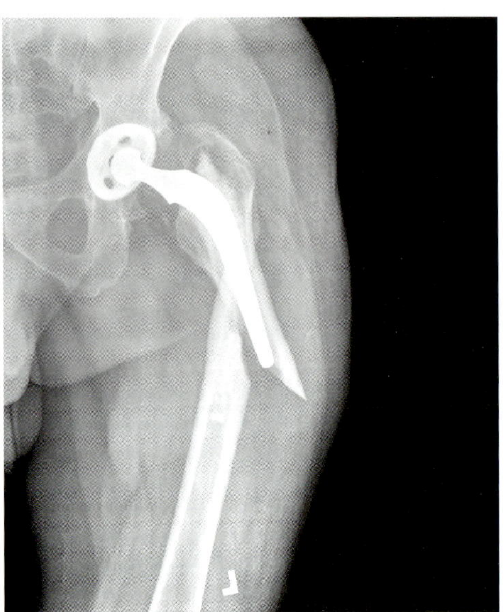

Fig. 11.47 Periprosthetic fracture

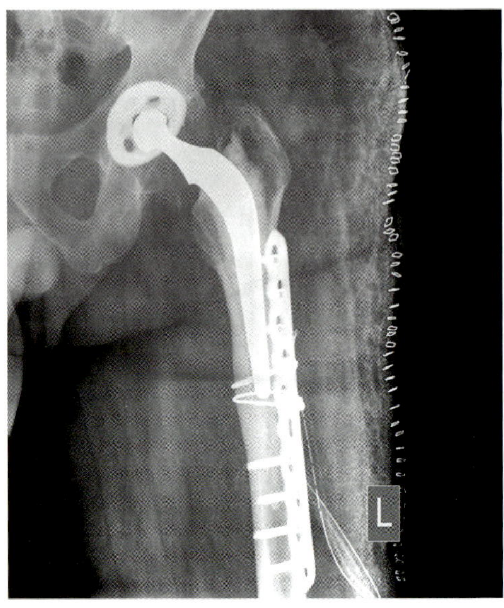

Fig. 11.48 Fixation by LCP with bicortical screws in distal fragments, unicortical screws in proximal fragments, cerclage wires with wire mounts

Type B1—Open the fracture site. Reduce and fix the fracture by locking compression plate (LCP) or dynamic compression plate (DCP) or low contact dynamic compression plate (LCDCP). Use unicortical screws and/or circlage wires with wire mounts in the area of prosthesis **(Figs 11.47 to 11.55)**.

Type B2—Expose the hip and remove the loose implant. Implant the cemented or uncemented acetabular cup. Expose the fracture site. Reduce the fracture and fix with LCP (locking compression plate) and unicortical screws (usually 12 mm length) and cerclage wires for extra support. Prepare the femoral canal by reaming and broaching. Apply the trial femoral stem. Do trial reduction. Remove the trial stem. Implant the long cemented C-stem to bridge the fracture site as shown in **Figures 11.56 to 11.62**.

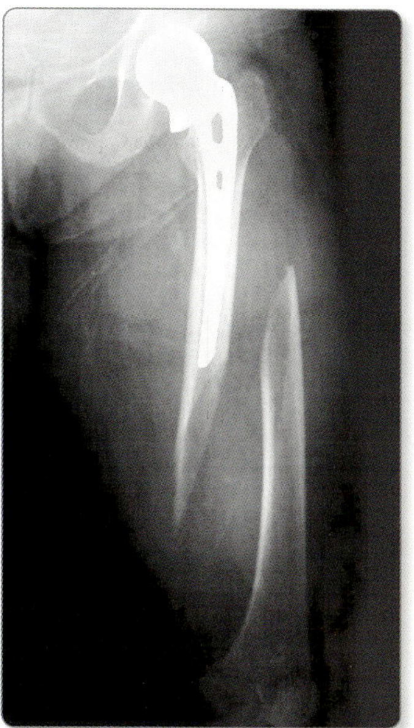

Fig. 11.49 Periprosthetic fracture

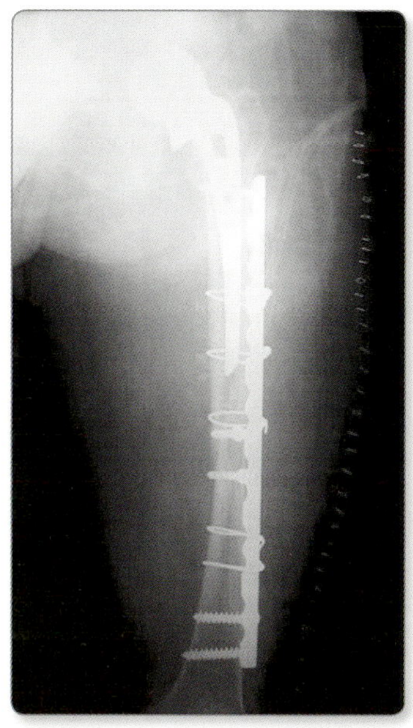

Fig. 11.50 Fixed with LCDCP, screws, cerclage wires with wire mounts

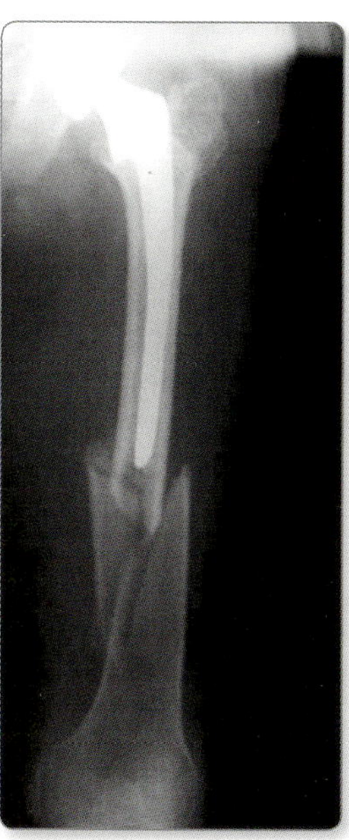

Fig. 11.51 Periprosthetic fracture

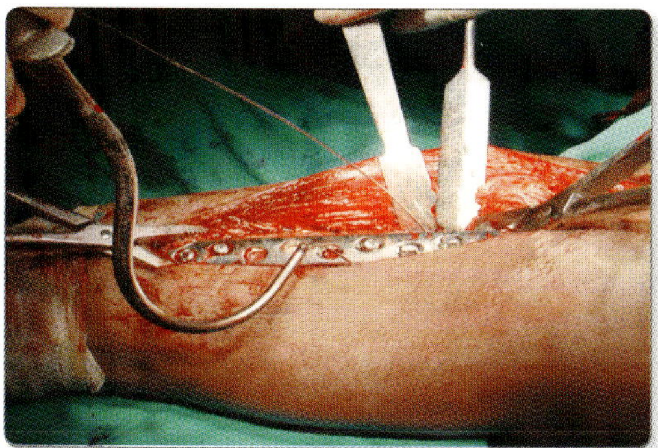

Fig. 11.52 Passing cerclage wire by wire passer

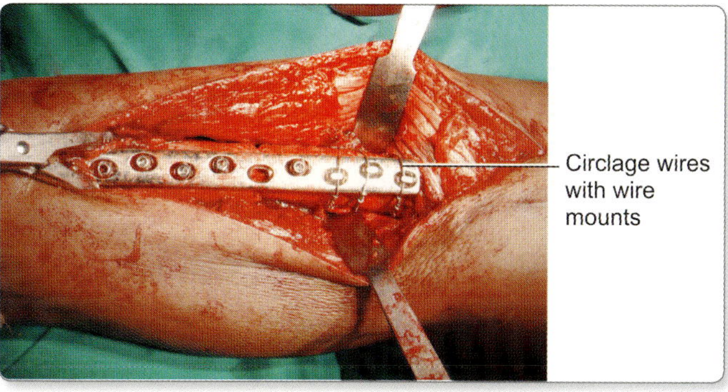

Fig.11.53 ORIF with broad LCDCP, screws, cerclage wires and wire mounts

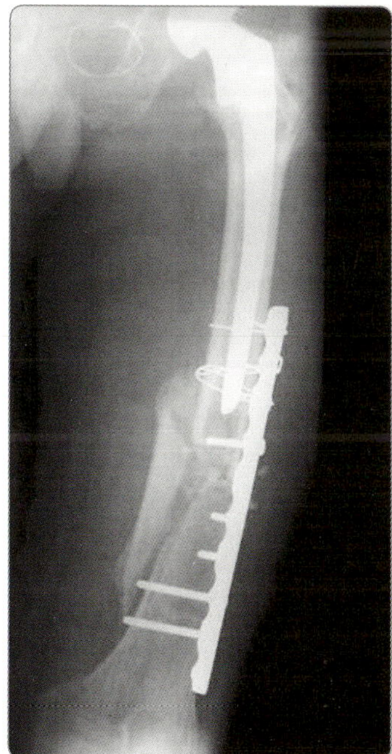

Fig. 11.54 Postoperative X-ray showing fixation by LCDCP, screws, cerclage wires with wire mounts

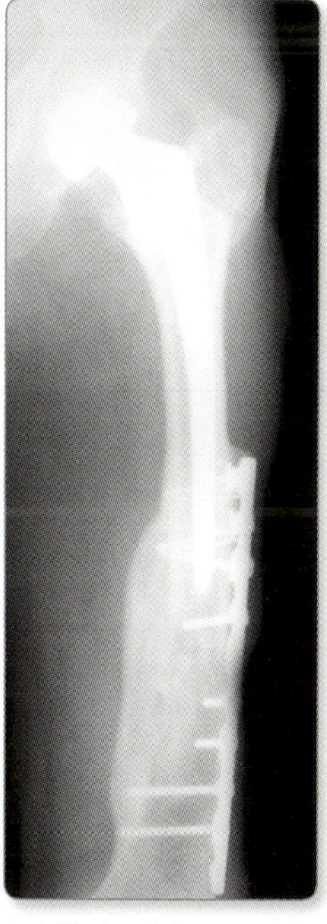

Fig. 11.55 Consolidation at 4 months

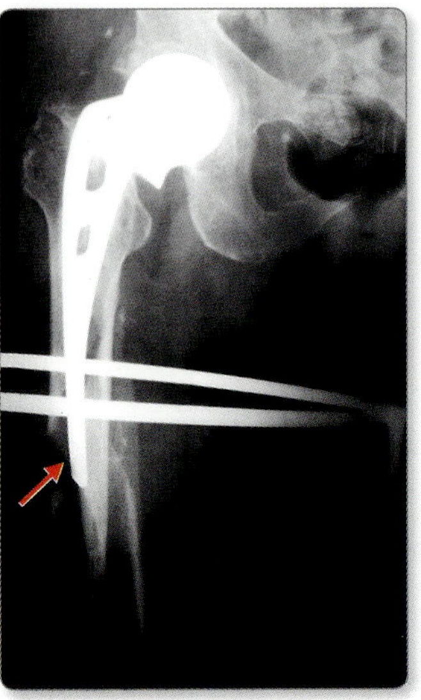

Fig. 11.56 Periprosthetic fracture

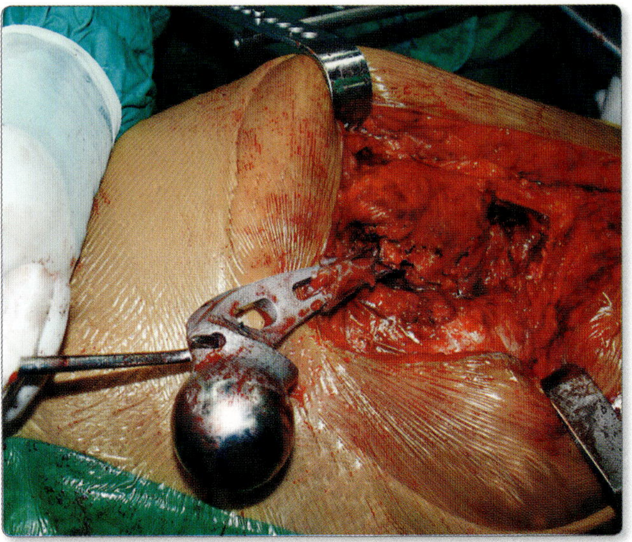

Fig. 11.57 Removal of loose implant

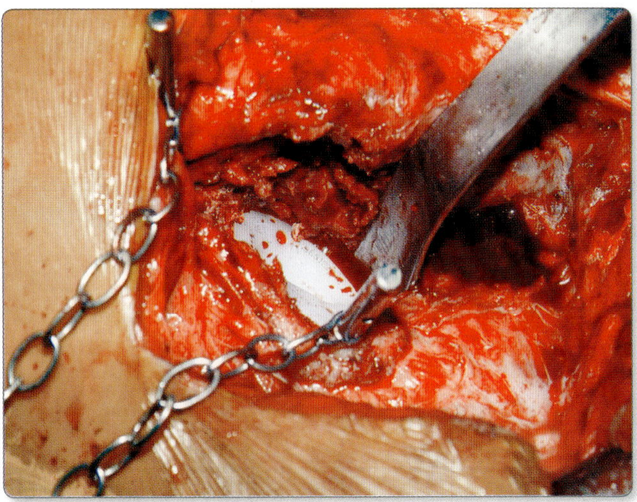

Fig. 11.58 Cemented cup

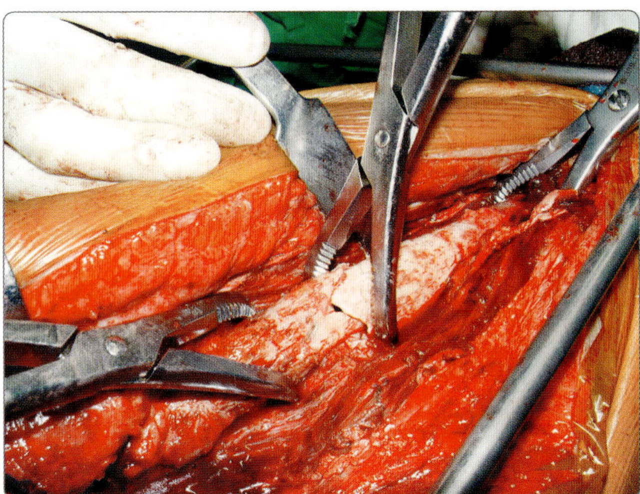

Fig. 11.59 Fracture reduction

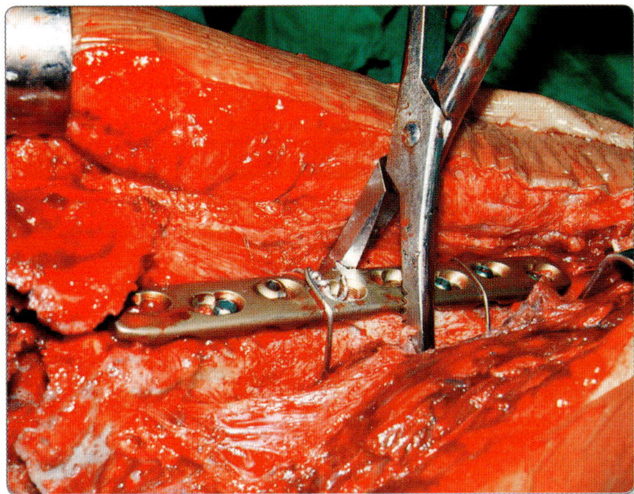

Fig. 11.60 Fracture fixation by LCP and cerclage wire

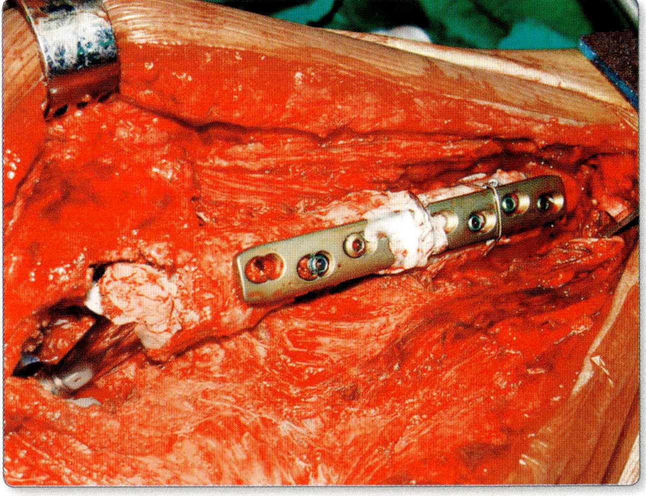

Fig. 11.61 Implantation of 240 mm long C-stem (Cemented)

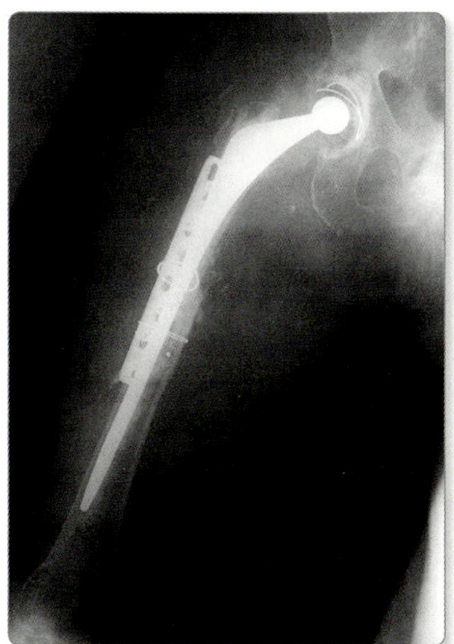

Fig. 11.62 Postoperative X-ray AP view

Alternatively uncemented long solution stem may be applied to bridge the fracture site **(Figs 11.44 and 11.46)**.

Type B3—Remove the loose implant and cement by ultrasonic cement removal system and apply distal fixation stem (revision solution stem) and fill up the gap with allograft **(Figs 11.63 to 11.67)**.

Infection

It is diagnosed by the symptoms, signs **(Fig. 11.68)** and investigations as described for infection in total knee replacement (Chapter 5). Periprosthetic osteolysis is the most frequent radiological finding **(Figs 11.69 and 11.77)**.

Two-stage revision surgery is the most common method for treating infected endoprostheses. The advantage of two stage revision is that the surgical debridement is carried out twice, hence, there is eradication of residual organisms.

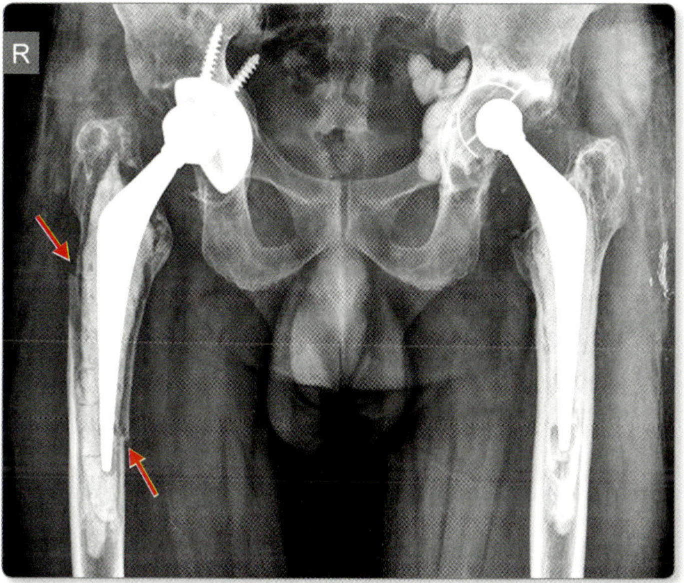

Fig. 11.63 Periprosthetic fracture with loosening of femoral prosthesis and poor bone stock of right femur

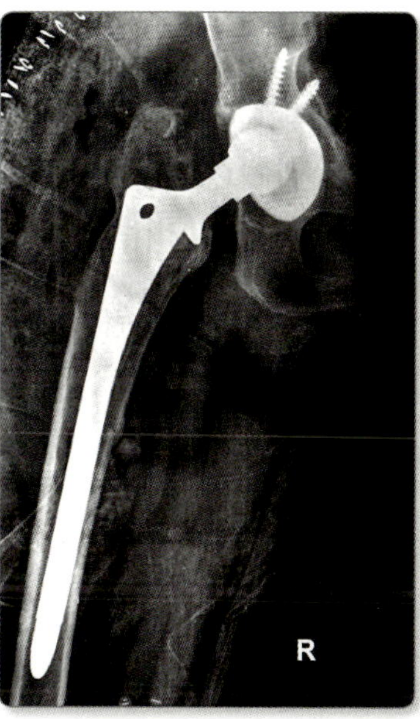

Fig. 11.64 After revision THR (removal of loose C-stem, bone right femur cement and insertion of solution stem), distal part of cement was removed by ultrasonic cement removal system and filling of allograft in gap

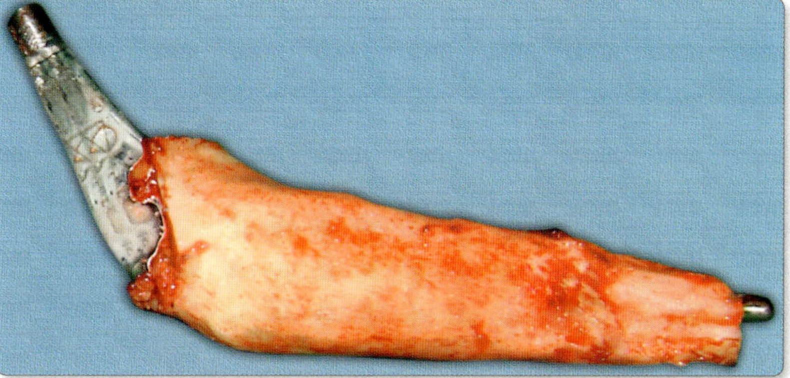

Fig. 11.65 Removal of loose C-stem

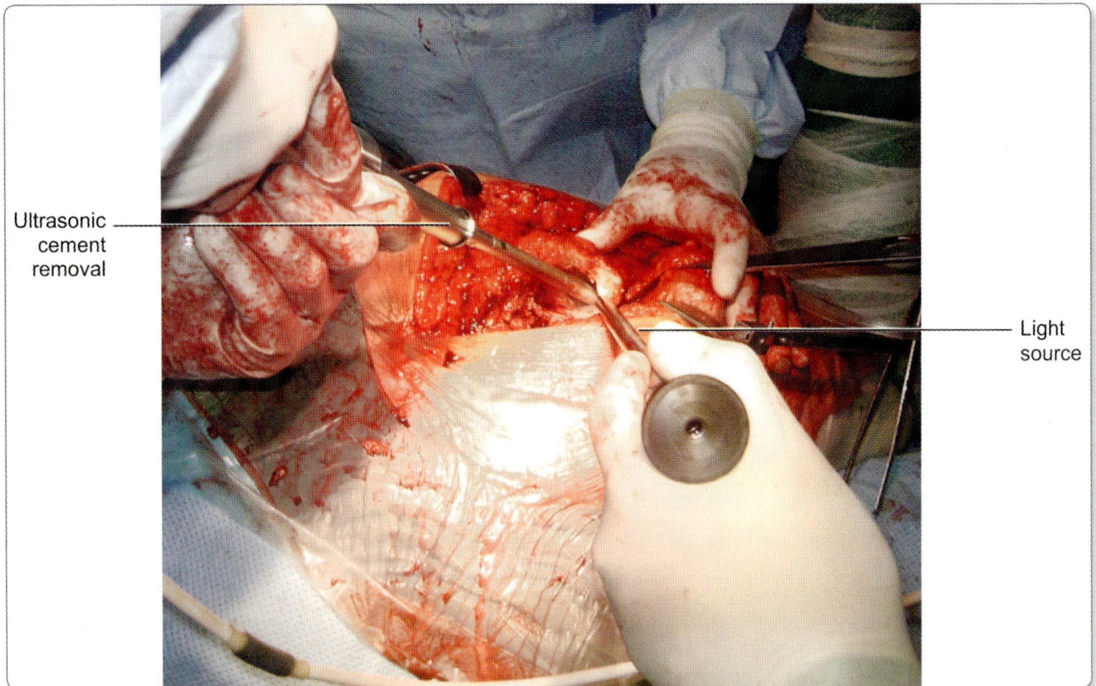

Fig. 11.66 Removal of bone cement from medullary canal by using ultrasonic cement removal system with help of light source

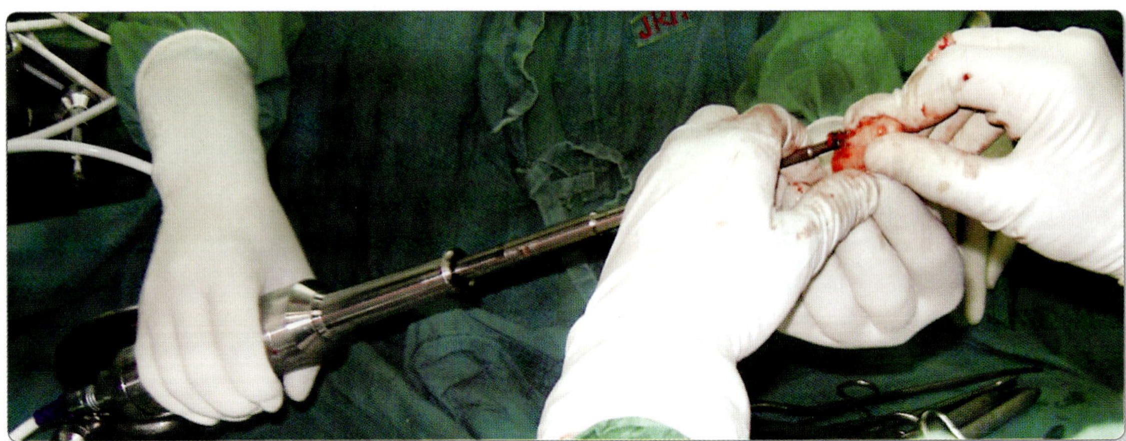

Fig. 11.67 Distal bone cement piece removed from medullary canal by ultrasonic cement removal sysytem

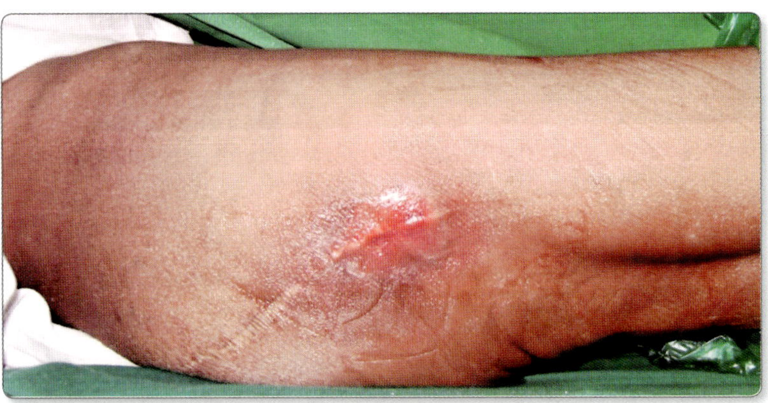

Fig. 11.68 Late infection showing redness, swelling, indurations and pus discharge

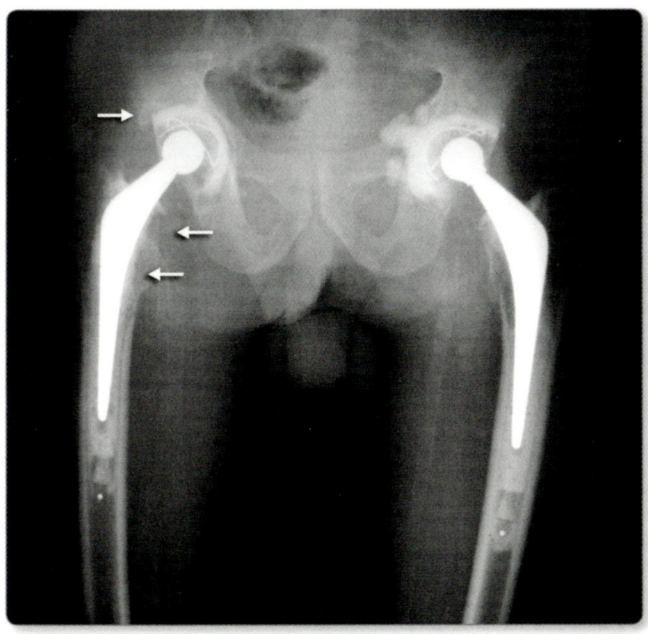

Fig.11.69 Periprosthetic osteolysis right hip due to infection (Compare from left hip)

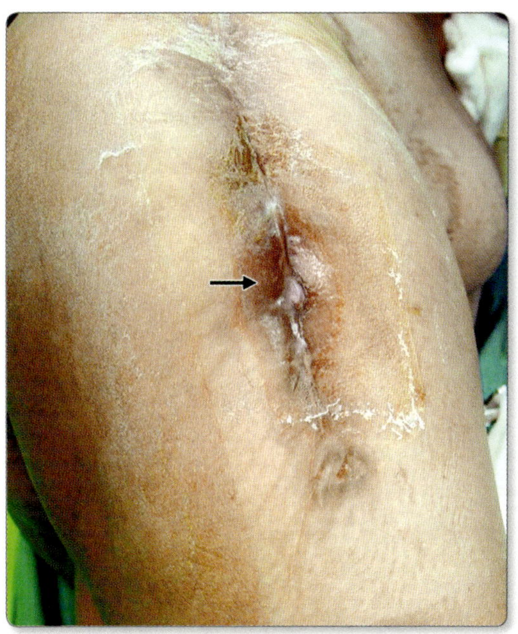

Fig. 11.70 Infection (discharging sinus)

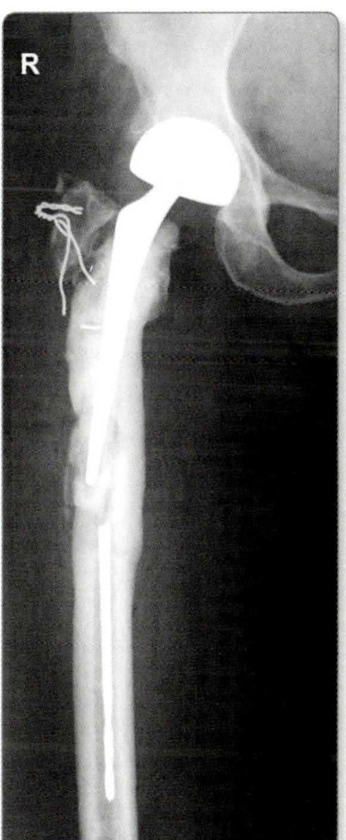

Fig. 11.71 Bipolar hip with non-union greater trochanter with wire and broken drill bit in the medullary canal

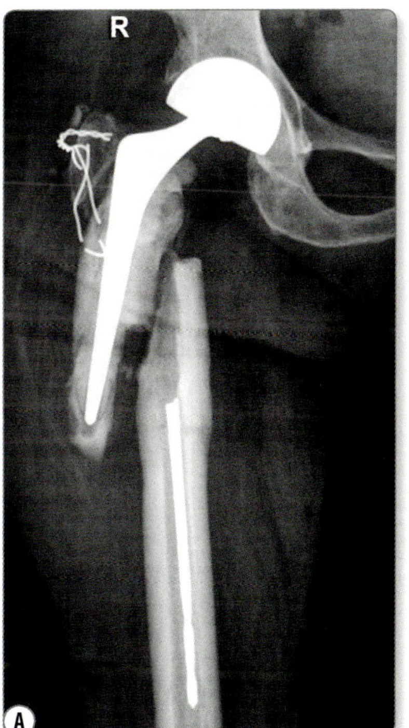

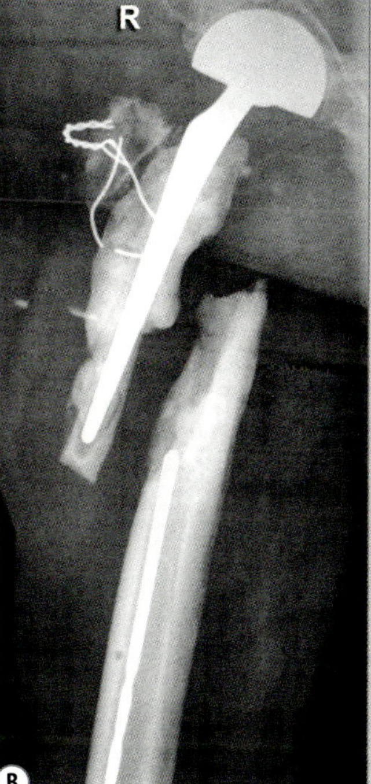

Figs 11.72A and B Patient presented with infection and periprosthetic fracture femur (AP and lateral views)

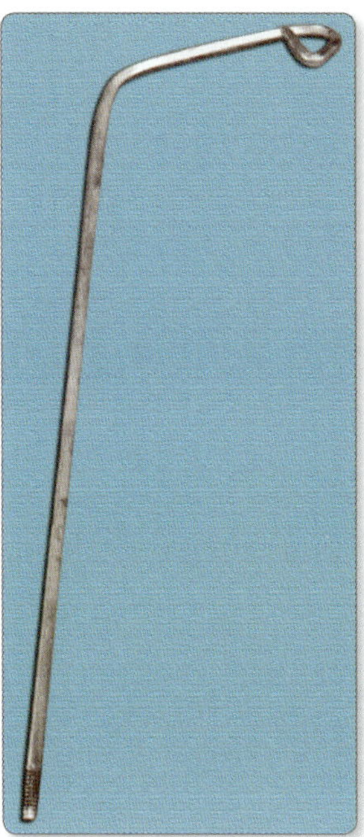

Fig. 11.73 Bent radial nail

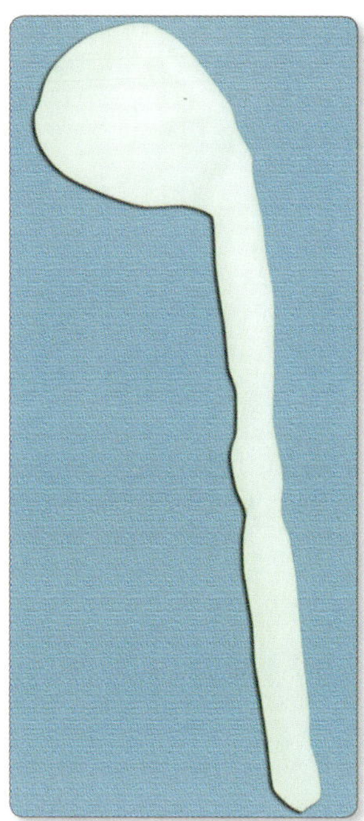

Fig. 11.74 Antibiotic-loaded bone cement to make customized cement spacer applied on radial nail in the shape of prosthesis

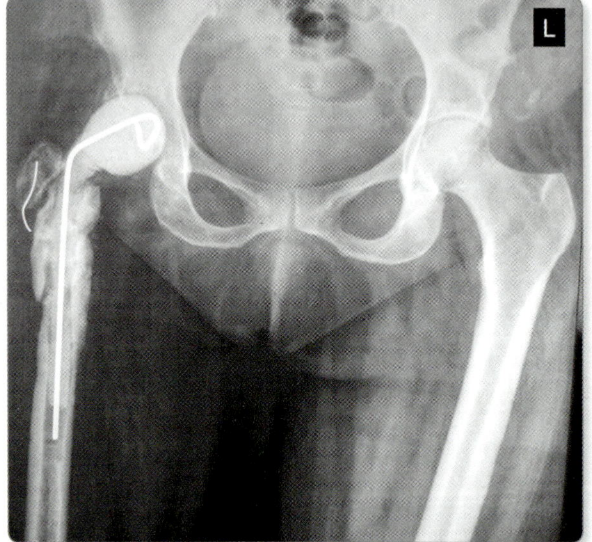

Fig. 11.75 Stage I, application of customized antibiotic-loaded cement spacer in the medullary canal after thorough debridement, removal of femoral stem, other hardware and bone cement

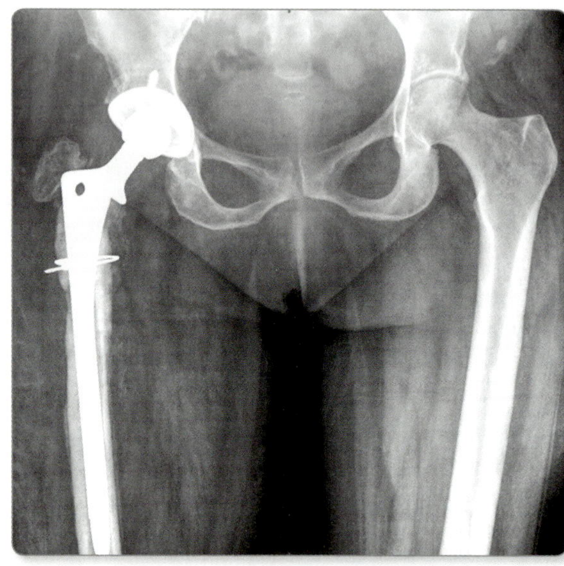

Fig. 11.76 Stage II revision THR, uncemented Duraloc acetabular shell and solution revision stem after removal of antibiotic-loaded cement spacer at 2 months of control of infection

Two Stage Revision THR

Stage I—Removal of bone cement, all hardware, thorough debridement and application of antibiotic loaded cement spacer.

Stage II—Removal of cement spacer after control of infection and revision THR cemented or uncemented (modular revision stem with distal fixation). Both are having 82% to 100% eradication rate of infection.

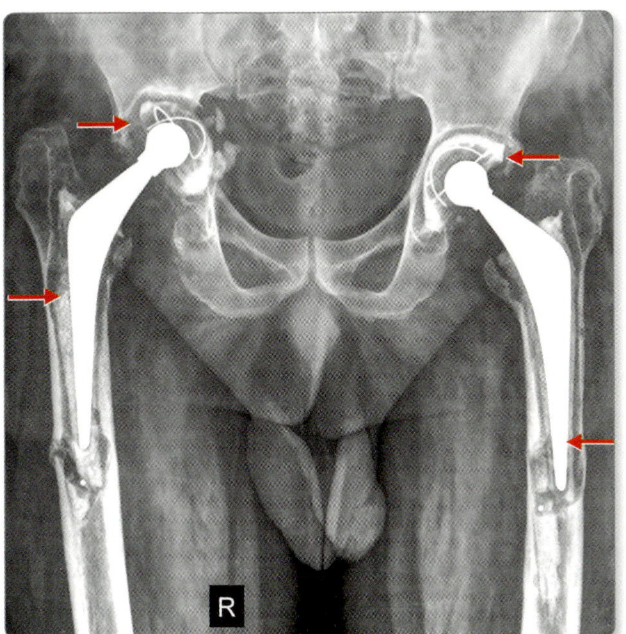

Fig. 11.77 Periprosthetic osteolysis and loosening of both hip joints due to infection

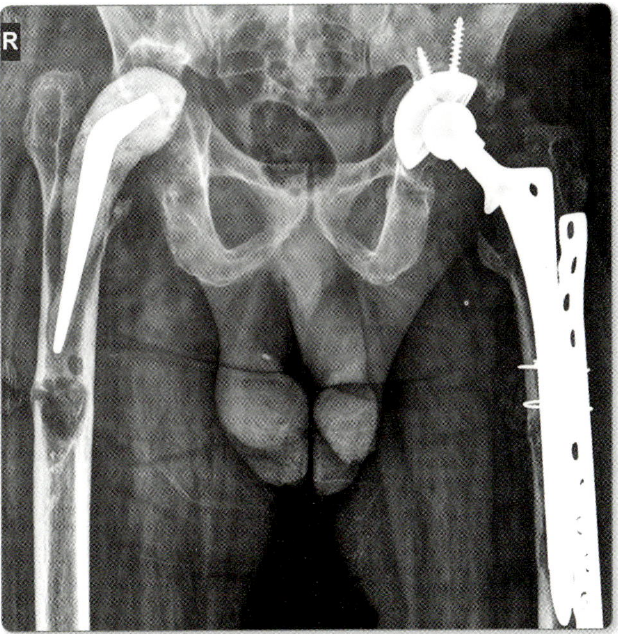

Fig.11.78 Stage I THR (antibiotic impregnated cement spacer) on right side and one stage THR (uncemented cup and solution stem) with fixation by plate of fracture occurred during removal of loose implant on left side

In the first stage, total hip prosthesis and all infected tissues and cement are removed **(Figs 11.70 to 11.72)**. Take swab for pus culture and sensitivity test. Antibiotic loaded articulating cement spacer is placed in position. The purpose of cement spacer is not to fix the prosthesis, so large amount of antibiotics can be mixed into the cement before the spacer is formed. If any bacteria remain in this space after extraction of the infected prosthesis, it will be killed by the high concentration of antibiotics. The function of cement spacer is to release the antibiotic into the infected bed of the prosthesis and to minimize soft-tissue contractures, retain soft tissue tension and so maintain reasonable functionality until a prosthesis can be reimplanted. There are several different types of spacers: Monoblock and two-part spacers, commercially available and customized spacer made in the operation theater.

We are using customized cement spacer made in operation theater. First determine the diameter of the medullary canal of femur after reaming by gradually increasing size of the reamer. Determine the size of head either by measuring the head of removed prosthesis or by acetabular trial. Take radial nail and bend it in shape of proximal femur **(Fig. 11.73)**. Prepare the antibiotic loaded bone cement spacer. Take 2 packets of 40 g gentamicin impregnated bone cement (CMW1 gentamicin) in a stainless steel bowl and mix 4 g vancomycin powder (2 g/40 g). Apply the bone cement liquid and mix slowly by spoon. Apply this antibiotic loaded bone cement over the pre-bent nail/stem and make the shape of head and stem similar to prosthesis **(Fig. 11.74)**. The diameter of stem is slightly lesser than the size of last reamer. The size of head is also slightly lesser than the determined size. After setting of the cement, apply this cement spacer in the femoral stem by gentle punching in 20° anteversion and reduce the head in the acetabulum as shown in **Figures 11.75 and 11.78**. Give intravenous suitable antibiotic (according to pus culture and sensitivity test) for 3 weeks (from 2 weeks to 6 weeks) and oral antibiotic for 6 weeks. If there is no sign of infection plan to do second stage revision total hip replacement **(Fig. 11.76 and Figs 11.79 to 11.89)**. The period of time between the two operations of a two-stage revision is very variable, ranging from a few days to several years, usually an interim phase of 6–12 weeks either left as Girdlestone situation or with the implantation of a cement spacer.

In stage II, bone defect of femur (Figs 11.82 to 11.87) or acetabulum **(Figs 11.88 and 11.89)** will require reconstruction by fresh frozen allograft.

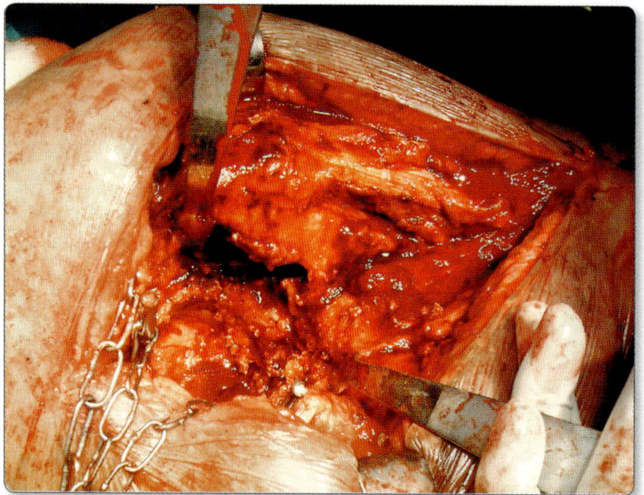

Fig. 11.79 Preparation of acetabulum during stage II revision right hip

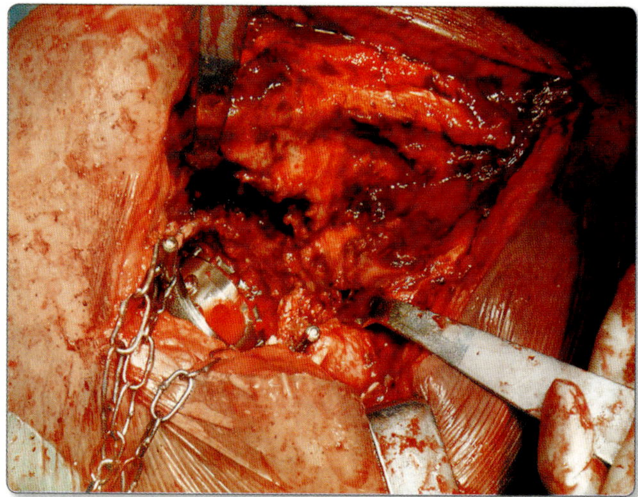

Fig. 11.80 Insertion of multiholes pinnacle cup after applying allograft in the acetabular bone defect

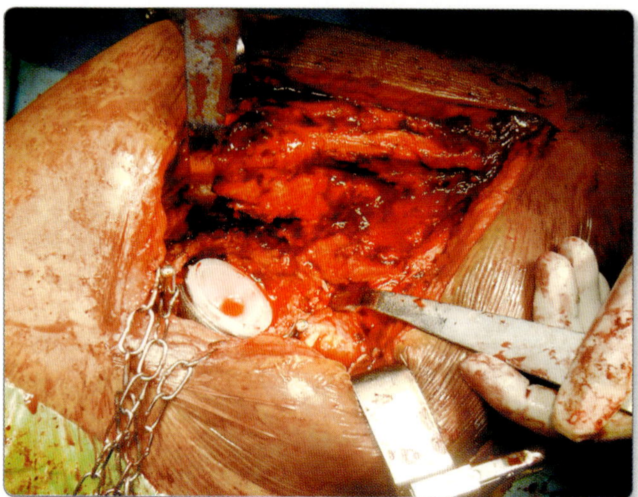

Fig. 11.81 Application of 36 mm ceramic acetabular liner

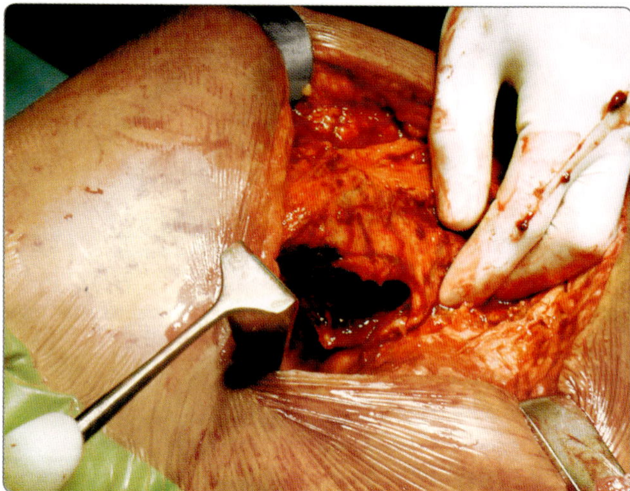

Fig. 11.82 Bone defect in femoral canal during stage II revision right hip

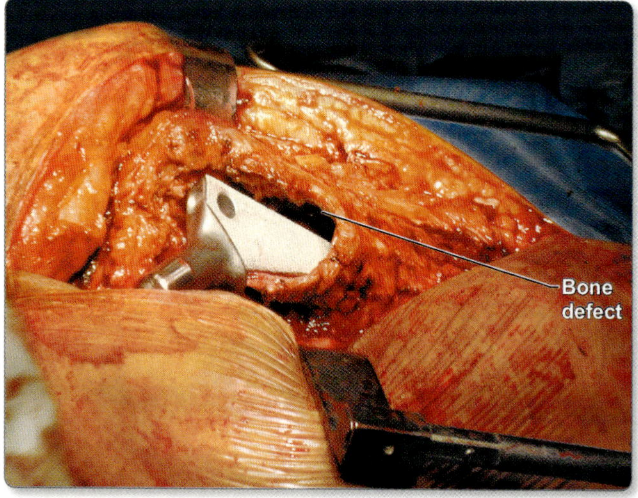

Fig. 11.83 Bone defect in femoral canal after insertion of solution stem during stage II THR

In the second stage, antibiotic loaded cement spacer is removed. Thorough debridement is done and revision THR is done, preferably uncemented modular revision stem with distal fixation (solution revision stem) **(Figs 11.76 to 11.89)**.

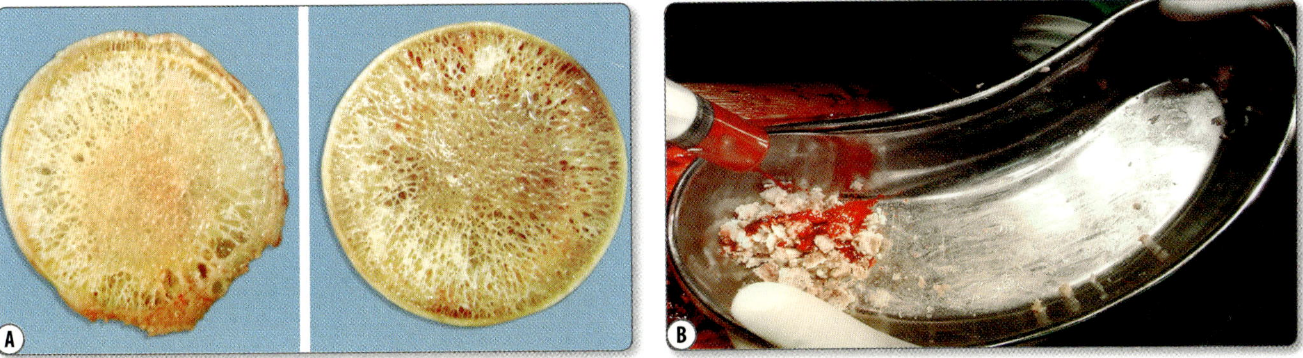

Figs 11.84A and B Fresh frozen allograft (femoral head)

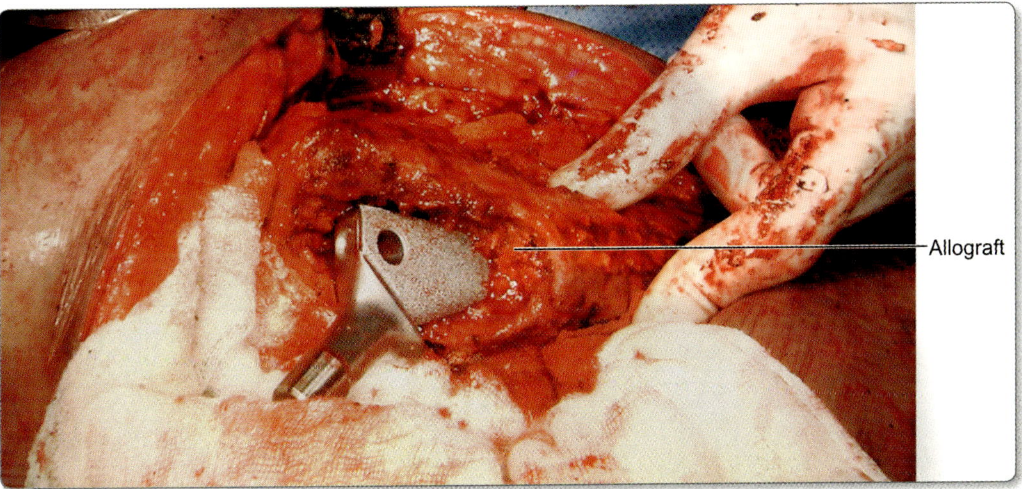

Fig. 11.85 Bone defcct filled up by fresh frozen allograft

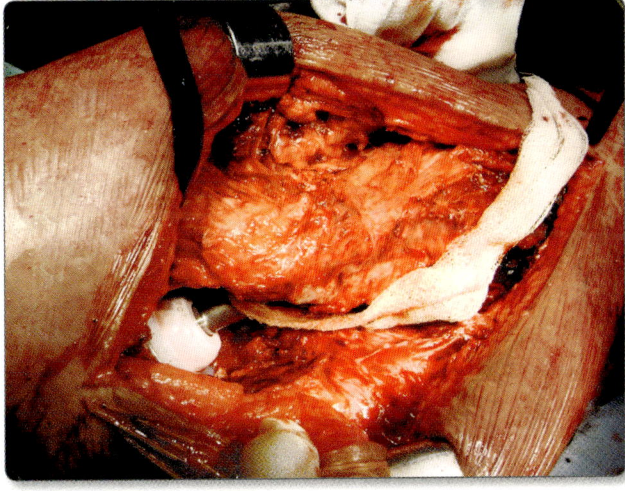

Fig. 11.86 After final reduction

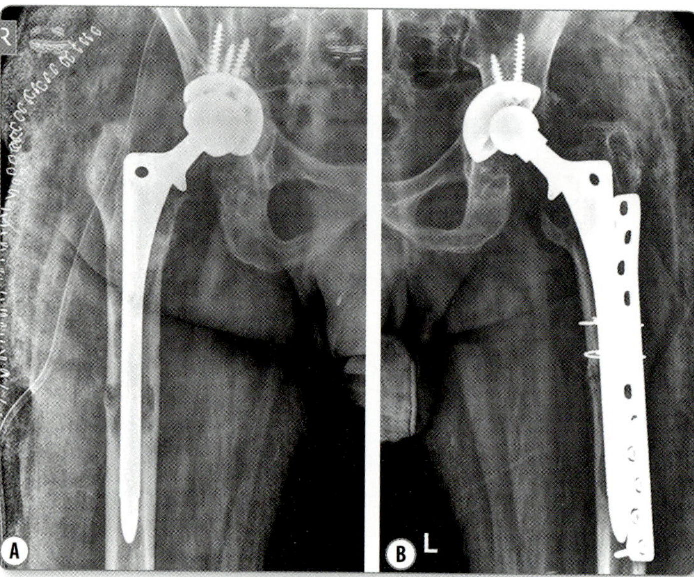

Figs 11.87A and B Stage II revision THR (pinnacle cup, ceramic on ceramic liner) of right hip and one stage revision of left hip (Duraloc, metal on polyethylene liner) with fixation by LCDCP, screws and cerclage wires for peroperative fracture

Reconstruction of superior acetabular defect by fresh frozen allograft:

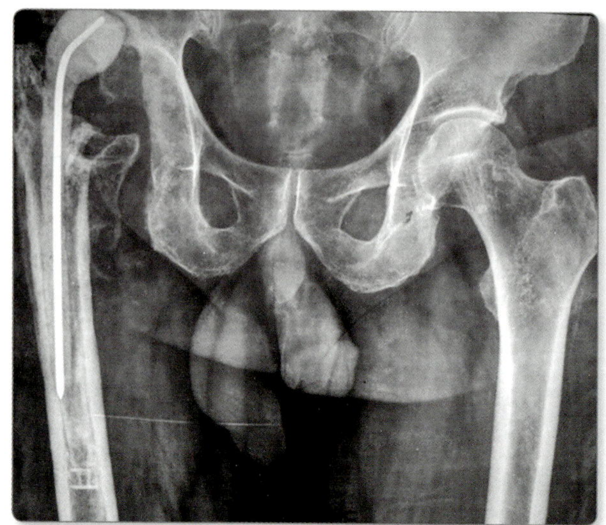

Fig. 11.88 Stage I revision with false acetabulum (Superior migration) for infection THR

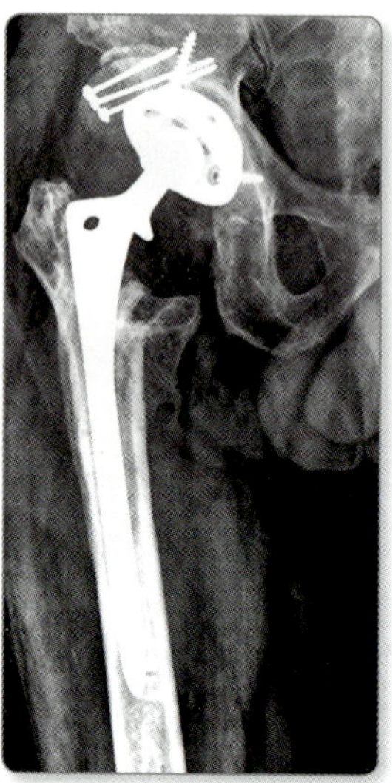

Fig. 11.89 Stage II revision with reconstruction of acetabulum by fresh frozen femoral head allograft and distal fixation solution stem

Implants Required For Revision THR

Revision Acetabular Cup

Cemented—Protrusio large acetabular reconstruction cup—right and left

OD—52, 56, 60 mm	OD—outer diameter
↓ ↓ ↓	
ID—49, 53, 57 mm	ID—inner diameter

Uncemented—

A. Duraloc shell (3 holes and multiholes)—48, 50, 52, 54, 56, 58, 60, 62, 64 and 66 mm OD
B. Pinnacle cup (3 holes and multiholes)—sizes—
   44 and 46 mm (for 28 mm liner and head)
   48 and 50 mm (for 32 mm liner and head)
   52, 54, 56, 58, 60, 62, 64 and 66 mm (for 36 mm liner and head)
   Cancellous bone screws 6.5 mm—15, 20, 25, 30, 35, 40 and 45 mm

Pinnacle liner—
Ceramic or polyethylene—sizes—
44, 46 mm (ID 28 mm)
48, 50 mm (ID 32 mm)
52, 54, 56, 58, 60, 62, 64, 66 mm (ID 36 mm)

C. Octopus acetabular reconstruction system
1. Octopus ring—50, 55 mm (right and left)
2. Octopus HA coated cup—50, 55 mm
3. Insert—
   i. Octopus hooded liner—28 mm—50, 55 mm
   ii. Octopus reorientation liner—28, 50, 55 mm
4. Octopus screws 6.5 mm—15, 20, 25, 30, 35, 40, 45, 50, 55, 60 and 65 mm.

Available Solution Revision Stems—12/14 Taper

This is extensively coated cementless implants and available in 8, 9 and 10 inch lengths, with either standard or calcar neck options, in straight and bowed variants.

1. 200 mm (8") straight stems—Diameters 10.5 mm, 12 mm, 13.5 mm, 15 mm, 16.5 mm.
2. 225 mm (9") bowed calcar replacement stems, 2.25 cm platform, right and left—Diameters 13.5 mm, 15 mm, 16.5 mm, 18 mm.
3. 250 mm (10") bowed stems, right and left—Diameters 13.5 mm, 15 mm, 16.5 mm, 18 mm.

Available REEF components (Fig. 11.90)

1. Distal stems (metaphyseal part 100 mm with proximal diameter 26 mm and diaphyseal part in two lengths—125 mm and 175 mm with 2 holes for interlocking screws).
   Distal stem lengths—
   i. 225 mm—Diameters 12 mm, 14 mm, 16 mm, 18 mm
   ii. 275 mm—Diameters 12 mm, 14 mm, 16 mm, 18 mm
2. Trochanteric components (collarless)—12/14 taper, 25 mm and 35 mm heights.
   Total length (length of trochanteric component + length of distal stem)
   i. 225 mm + 25 mm = 250 mm
   ii. 225 mm + 35 mm = 260 mm
   iii. 275 mm + 25 mm = 300 mm
   iv. 275 mm + 35 mm = 310 mm
3. Locking screws—lengths 16 mm and 26 mm
4. Lateral wings—
   i. Size 1–14 mm
   ii. Size 2–16 mm
   iii. Size 3–18 mm
5. Interlocking screws—Diameter 5 mm, length 20 mm, 25 mm, 30 mm, 35 mm, 40 mm, 45 mm, 50 mm, 55 mm, 60 mm, 65 mm, 70 mm, 75 mm, 80 mm.

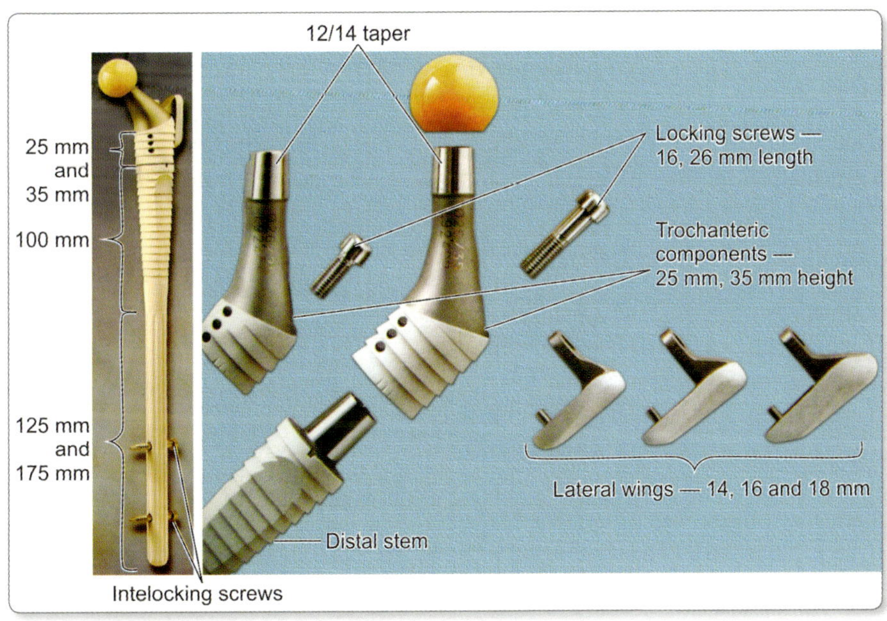

Fig. 11.90 Parts of REEF

Moreland Instruments Required for Removal of Bone Cement and Failed Implants (Figs 11.91 to 11.94)

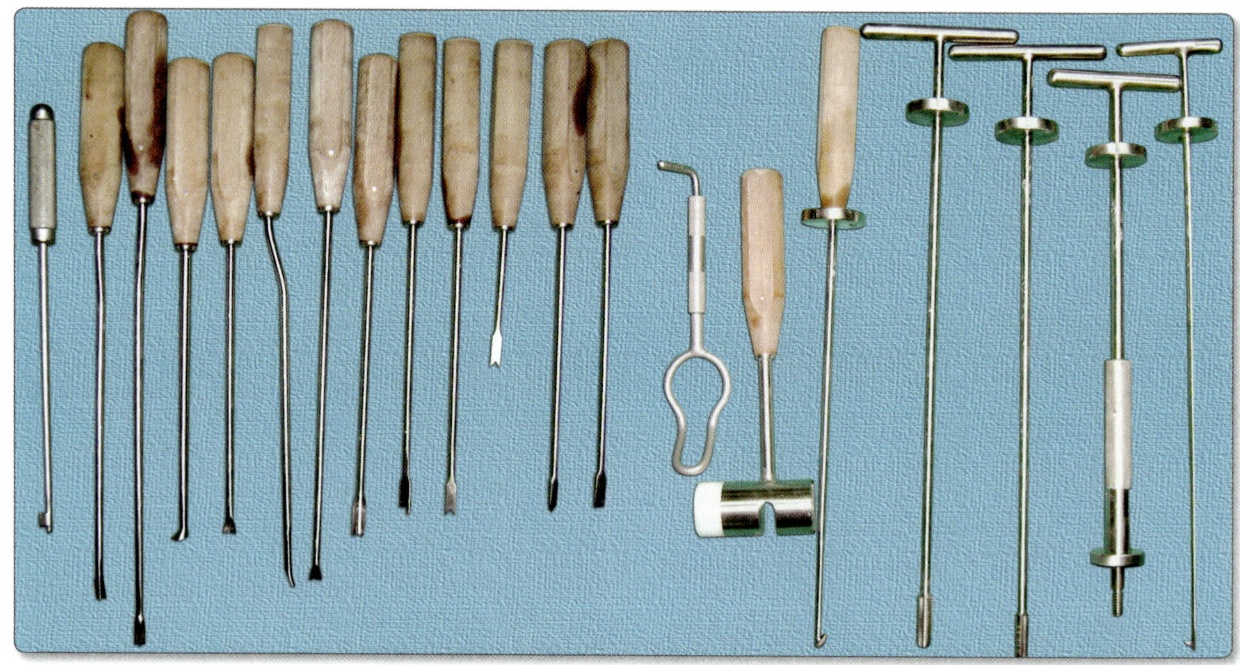

Fig. 11.91 Instruments for removal of bone cement and implants

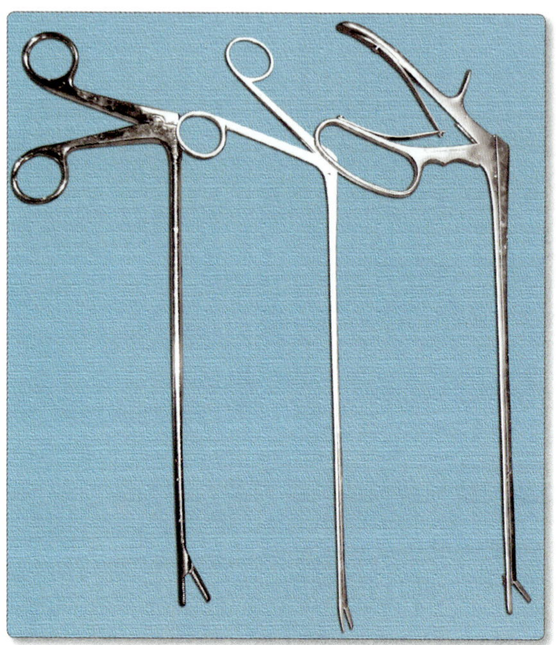

Fig. 11.92 Cement grasping forceps

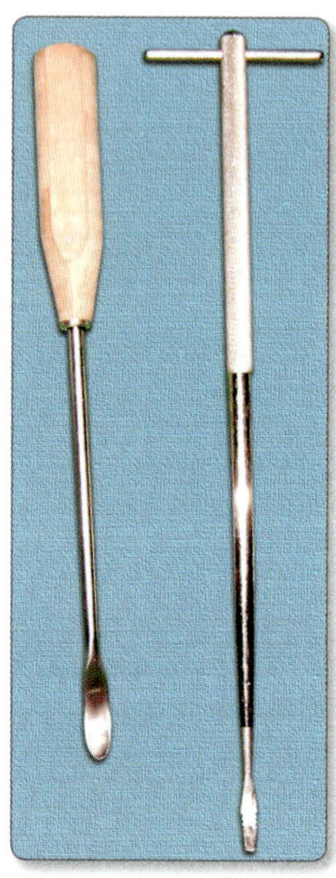

Fig. 11.93 Instruments for cup removal

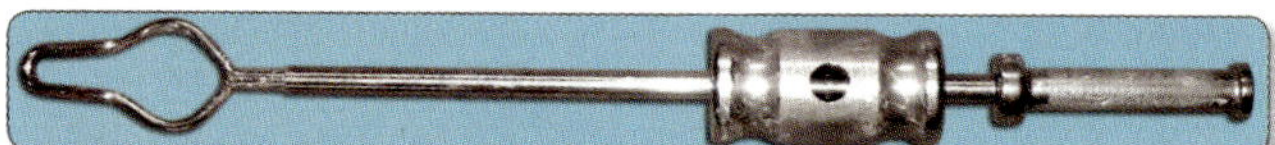

Fig. 11.94 Femoral stem remover

12 CHAPTER

Physiotherapy in TKR and THR

CHAPTER OUTLINE

- TKR
- THR

TKR

In preoperative phase, knee strengthening program is started. Special emphasis is given on getting full extension or reducing fixed flexion deformity (FFD) by means of splintage (knee brace) and quadriceps strengthening. This decreases intraoperative soft tissue release. Explain do's and don'ts to patient.

Do's:

1. Use western style toilet.
2. Walk with moderate speed.
3. Climb up and down stairs.
4. Sit on high chair approximately 20 inches height.
5. Regular exercises as explained.
6. Control of weight.
7. Watch to prevent infection of any kind, particularly urinary and dental infection.
8. Regular visit to operating surgeon.
9. Follow the instructions as explained.

Don'ts:

1. No squatting or sitting on floor.
2. No jogging or running.
3. No contact sports and other impact activities.
4. No local massage or heat therapy.
5. No cross-legged sitting.

In postoperative stage, emphasis is given to overcome quadriceps inhibition. Static quadriceps and ankle toes movements (ATM) are encouraged as early as possible in first 24 hours. About 10 to 15 repetitions every hour will minimize hematoma collection and edema of leg and foot. Once drain is removed, gradually increase the knee flexion exercise, isometric quadriceps exercise and vastus medialis obliquus (VMO) exercise. Usually by 4th postoperative day, most patients achieve 80–90° of knee flexion. Use of CPM is usually not required unless patient is confined to bed in initial few days for some other postoperative complication or in cases where preoperative movement of knee is limited. Knee flexion is guarded in 1st week if there is extensive soft tissue release especially with knee valgus and gross flexion deformity. As soon as the drain is out, patient can be mobilized with walking aids (walker/crutches) with knee brace on operated side. If other knee is having gross flexion and varus deformity, patient may have limb length discrepancy. In such cases, other knee is operated as soon as possible to encourage ambulation. Patient increases distance of walking on day to day basis as per his/her comfort. Short equidistance steps are encouraged. Poor quadriceps strength in preoperative phase requires longer time for recovery in postoperative phase. Sometimes eccentric quadriceps training is required before progressing to concentric strengthening program. It is important to note that sometimes nonweight bearing (NWB) gait training is required if fracture occurs during surgery below prosthetic fitting, even though it is fixed with bone cement. Considering bone quality, weight bearing may be delayed in certain specific cases. Patients are encouraged to do partial-weight bearing (PWB) walking with knee brace and walker till soft tissue healing occurs, i.e. 3 weeks. In this stage, emphasis is given on restoring heel toe gait pattern. As waddling gait has become patient's gait pattern for many days in preoperative stage and patient has to relearn normal gait pattern. Usually after one month from date of surgery, independent gait is advised along with stair climbing. By this time, patient is able to perform his activities of daily living (ADL) comfortably.

THR

Preoperative physiotherapy begins 1 to 2 weeks prior to surgery. Exercise program is introduced to the patient like static glutei, quadriceps, hip abduction and extension training and ankle pumps (ankle toe movements). Patient is made to learn transfer technique from bed to assume erect position without flexion at hip. Explain do's and don'ts.

Do's:

1. Use western style toilet (height should be according to tibial length of the patient).
2. Walk with moderate speed.
3. Climb up and down stairs.
4. Sit on high chair approximately 20 inches height.
5. Go in and out of car by keeping legs together and advancing legs first.
6. Regular exercises as explained.
7. Control of weight.
8. Watch to prevent infection of any kind particularly urinary and dental infection.
9. Regular visit to operating surgeon.
10. Follow instructions as explained.

Don'ts:

1. Not to cross legs in sitting or lying.
2. Avoid squatting and crossed legged sitting.
3. Avoid sitting on low stool or sagging chair.
4. Avoid hip adduction (use wedge pillow between legs).
5. Prevent hip rotation in early stage (use derotation bar).
6. Avoid flexion beyond 90°, adduction and internal rotation at hip or combination of these movements.
7. No jogging or running.
8. No contact sports and other impact activities.
9. No local massage or heat therapy.

Postoperative exercise program consists of static hip extension and abduction exercise, ankle toes movements, static quadriceps and breathing exercise.

Bridging can be started with operated leg in complete extension. This will be helpful for toilet activities and gives some pressure relief to gluteal region. Patient will be confined to bed for minimum 2 weeks except for gait training, if permissible. Resuming erect position may lead to postural hypotension on day one as patient is confined to bed for longer time. Keep a close watch on pulse and progression to walking is done gradually. Usually after stitch removal, i.e. 2 weeks postoperative, hip flexion is gradually progressed to 90° and further sitting at the edge of bed is permitted. Ambulation is done with walker either non-weight bearing (NWB) or partial weight bearing (PWB) depending upon cemented or uncemented THR. In cemented THR, partial weight bearing can be started from 2nd postoperative day and full weight bearing after one month. In uncemented THR, patient starts non-weight bearing walking for initial 6 weeks then partial weight bearing walking for 3 months. After completion of 3 months, patient starts full weight bearing (FWB) walking. However, depending on intraoperative stability of prosthesis, soft tissue release, 1st surgery or revision surgery, weight bearing and hip joint mobilization vary.

Hip extension, abduction training continues as home exercise program post discharge. Between 6 and 12 weeks, patient is mobilized with stick in opposite hand. It increases base of support, gives leverage to abductors, thereby decreasing joint reaction force. Full weight bearing walking and most of normal activities are allowed after 3 months.

Patient's Guide to Arthritis and Joint Replacement

13

CHAPTER

CHAPTER OUTLINE

- Suggestions to the Patients
- Job Recommendation for Person who has Undergone TKR and/or THR

Introduction

Arthritis is a painful disabling condition of joints which cripples millions of people around the world every year. In advanced stage, it leads to severe disability and makes a person dependent on others even for his routine essential activities. This adversely affects the quality of life. But now, total joint replacement offers relief from pain and improved quality of life.

Arthritis is the wearing away of smooth surface (cartilage) of a joint. This causes pain and swelling of the joint. In advanced stage, the cartilage is completely worn out and bone ends rub together producing severe pain and disability **(Figs 13.1 to 13.3)**.

Arthritis can develop because of old age, previous injuries, fractures, infections and diseases like rheumatoid arthritis. There are over one hundred types of arthritis. Some common types are osteoarthritis, rheumatoid arthritis, ankylosing spondylitis and gout. Most common type, also called degenerative, aging arthritis or osteoarthritis, starts in middle age due to wear and tear of the joints. In the beginning, there is mild pain but in advanced stage cartilage is completely worn out causing severe pain and disability. Rheumatoid arthritis is more crippling chronic condition affecting immune system of body. It can affect at any age and is more common in females. Ankylosing spondylitis affects the spine and joints which get inflamed and loose their flexibility and become stiff. Arthritis is probably due to a combination of many factors which include age, heredity, overweight, injury or overuse, occupation or lifestyle and infection.

Arthritis is diagnosed by patient's symptoms (pain, crackling sound in joints, difficulty in walking up and down stairs), clinical examination, X-ray, and blood tests. Once the surface of joint is damaged, it is not usually possible to prevent arthritis from progressing. However, most forms of arthritis can be controlled with appropriate treatment. In

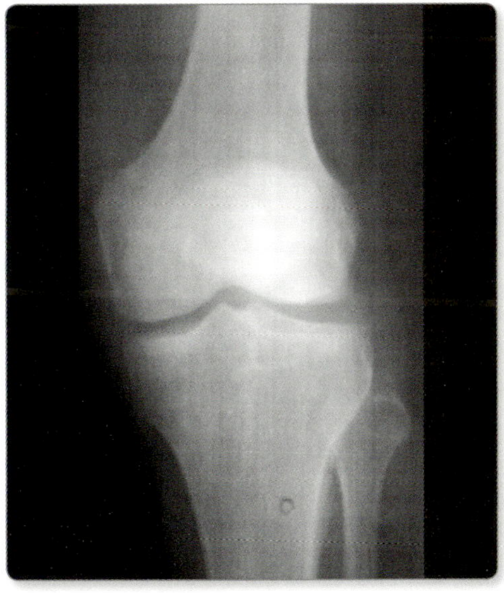

Fig. 13.1 Normal knee

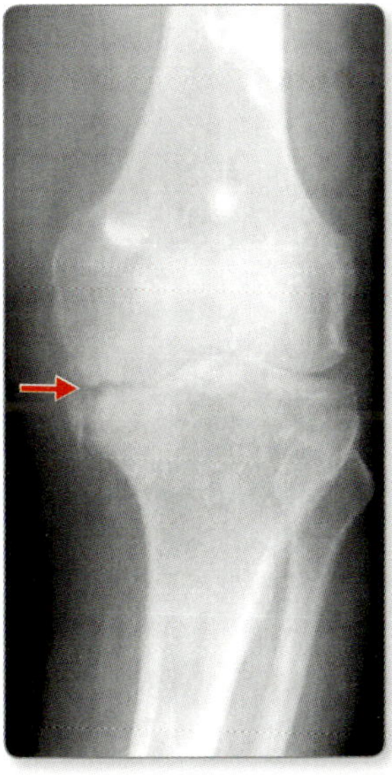

Fig. 13.2 Arthritic knee

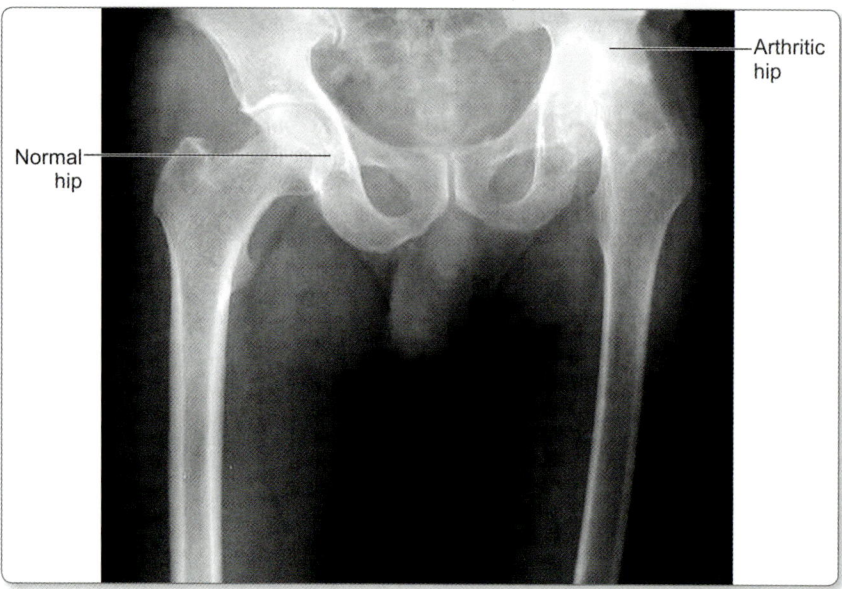

Fig. 13.3 Normal and arthritic hip

early stages, medicines, physiotherapy, weight reduction, heat therapy, splints, use of walking stick can give relief in pain. In advanced stages where these methods are unable to give relief, patients need total joint replacement surgery. A person will need joint replacement when pain becomes chronic and constant, not getting relieved with medicines, pain does not allow walking even short distances, pain disturbs sleep and adversely affecting social, professional and personal life. The benefits of joint replacement are freedom from pain, easier movement and mobility, better quality of life through greater independence, ability to perform most of the routine essential activities.

In total joint replacement surgery, the damaged bone ends and cartilage are replaced with artificial surfaces, which are designed like normal bone ends called artificial joints to restore normal functions and movements.

An artificial joint can last for 15–20 years. It is made up of specialized steel, titanium, cobalt, chromium alloy and plastic (high density polyethylene). The hip and knee joints are commonly affected and replaced. Hip is a ball and socket joint. The ball is removed and replaced with a metal ball fixed to the thighbone. The socket is cleaned and fitted with a plastic cup with bone cement or uncemented metallic cup with plastic, metal or ceramic liner. The damaged surfaces of knee bones are removed and replaced with metal surfaces and fixed to bone with bone cement and plastic inserted in between. The surface of knee cap is also replaced with plastic implant.

Before surgery, patient has to undergo complete medical checkup, blood tests, ECG, etc. Patient has to learn specific exercises to speed up the recovery, loose excessive weight and stop smoking. Patients having medical problems like diabetes, hypertension can also undergo total joint replacement under medical supervision.

Surgery is usually performed under spinal or epidural anesthesia where only lower part of the body is anesthetized. In some cases, general anesthesia is also given to make patient fully unconscious. Modern anesthetic techniques are quiet safe. The average time taken for surgery is 2 hours. After total hip or total knee surgery, patient is in bed for 2 days. On 1st day, regular active and passive exercises of the operated leg are started. On 3rd day, the drain is removed and the patient is made to stand and walk, initially with walker or crutches. After 4–6 weeks, the patient can walk independently without support and can climb steps up and down. Hospital stay is approximately 2 weeks.

Any major operation involves certain risks and complications. With advanced anesthetic and surgical techniques, these risks and complications are very low. Patient, however, should be aware of these. Infection is a serious complication. All precautions are taken to avoid the risk of infection. Despite all the care, about 1% patients may have the risk of developing infection which can be treated with antibiotics. If no response, then removal of implant is required to clear out the infection. Another joint can be implanted later on. Thrombosis (blood clots) may occur in veins of legs in 8–10% of patients. Various techniques are used to prevent it. Death due to this is extremely rare (less than 0.1%). Wear-out or loosening of implant can happen after 10–15 years. It depends on design, quality, material and load on the joint. When excessive wear occurs, it needs revision. Limb length discrepancy (usually <2.5 cm) may occur following total hip replacement (THR) which is usually compensated at pelvis and spine in due course and rarely requires raising of the sole of shoe.

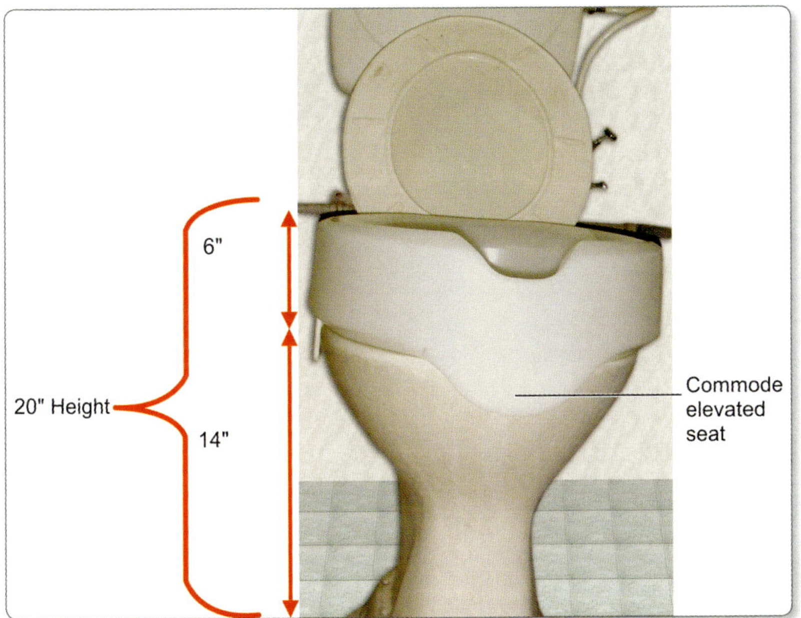

Fig. 13.4 Commode elevated seat

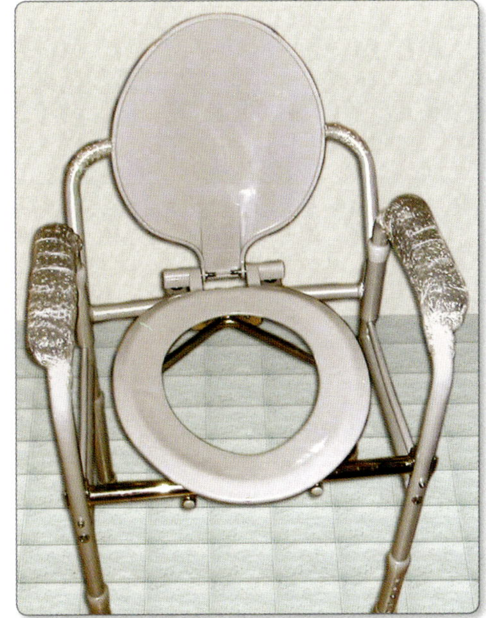

Fig. 13.5 Portable commode chair

To have a successful joint replacement, choose a surgeon who has adequate training and experience in joint replacement surgery, operation theater set-up is of highest standard for joint replacement surgery, good quality of implant, meet and talk to several other patients who have been operated by the surgeon, follow the instructions given by the surgeon and understand the limitations. The instructions are use of Western style toilet, walk with moderate speed, sit on high chair—approximately 20 inches height, regular quadriceps exercises, control of weight, watch to prevent infection of any kind particularly urinary and dental infection, regular visit to surgeon. Limitations are to avoid squatting or sitting on floor, jogging or running, local massage or heat therapy and cross-legged sitting. Patient has to come for follow-up one month after surgery then 3 months, 6 months, 1 year and subsequently once a year or if there is any problem.

"A pain-free joint may not add years to life but it will certainly add life to years."

Suggestions to the Patients

1. Have a Western style toilet of 18–20 inches height. If the height is not adequate, an additional height can be added by commercially available commode elevated seat as shown in **Figure 13.4**.
2. Those who are not having Western style toilet, they can use the commercially available portable commode chair with Indian style toilet as shown in **Figure 13.5**.
3. A horizontal bar fixed in the wall near the toilet at approximately 28–30 inches height is useful support for the elderly patient in sitting and standing from Western style toilet.

Job Recommendation for Person who has Undergone TKR and/or THR

Recommended for permanent change of job not involving heavy manual work, lifting heavy weight, prolonged walking, frequent climbing up and down stairs, running, jogging, jumping, playing, parade, squatting and cross-legged sitting.

The purpose of such recommendation is to prevent early wear and tear of cup and head, loosening of implant and dislocation of joint.

"If you take care of replaced joint, the joint will take care of you for longer period."

Operation Theater Setup for Joint Replacement Surgery

14
CHAPTER

Introduction

Most meticulously and technically well-performed joint replacement surgery can give catastrophic results if complicated by infection which will cause anguish and misery to the patient and relatives, financial loss, litigation, bad reputation to surgery, surgeon and institution. According to Whyte et al, most postoperative infections are due to intraoperative contamination in operation theater (OT). Ninety-eight percent contamination is from airborne source in OT. As per Lord Lister, when surgeon operates on a previously unbroken integument, he has the opportunity of preventing the septic particles from entering. Sir John Charnley introduced the concept of unidirectional airflow system to eliminate source of wound contamination and reduce overall infection rate. Incidence of joint sepsis following total joint replacement surgery significantly reduced when performed in ultraclean air system. As per Lidwell et al., results of randomized study of 8,056 patients undergone THR and TKR with follow-up for 2 or more years, the incidence of deep infection was found to be 1.5% in conventional and 0.6% in ultraclean OT. Further reduction in infection rate was found when whole body exhaust suits were used. In conventional OT, there is uncontrolled air pattern and bacteria count is reduced just by air dilution. In ultraclean ventilation system, positive pressure zone of unidirectional airflow gives effect of air dilution and room air displacement which markedly reduces bacterial count in operating field.

Objectives of Laminar Flow Ventilation

- To provide bacteria-free environment at operation site
- To provide a comfortable environment for operating team and patient with controlled temperature, humidity and ventilation.

Specifications for Joint Replacement Operation Theater

(Ref: "Design and utilization of operation theaters" by Ivan DA Johnston, University of Manchester)

Temperature	20–22°C
Relative humidity	50–60%.
Air velocity	0.1–0.3 m/s, pressure highest (25 Pa) over OT table and lowest in sterile corridor.
Column spacing	7.2 m × 7.2 m.
Height	Minimum 2.8 m.
Main Structure	Steel or reinforced concrete.
Artificial lighting	Minimum 80,000 lux.
Air supply	- Ultraclean vertical laminar flow system. - filtering of 0.5 micrometer to prevent contamination. - should not carry more than one bacteria carrying particle per 6 liters (150/cubic meter) of air.

Vertical Laminar Flow Ventilation

Principle

No contaminated air can penetrate a clean air flow moving vertically downward then outward from the clean zone in all direction.

Air supplied from AC plant or AHU (air handling unit) at a particular temperature and humidity is passed through system of filters—the prefilter, microvee filter and the HEPA filters (high efficiency particulate air filters). Air after passing through the first two filters is brought into SS (stainless steel) plenum which contains HEPA filters in a banking arrangement. The air inside the plenum gets

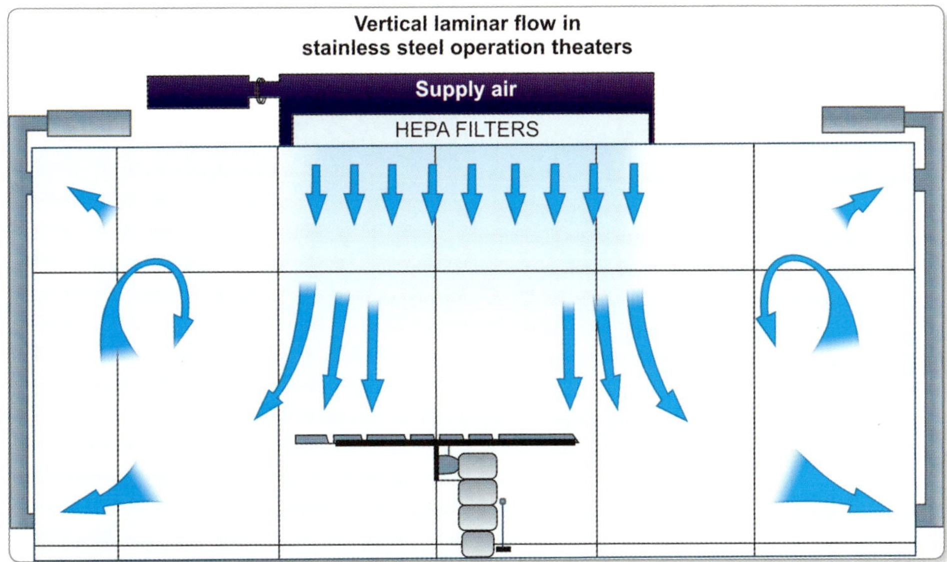

Fig. 14.1 Vertical laminar flow

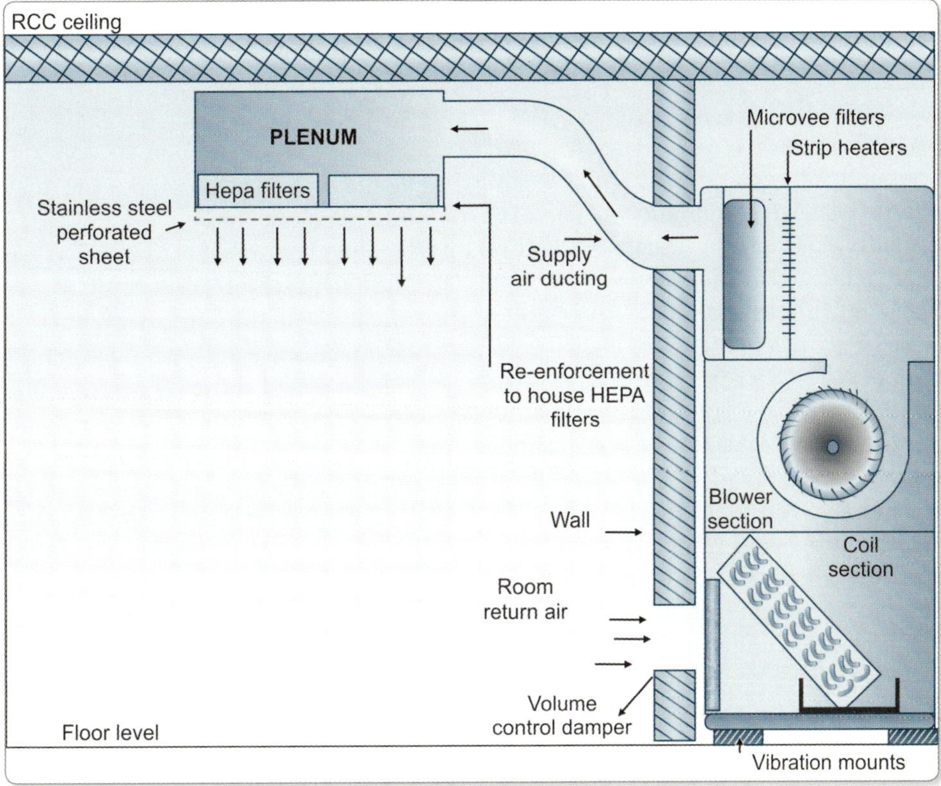

Fig. 14.2 AHU and air filters

pressurized and passes through the HEPA filters in uniform pattern vertically downward and outward **(Figs 14.1 and 14.2)**. It provides 99.97% ultraclean bacteria-free air in operating field. It filters particles up to 0.3 micron size (particles above 10 micron size carry cluster of organisms). About 50 to 60 air changes per hour reduce bacterial stagnation. Positive pressure is always maintained inside the theater preventing entry of contaminated air from adjoining areas. It effectively controls infection. Twenty-five percent of air is exhausted via doors and rest (75%) taken back to AHU through air gills.

Regular Maintenance

Change of pre- and microvee filter every 3 months.

Change of HEPA filters once in 2 years or whenever pressure drops. DOP test efficiency 99.97% should be maintained. DOP (di-octyl phthalate) is condensed into a mist with a high concentration of particles of 0.3 micron diameter. Filtration efficiency is determined by measuring and comparing the concentration of DOP in the inlet and outlet air streams. Periodical culture of air sample.

Body Exhaust System

Human body sheds 30 million particles and 3000 to 5000 micro-organisms per minute which can be reduced to 50% by using body exhaust system.

Prevention of Infection

Contamination of wound by bacteria usually occurs from:

1. Airborne
2. Surgical team
3. Patient's skin
4. Hematogenous spread.

Infection from airborne can be controlled by laminar flow ventilation, use of ultraviolet light, minimum movement of persons inside OT, multiple barrier doors, change of clothes by surgical team and patient, change of shoes by surgical team, weekly washing and fumigation of OT. OT discipline must be maintained.

Infection from surgical team can be controlled by proper scrubbing of hands with betadine scrub and keeping a thin layer of betadine scrub, wearing impervious gown and body exhaust system.

Infection from patient's skin can be controlled by proper bath with antiseptic soap from 2 days prior to surgery, betadine scrubbing of the operating limb 1 day before and on the day of surgery before sending the patient in OT, betadine scrubbing of operating limb on OT table and application of spirit, scrubbing of limb by betadine solution, application of InteguSeal (sterile, film-forming cyanoacrylate liquid, provided in a ready-to-use applicator) microbial sealant to the operative field to lock the skin pathogens and thus prevent contamination of the incision site, complete covering of limb with impervious stockinet and Ioban (iodophore impregnated adhesive drape). Shaving of the part is done on the day of surgery just before sending the patient to OT to avoid colonization of the bacteria.

Infection from hematogenous spread can be controlled by curing hidden infections (like dental caries, UTI, etc.) before surgery, use of preoperative, peroperative and postoperative broad spectrum antibiotics.

Factors Responsible for Contamination in OT

1. Design of OT.
2. Ventilation.
3. Temperature and humidity.
4. Staff discipline.
5. Use of protective clothing and footwear.
6. Cleaning program.

Recommendation by British Medical Council for OT Setup

Location—separate from general traffic and air movement of hospital.

1. Zoning—sequence of increasing clean zones from entrance to the operating area with aim of absolute asepsis at operating site.
2. Easy movement of staff from one clean area to another without passing through dirty area.
3. Removal of dirty material, used linen without passing through clean area.
4. Laminar flow system to provide clean air.
5. Purified water for hands scrubbing.
6. Air curtain at the entry of OT.
7. Drainage, sewage pipes and water line to be avoided at least near and above OT roof.
8. OT should not be used as store room.

Nano TiO_2 (Titanium Dioxide) Enviro-shield

It is a coating applied with a specialized sprayer (spray gun) and can be sprayed on almost any surface—windows, walls, ceilings and floors, etc. When these surfaces are exposed to light (either natural or artificial), the nano TiO_2 is activated (photo-catalytic oxidation, PCO) which then acts as an anti-microbial agent by continuously killing bacteria (*Staphylococcus* spp. including MRSA, *Pseudomonas aeruginosa*, etc.), molds (*Aspergillus, Penicillium, mucor* spp., etc.) and viruses (influenza, SARS, Avian flu, etc). "Enviro-shield" is a one-step disinfecting solution along with its additional features, by which nano TiO_2 deodorizes indoor air (VOCs, volatile organic compounds and other organic smells) and provides antistatic and self-cleaned surfaces as dirt and water just would not act.

Bibliography

1. Aggarawal VK, Rasouli MR, Parvizi J. Periprosthetic joint infection: Current concept. Ind JOrthopaed. 2013;47:10-7.
2. Altcheck D, Sculco TP,Rawling B. Autogenous bone grafting for severe angular deformity in total knee arthroplasty. J Arthroplasty. 1989;4:151-6.
3. Altimate Envirocare Asia Pvt. Ltd.: www.altimategogreen.com, altimate enviro-shield, Nano Titanium Dioxide PCO (photo-catalytic oxidation) technology.
4. Aribindi R, Paprosky W, Nourbash P, Kronick J, Barba M. Extended proximal femoral osteotomy. Instr Course Lect. 1999;48:19-26.
5. Barrack R, Wolfem. Diagnosis of the infected total knee replacement: In: Engh G, Rorabeck C (Eds.) Revision total knee arthroplasty. Baltimore: Williams and Wilkins. 1997:355-70.
6. Barrack RL, Mulroy RG Jr, Harris WH. Improved cementing techniques and femoral component loosening in young patients with hip arthroplasty: A twelve year radiographic review. J Bone Joint Surg Br. 1992;74:385-9.
7. Bengston S, Knuston K, Lidgrel L. Revision of infected knee arthroplasty. Acta orthop Scand. 1986;57(6):489-94.
8. Bengston S, Knutson K, Lidgren L. Treatment of infected knee arthroplasty. Clin Orthop. 1989;245:173-8.
9. Berger RA, Rubash HE, Seel MJ, et al. Determining the rotational alignment of the femoral component in total knee arthroplasty using the epicondylar axis.
10. Berry DJ. Emerging fixation modalities: It's a changing world. Presented at the 9th Annual Current Concepts in Joint Replacement Spring 2008 Meeting. May 18-21, 2008. Las Vegas.
11. Berry DJ. Metaphyseal cones and sleeves help surgeons over many revision TKA hurdles. ORTHOPEDICS TODAY. December 1, 2008.
12. Bhan S. Extensile exposure for total knee arthroplasty. Orthopaedics today. 2001;III:232-5.
13. Bourne RB, Crawford HA. Principles of revision total knee arthroplasty. Orthop Clin North Am. 1998;29(2):331-7.
14. Brand MG, Daley RJ, Ewald FC, and Scot RD. Tibial tray augmentation with modular metal wedges for tibial bone stock deficiency. Clin Orthop. 1989;248:71-9.
15. Brooks AT, Nelson CL, Hofmann OE. Minimal femoral cortical thickness necessary to prevent perforation by ultrasonic tools in joint revision surgery. J Arthroplasty. 1995;10:359-62.
16. Caillouette JT, Gorab RS, Klapper RC, Anzel SH. Revision arthroplasty facilitated by ultrasonic tool cement removal, I: In vitro evaluation. Orthop Rev. 1991;20:353-7.
17. Callaghan JJ, Elder SH, Stranne SK, Fulghum CF, Seaber AV, Myers BS. Revision arthroplasty facilitated by ultrasonic tool cement removal: An evaluation of whole bone strength in a canine model. J Arthroplasty. 1992;7:495-500.
18. Campbell's Operative Orthopaedics: Arthroplasty of knee and hip.
19. Chen F, Mont MA, Bachner RS. Management of ipsilateral supracondylar femoral fractures following total knee arthroplasty. J Arthroplasty. 1994;9:511-26.
20. Colwell CW. Low molecular weight heparin prophylaxis in total knee arthroplasty. Clin Orthop. 2001;392:245-8.
21. Conditt MA, Stein JA and Noble PC. Factors affecting the severity of backside wear of modular tibial inserts. Journal of Bone and Joint surgery. February 2004;86A(2):305-11.
22. Conway JD, Mont MA, Bezwada HP. Arthrodesis of the Knee J Bone Joint Surg (Am). 2004;86:835-48.
23. Costerton JW, Montanaro L, Arciola CR. Biofilm in implant infections: Its production and regulation. Int J Artif Organs. 2005;28:1062-8.
24. Delank KS, Schmidt M, Michael JW, Dietlein M, Schicha H and Eysel P. The implications of 18F-FDG PET for the diagnosis of endoprosthetic loosening and infection in hip and knee arthroplasty: Results from a prospective, blinded study. BMC Musculoskeletal Disorders. 2006;7:20.
25. Dennis D. Wound complications in total knee arthroplasty. Instr Course Lect. 1997:46:165-9.
26. DePuy implants and bone cement literatures.
27. DePuy Surgical Technique for Total Knee and Total Hip Replacement.
28. Dorr LD, Ranawat CS, Sculco TP, McCaskill B. Bone grafts in total knee arthroplasty. Clin Orthop. 1986; 205:153-65.
29. Ellington JK, Reilly SS, Ramp WK, Smeltzer MS, Kellam JF, Hudson MC. Mechanism of Staphylococcus aureus invasion of cultured osteoblast. Microb Pathog. 1999;26:317-23.
30. Elson R, Jephcott A, et al. Antibiotic loaded acrylic cement. JBJS Br. 1977; 59:197.
31. Engh G. Bone defect classification.In: Engh GA, Rorabeck CH Eds). Revision total knee arthroplasty. Williams and Wilkins. 1997:63-120.
32. Fehring TK, Odum S, Calton TF, Mason JB. Articulating versus static spacers in revision total knee arthroplasty for sepsis. Clin Orthop. 2000;380:9-16.
33. Fehring TK, Odum SM, Griffin WL, McCoy TH, Masonis JL. Surgical Treatment of Flexion Contractures After Total Knee Arthroplasty: The journal of Arthroplasty. 2007;22(6):62-6.
34. Felix NA, Stuart MJ, Hansen AD. Periprosthetic fractures of the tibia associated with total knee arthroplasty. Clin Orthop 1997;345:113-124.
35. Fink B. Revision of late periprosthetic infections of total hip endoprostheses: Pros and cons of different concepts. Int J Med Sci. 2009;6:287-95.
36. Firestone TP, Krackow KA, Davis JD IV, Tiny SW, Hungerford DS. The management of fixed flexion contracture during total knee arthroplasty. Clin Orthop. 1992;284;221-7.
37. Gallo J, Kolar M, Novotny R, Rihakova P, Ticha V. Pathogenesis of prosthesis-related infection. Biomed Pap Med Fac Univ Palacky Olomouc Czech Re pub. 2003;147:27-35.
38. Gardiner R, Hozack WJ, Nelson C, Keating EM. Revision total hip arthroplasty using ultrasonically driven tools. A clinical evaluation. J Arthroplasty. 1993;8:517-21.
39. Goldberg SH, Studders EM, Cohen MS. Ultrasonic Cement Removal in Revision Arthroplasty. Orthopaedics. August 2007;30(8):632.
40. Goldman R, Scuderi G, Insall J. Two-stage reimplantation for infected total knee replacement. Clin Orthop. 1996;331:118-24.
41. Gristina AG, Costerton JW. Bacterial adherence and glycocalyx and their role in musculoskeletal infection. Orthop Clin North Am. 1984;15:517-35.

42. Hak DJ, Leiberman JR, Finerman GA. Single plane and biplane external fixators for knee arthrodesis. Clin Orthop. 1995;316:134-44.
43. Hartman MB, Ferhling TK, Jordan L, Norton HJ. Periprosthetic knee sepsis: The role of irrigation and debridement.
44. Healy WL, Siliski JM, Incavo SJ. Operative treatment of distal femoral fractures proximal to total knee replacements. J Bone Joint Surg Am. 1993;75:27-34.
45. Henderson MH Jr, Booth RE Jr. The use of an antibiotic-impregnated spacer block for revision of the septic total knee arthroplasty. Semin arthroplasty. 1991;2(1):34-9.
46. Hernandez-Martinez A, Flores-Sanchez X, Joshi-Jubert N, Escudero-Gonzalez O, Soldado-Carrera F. Knee arthrodesis in total prosthesis of the septic knee joint using a bone transport system, Spanish Society of Orthopaedics and Traumatology (SECOT), Journal of Bone and Joint Surgery - British Volume, Orthopaedic Proceedings . October 2003;86B(SuppII):132.
47. Hofmann AA, Kane KR, Tkach T K, Plaster RL, Camargo MP. Treatment of infected total knee arthroplasty using an articulating spacer. Clin Orthop. 1995;321:45-54.
48. Huiskes R. Some fundamental aspects of human joint replacement. Analyses of stresses and heat conduction in bone-prosthesis structures. Acta Orthop Scand Suppl. 1980;185:1-208.
49. Hull Rd, Pineo GF, Francis C, et al. Low molecular weight heparin prophylaxis using dalteparin in dose proximity to surgery vs warfarin in hip arthroplasty patients. A double blind randomized comparison. The North American Fragmin Trial Investigators. Arch Int Med. 2000: 160:199-207.
50. Insall J, Scot W, Windsor R. Surgical approaches in surgery of the knee, Insall J, Scot W, Windsor R (Eds). New York, Churchill Livingstone. 1993:135.
51. Insall JN, Thompson FM, Brause BD. Two-stage reimplantation for the salvage of infected total knee arthroplasty. J Bone Joint Surg Am. 1983;65(8):1087-98.
52. Insall JN. Total knee replacement in surgery of the knee Insall JN (Ed): New York, Churchill Livingstone. 1984:587-695.
53. Jakob RP, Murphy SB. Tibial osteotomy for varus gonarthrosis: Indication, planning and operative technique. Instr Course Lect. 1992;41:87-93.
54. Janet D Conway, Michael A Mont, Hari P Bezwada. Arthodesis of the knee. J Bone and Joint Surg (Am). 2004;86:835-48.
55. Jones RE, Barrack RL and Skedros J. Modular, mobile-bearing hinge total knee arthropalsty. Clinical orthopaedics and related research. 2001 Nov;(392):306-14.
56. Jones RE, Skedros JG, Chan AJ, Beauchamp DH and Harkins PC. Total knee arthroplasty using the S-ROM Mobile -bearing Hinge prosthesis. J Arthroplasty. 2001;16(3).
57. Jones RE. Total knee arthroplasty with modular rotating-platform hinge. ORTHOSuperSite. Sept 2006.
58. Keyes GW, Carr AJ, Miller RK, Goodfellow JW. The radiographic classification of medial gonarthrosis. Acta Orthop Scand. 1992;63(5):497-501.
59. Klapper RC, Caillouette JT, Callaghan JJ, Hozack WJ. Ultrasonic technology in revision joint arthroplasty. Clin Orthop Relat Res. 1992;285:147-54.
60. Klapper RC, Caillouette JT. The use of ultrasonic tools in revision arthroplasty procedures. Contemp Orthop. 1990;20:273-9.
61. Krackow KA, Jones MM, Teeny SM, Hungerford DS. Primary total knee arthroplasty in patients with fixed valgus deformity. Clin Orthop. 1991;273:9.
62. Laskin RS, Schob CJ. Medial capsular release for severe varus deformities. J. Arthroplasty. 1987;2:313-6.
63. Levitsky KA, Hozack WJ, Balderston RA, et al. Evaluation of the painful prosthetic joint: Relative value of bone scan, sedimentation rate and joint aspiration. J Arthroplasty. 1991;6:237-44.
64. Lewis PL, Rorabeck CH. Periprosthetic fractures. In Engh GA, Rorabeck CH (Eds): Revision Total Knee Arthroplasty. Baltimore, Williams & Wilkins. 1997:275-95.
65. Lidwell OM, Lowbury EJL. Multihospital trial on the use of ultraclean air in orthopaedic operating rooms to reduce infection: Preliminary communication. JR Soc Med. 1978:71.
66. Lonner JH, Barrack R, Fitzgerald RH jr, Hanssen AD, Windsor ER. Infection in total knee arthroplasty: Part1. Classification, prophylaxis and diagnosis. Am J Orthop. 1999;28(9):530-5.
67. Lotke PA, Wong R, Ecker ML. Use of methylmethacrylate in primary total knee replacement with large tibial defects. Clin Orthop. 1991;270:288-94.
68. Mangram AJ, Horan TC, Pearson ML, Silver LC,Jarvis WR. Guideline for Prevention of Surgical Site Infection, 1999. Infection Control and Hospital Epidemiology. April 1999;20(4):250-78.
69. Nicoll BK, Peters RJ. Heat generation during ultrasonic instrumentation of dentin as affected by different irrigation methods. J Periodontol. 1998;69:884-8.
70. Orthosonics literatures for ultrasonic system of cemented and uncemented revision arthroplasty.
71. Parvizi J, Jacovides CL, Adeli B, et al. CRP in joints: A molecular marker for periprosthetic joint infection? Paper #124. Presented at the 2011 Annual Meeting of the American Academy of Orthopaedic Surgeons. Feb. 15-19. San Diego.
72. Poilvache Pl, Insall JN, Scuderi GR, et al. Rotational landmarks and sizing of distal femur in total knee arthroplasty. Clin Orthop. 1996; 331:35.
73. Rand J, Bryan R. Revision after total knee arthroplasty. Orthop Clin. North Am. 1993;75:158-63.
74. Rand JA, Fitzgerald RH Jr. Diagnosis and management of the total knee arthroplasty. Orthop Clin North Am. 1989;28(9):530-5.
75. Rand JA. Alternatives to reimplantation for salvage of the total knee arthroplasty complicated by infection. J Bone Joint Surg. 1993;75A:282-9.
76. Reconstruction of a Medial Tibial Plateau Defect Using a "Pillar" Bone Graft – A Report of Two Knee Reconstructions, SRE Sayampanathan, MA Ali, Singapore Medical Journal.
77. Rhoads DD, Noble PC, Reuben JD, et al. The effect of femoral component position on patellar tracking after total knee arthroplasty. Clin Orthop. 1990; 260:43.
78. Ritter M. Intraoperative controls of bacterial infection during total knee replacement. Orthop Clin North Am. 1989;20:49-53.
79. Ritter M. Screw and cement fixation in large defects in total knee arthroplasty. J arthroplasty. 1986;1:125-30.
80. Ritter MA, Eitzen H, French MLV, et al. The operating room environment as affected by people and the surgical face mask. Clin Orthop. 1975; 111:147-50.
81. Schoifet SD, Morrey BF. Treatment of infection after total knee arthroplasty by debridement with retention of the components. JBJS. 1990;72A:1383-90.
82. Stulberg SE. Arthrodesis in failed total knee replacements. Orthop Clin North Am. 1982;13:213-34.
83. Teeny SM, Krackow KA, Hungerford DS, Jones M. Primary total knee Arthroplasty in patients with severe varus deformity. Clin Orthop. 1991;273:19-31.
84. Tew M, Forster IW. Effect of knee replacement on flexion deformity. JBJS Br. 1987; 69(B):395-9.

85. Vince K. Revision knee arthroplasty technique. Instructional course lectures—AAOS, Heckman JD (Edn). 1993:325.
86. Walker PS, Isieh H. Conformity in condylar replacement knee prostheses. JBJS (Br) 1977;59:222-8.
87. Watanabe W, Sato K, Itoi E. Autologous bone grafting without screw fixation for tibial defects in total knee arthroplasty. J Orthop Sci. 2001;6:481-6.
88. Webster J, Alghamdi AA. Use of plastic drapes during surgery for preventing surgical site infection. Cochrane Database Syst Rev. 2007;(4):CD006353.
89. Whiteside LA, Kasselt MR, Haynes DW. Varus-valgus and rotational stability in rationally unconstrained total knee arthroplasty. Clin Orthop. 1987;219:147-57.
90. Whittaker JP, Dharmarajan R, Toms AD. The management of bone loss in revision total knee replacement. J Bone Joint Surg (Br). 2008;90-B:981-7.
91. Windsor R, Bono J. Infected total knee replacement. J Am Acad Ortho Surg. 1994; 2; 44-53.
92. Windsor R, Insall J, Vince K. Technical consideration of total knee arthroplasty after proximal tibial osteotomy. J Bone and Joint Surg (Am). 1988;70:547-51.
93. Windsor RE, Insall JN, Sculco TP. Bone grafting of tibial defects in primary and revision total knee arthroplasty. Clin Orthop. 1986;205:132-7.
94. Windsor RE, Insall Jn, Urs WK, Miller DV Brause BD. Two-stage reimplantation for the salvage of total knee arthroplasty complicated by infection. JBJS. 1990;72A:272-8.
95. Wongchaissuwat C, Hemami H, Buchner H. Control of sliding and rolling at natural joints. J Biomech Eng. 1984;106:368-75.
96. Write JA, Nair SP. Interaction of Staphylococci of bone. Int J Med Microbiol. 2010;300:193-204.
97. Yeager MP, Glass DD, Neff RK, Brinck Johnson T. Epidural anaesthesia and analgesia in high risk surgical patients. Anaesthesiology. 1987; 66:729-36.
98. Zoccali C, Teori G, Salducca N. The role of FDG-PET between septic and aseptic loosening in hip prosthesis: A review of literature, International orthopaedics (SICOT). 2009:33:1-5.

Index

Page numbers followed by *f* refer to figure